Epilepsy and the Ketogenic Diet

NUTRITION ◊ AND ◊ HEALTH

Adrianne Bendich, Series Editor

EPILEPSY

AND THE

KETOGENIC DIET

Edited by

CARL E. STAFSTROM, MD, PhD

Department of Neurology
University of Wisconsin, Madison, WI

JONG M. RHO, MD

The Barrow Neurological Institute
and St. Joseph's Hospital and Medical Center, Phoenix, AZ

Foreword by

PHILIP A. SCHWARTZKROIN, PhD

Department of Neurological Surgery
University of California, Davis, CA

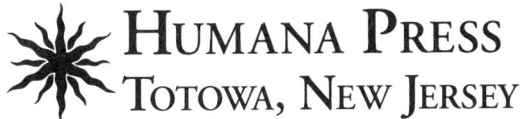

HUMANA PRESS
TOTOWA, NEW JERSEY

© 2004 Humana Press Inc.
999 Riverview Drive, Suite 208
Totowa, New Jersey 07512

www.humanapress.com

Cover design by Patricia F. Cleary.

For additional copies, pricing for bulk purchases, and/or information about other Humana titles, contact Humana at the above address or at any of the following numbers: Tel.: 973-256-1699; Fax: 973-256-8341; E-mail: humana@humanapr.com; or visit our Website: www.humanapress.com

Printed in the United States of America. 10 9 8 7 6 5 4 3 2 1

eISBN 1-59259-808-0

Library of Congress Cataloging-in-Publication Data

Epilepsy and the ketogenic diet / edited by Carl E. Stafstrom and
Jong M. Rho ; foreword by Philip A. Schwartzkroin.
     p. ; cm. -- (Nutrition and health)
  Includes bibliographical references and index.
  ISBN 1-58829-295-9 (alk. paper)
  1. Epilepsy--Diet therapy. 2. Ketogenic diet.
  [DNLM: 1. Epilepsy--diet therapy. 2. Dietary Fats--therapeutic
use. 3. Ketone Bodies--biosynthesis. 4. Models, Animal. WL 385
E607 2004] I. Stafstrom, Carl Ernest. II. Rho, Jong M. III. Series:
Nutrition and health (Totowa, N.J.)
  RC374.K46E64 2004
  616.8'530654--dc22

                                                        2004008391

SERIES EDITOR'S INTRODUCTION

The *Nutrition and Health* series of books has an overriding mission to provide health professionals with texts that are considered essential because each includes: (1) a synthesis of the state of the science, (2) timely, in-depth reviews by the leading researchers in their respective fields, (3) extensive, up-to-date, fully annotated reference lists, (4) a detailed index, (5) relevant tables and figures, (6) identification of paradigm shifts and the consequences, (7) suggestions of areas for future research, and (8) balanced, data-driven answers to patient /health professionals questions that are based upon the totality of evidence rather than the findings of any single study.

The series volumes are not the outcome of a symposium. Rather, each editor has the potential to examine a chosen area with a broad perspective, both in subject matter as well as in the choice of chapter authors. The international perspective, especially with regard to public health initiatives, is emphasized where appropriate. The editors, whose trainings are both research- and practice-oriented, have the opportunity to develop a primary objective for their book; define the scope and focus, and then invite the leading authorities from around the world to be part of their initiative. The authors are encouraged to provide an overview of the field, discuss their own research, and relate the research findings to potential human health consequences. Because each book is developed *de novo*, the chapters are coordinated so that the resulting volume imparts greater knowledge than the sum of the information contained in the individual chapters.

Epilepsy and the Ketogenic Diet, edited by Carl E. Stafstrom and Jong M. Rho is a unique addition to the Nutrition and Health Series and fully exemplifies the potential for this Series to include clinically relevant texts that are valuable to practitioners as well as cutting-edge researchers. Moreover, this text fills a critical gap because at present, there is no work that addresses both the clinical and basic aspects of the ketogenic diet (KD) in a comprehensive, up-to-date manner. The volume includes a detailed description of the KD, which is a high-fat, low-carbohydrate, adequate-protein diet that has been used for more than 80 years for the treatment of medically intractable epilepsy. Initiation of the diet has consistently resulted in effective seizure control in a high proportion of both children and adults when patients' seizures fail to be controlled by standard anticonvulsant drugs. The diet is now an indispensable part of the armamentarium of epilepsy treatments; however, its mechanism of action is still not completely understood. Stafstrom and Rho have thus developed this book to capture the practical aspects of administering the KD as well as to examine the consequences of the biochemical changes that result from its initiation in humans and in animal models of epilepsy.

Drs. Stafstrom and Rho are internationally recognized leaders in the field of epilepsy treatment and the exploration of the biochemical mechanisms of action of the KD at the molecular level. Both are excellent communicators; they have worked tirelessly to develop a comprehensive book that is destined to be the benchmark in the field because of its extensive, in-depth chapters covering the most important aspects of the complex interactions between the KD and its nutrient components, neurodevelopment, brain biochemistry and physiology. The editors have chosen the most well-recognized and respected authors from around the world to contribute the 22 informative chapters. Key features of this comprehensive volume include an exhaustive list of more than 30 pages that provides the reader with the only documented information on the carbohydrate and calorie content of hundreds of commonly used drugs. This is a critical and excellent source of detailed information that is required by parents and caregivers to accurately calculate the intakes of patients on the KD who also require medications that could affect the diet's efficacy. The editors have also included a list of reputable resources on the KD as well as epilepsy that is invaluable to both the patient and health professional. A significant resource for families with children that have seizure disorders is the Charlie Foundation. The founder, Jim Abrahams, Charlie's father, has provided an Afterword at the end of this volume that traces his struggle to find an effective solution to his son's seizures. Fortunately, the KD was of great help. This chapter will be very valuable to parents, students as well as health practitioners.

The editors of the volume, Stafstrom and Rho, clearly understand the seriousness of the issue of epilepsy, drug effects and the complexity of initiating and maintaining a patient on the KD. They have included individual comprehensive chapters by a number of hands-on physicians as well as nurses and dietitians who carefully review the programs that are put in place to help assure a successful KD intervention. Emphasis is placed on the need for a team of health providers that are made aware of the complexities of treating patients with epilepsy who are placed on the KD; this includes emergency room physicians, social workers, teachers and others who will have routine contact with epileptic patients. As an example of the practical information contained within this volume, there are detailed equations that permit the caregiver to calculate the actual amounts of different types of foods that can be included in daily diet plans. Since many of the individuals who use the KD are young children, it is important that such practical information is presented in detailed tables that are easily understood, thus providing a critical resource to both healthcare providers and parents.

The book chapters are logically organized in three major sections. The first section provides the reader with the basics of brain structure and physiology including a review of the triggers for electrical activity within the central nervous system. This section also contains a well organized chapter that outlines the historic beginnings of the KD and its establishment as a treatment for epilepsy. Unique chapters in the second section include individual chapters covering the perspectives of the physician, dietician and nurse in the use of the KD followed by detailed chapters on its efficacy in children as well as in adults. A hallmark of the second section is the detailed assessment of the indications for and the contraindications and/or complications that arise from using the KD. Thus, this volume provides the full range of information concerning the treatment of seizures with the KD. Another advantage of this volume is the inclusion of specific chapters on the metabolic changes that are the consequence of consuming the KD and the changes that can be visualized using neuroimaging techniques. There is also a chapter on the potential for the KD to be useful in conditions other than epilepsy based currently on theoretical grounds. Hopefully, spurred by information provided in this volume, there may prove to be greater uses for the KD in conditions such as obesity, bipolar disorder and other metabolically-related disorders. The completeness of this volume is further exemplified by a full chapter that discusses other dietary treatments for the epileptic patient.

Although dietary modifications have been used for more than 100 years in the treatment of epilepsy, many outstanding questions remain concerning its mode(s) of action. The third section contains ten chapters that examine the effects of the KD on the metabolism of fats, amino acids and carbohydrates in the central nervous system at the macro level and also at the cellular level. Specialized topics in the third section include discussions of the effects of ketones (beta-hydroxybutyrate, acetoacetate, acetone) on brain energy reserves, handling of glucose, excitatory and inhibitory neurotransmitters, specific analyses of the importance of glutamate, genes and gene-encoding enzymes that are turned on and off as a result of ketosis, interactions with insulin and glucagon and glucocorticoids. The critical role of animal models that include knock-out mice, chemically and/or electrically altered tissues, natural models of epilepsy, and other novel models is extensively reviewed. Of great importance are the discussions in these ten chapters of the areas where research is critically needed to further our understanding of the multiple effects of the KD on brain function.

Of great importance, the editors and authors have balanced the most technical information with discussions of its value for parents and patients as well as graduate and medical students, health professionals and academicians. Hallmarks of the chapters include complete definitions of terms with the abbreviation fully defined for the reader and consistent use of terms between chapters. There are numerous relevant tables, graphs and figures as well as up-to-date references; all chapters include a conclusion section that provides the highlights of major findings. The volume contains a highly annotated index and within chapters readers are referred to relevant information in other chapters.

This important text provides practical, data-driven resources based upon the totality of the evidence to help the reader evaluate the critical role of nutrition, especially in children with epilepsy, in optimizing the efficacy of the KD. The overarching goal of the editors is to provide fully referenced information to health professionals so they may have a balanced perspective on the value of this dietary intervention to assure the KD's maximal benefits with minimal adverse effects. Finally, it must be noted that all of the authors and the editors agree that much more research is required to be able to give the best advice to patients with regard to the optimal administration of the KD and it biological mechanisms of action.

In conclusion, *Epilepsy and the Ketogenic Diet*, edited by Carl E. Stafstrom and Jong M. Rho provides health professionals in many areas of research and practice with the most up-to-date, well referenced and easy-to-understand volume on the importance of the ketogenic diet in optimizing the treatment of epilepsy, especially when antiepileptic drug treatments have failed. This volume will serve the reader as the most authoritative resource in the field to date and is a very welcome addition to the *Nutrition and Health* series.

Adrianne Bendich, PhD, FACN,
Series Editor

FOREWORD

The ketogenic diet (KD) has become a significant feature of many epilepsy treatment programs. Although there is no longer much question that the KD has beneficial effects in a substantial proportion of drug-resistant epilepsies, there remain a large number of uncertainties and mysteries regarding its application and mechanism(s) of action. These questions appear at both the clinical treatment level and in the basic research laboratory. Our need to better understand the KD—what it does, when, and how—is similar to historical efforts to understand the application alternatives and underlying mechanisms of any clinically useful treatment. Especially given the dramatic antiepileptic results that are sometimes achieved with the diet, the KD should be a major treatment option. Yet implementation and maintenance of the KD is often difficult, and so it tends to be a treatment of last resort. Further, absence of KD efficacy can often be traced to lack of compliance—owing to the difficulty of holding strictly to the necessary dietary regimen. An understanding of the principles on which KD anticonvulsant efficacy is based could and should lead to the development of more palatable treatments—or even more powerfully effective treatments. Such understanding is the basis for rational drug design. And that is the goal in investigations of the KD. The current volume summarizes the broad literature pertinent to the KD and attempts to paint the backdrop on which innovative research strategies can be formulated. The major questions are outlined below.

CLINICAL RESEARCH ISSUES

Which Patients/Epilepsies Are the Best Candidates for KD Treatment?

Patient sex or age: Current information suggests that sex is not a basis for patient selection. In general, KD has been used primarily as a pediatric treatment; recent studies suggest that it can be used in infants and in adults. Is there preferential efficacy based on age? Is the KD acting at a site, or on a mechanism, that is unique to the immature brain?

Seizure etiology or seizure/syndrome type: There is little information in the literature to indicate that KD is preferentially effective against certain types of seizures or syndromes. However, given that KD is often a treatment of last resort, it is unclear how effective it is on epilepsies that are not medically refractory. Do underlying pathologies or etiologies make any difference? What is the relatively efficacy of the KD (compared to "conventional" antieplieptic drugs [AEDs]) against catastrophic epilepsies, e.g., the Lennox-Gastaut syndrome?

Duration of epilepsy before treatment is started: Experimental animal data suggest that KD may be more effective when instituted soon after the initiation of seizure activity. Do seizures get more difficult to treat with KD as they progress? Should the KD be used as a "primary" treatment for childhood epilepsies—and if so, when? Why wait until several AEDs have been evaluated before the KD alternative is considered?

What Are the Key Strategies in Obtaining Optimal Results When Instituting the KD?

Fat/carbohydrate/protein ratios: Guidelines for clinicians and dietitians have been published, but the details of the KD procedure vary somewhat from institution to institution. Is there good evidence to identify the best fat/carbohydrate/protein ratios?

KD initation by fasting: What is the advantage of initiating the KD with a brief fasting period? What does that fasting period achieve other than to increase the rate of ketosis? And, to challenge the existing lore, does the KD really establish a "starvation"-like metabolic state?

Calorie restriction and/or regulation of fluid intake: Clinicians typically monitor calorie intake carefully for children on the KD—presumably to prevent unwanted weight gain with the high fat diet. However, laboratory studies have suggested that calorie restriction, per se, may have anticonvulsant results. How important is calorie restriction for clinical anticonvulsant efficacy? Also, how important is it to monitor fluid intake? Is KD efficacy related to dehydration? Certainly, brain water balance (i.e., osmotic shifts) greatly affects neuronal excitability.

What, and How Serious, Are Potential Adverse Side Effects of the KD?

Altered fluid balance: Investigators have reported potential problems with the development of kidney stones, as well as other possible reflections of fluid-intake dysregulation (e.g., cardiac irregularities). How common are such adverse consequences, and how serious?

Hyperlipidemia: Do children on such an abnormally high-fat diet have problems related to hyperlipidemia/high cholesterol? What are the long-term consequences for general health?

Growth defects: What are the consequences of the KD for normal growth? Slow growth might indeed be expected in the face of such low protein intake.

Are There Clinically Obtainable Markers of Likely Success or Failure?

Ketosis: Historically, KD efficacy has been linked to a critical level of ketonemia, although the measurements have typically been made on ketones in the urine. How do these measures relate to serum—or perhaps more critically, to brain (e.g., CSF, parenchymal)—ketone levels? Is there a threshold below which anticonvulsant efficacy is not seen? Is degree of KD efficacy related to the level of ketonemia?

Glucose regulation and related metabolism: What about other metabolic changes that are induced by KD, most notably alterations in glucose levels and the consequent change in insulin/glucagon metabolism?

Deviations from the diet: The clinical (and research) lore suggests that even mild/brief deviations from the KD regimen leads rapidly to loss of seizure control. What is the documentation for these observations? How is loss of seizure control related (temporally and in terms of magnitude) to metabolic markers?

What Are the Long-Term Treatment Considerations Related to KD Treatment?

Length of treatment: For many types of epilepsies, the patient would be expected to stay on AED medication for a lifetime. Is that also the case for KD? How long should a child be kept on the diet? What should be done when the patient comes off the diet—

especially because the usual drug "weaning" paradigm might not be applicable to the KD treatment?

Other medications: Is KD treatment alone sufficient to provide seizure protection? What are the preferred choices for secondary medication, and when should they be employed?

Effects of KD on other behaviors: How does the KD affect nonseizure function (e.g., mood, cognitive function, and so on), and how should those changes be factored into the determination of long-term KD treatment vs more traditional AED treatment?

Does the KD Provide Effective Treatment Beyond Its Anticonvulsant Action?

Antiepileptogenicity: Anecdotal reports, from both the clinic and the laboratory, suggest that the KD may (at least in some cases) do more than simply control seizure manifestations. Does KD treatment offer a potential "cure" or antiepileptogenic promise? Does seizure "blockade" persist beyond the period of treatment? Are such observations simply a result of treatment in a pediatric epilepsy context (i.e., where seizure phenomenology may change/remit in any case, with brain maturation), or does the KD induce a long-lasting change?

Neuroprotection: How might the KD have long-term consequences for seizure activity? for epileptogenesis? Preliminary evidence from the laboratory suggests a potential neuroprotective effect. Is that simply a function of reduced seizure severity, or is it relevant to other brain-damaging insults?

BASIC RESEARCH ISSUES

Which Consequences of KD Are Necessary and Sufficient to Produce Anticonvulsant Effects?

Ketosis: The KD profoundly alters normal metabolism. Most research into underlying mechanisms of KD have focused on the most obvious changes, i.e., the elevation of ketone bodies and their presumed substitution (for glucose) as the major metabolic substrate. That there is an elevation in ketone bodies is unquestionable; further, this rise is correlated with anticonvulsant efficacy. However, whether these ketones are the key elements in KD anticonvulsant efficacy has yet to be determined. Further, almost all blood ketone measurements have been made on β-hydroxybutyrate. Recent laboratory studies suggest that other ketones (e.g., acetone) may have a more profound anticonvulsant effect.

Alterations in glucose/insulin levels: Although less well studied, the KD also has significant effects on glucose levels, and as a consequence, on insulin and related metabolic factors. Such changes, associated with ketosis, have been extensively described in the diabetes literature. Insulin changes have dramatic effects on a number of hormonal and neurotransmitter systems, at least some of which can directly affect brain excitability.

Calorie restriction: Often correlated with KD is a reduction in total caloric intake. Indeed, clinical procedures often regulate calorie intake at less than 100% of the normal age-associated recommended allowance. And recent laboratory studies have found significant anticonvulsant effects of calorie restriction, independent of KD per se (although usually associated with at least some degree of ketonemia). Does calorie limitation play a significant role in KD-induced seizure control? If so, how?

Other: It is worth emphasizing that KD alters many metabolic pathways. Our challenge is to recognize the seizure-relevant pathway(s). These may not always be the most obvious (i.e., ketone elevations). Indeed, there may be multiple pathways and seizure-relevant effectors.

Why Are the KD-Induced Anticonvulsant Conditions So Sensitive to Noncompliance?

Metabolic perturbations that cause loss of seizure control: What stimuli disrupt the KD-established anti-seizure state? Is it only glucose? What about treatments that interfere with more "distal" or downstream KD-related pathways?

Markers that change rapidly with noncompliance: One potential approach to identify key seizure-relevant factors is to examine KD-related markers that change rapidly, in parallel with loss of seizure control.

What KD "Products" Have Direct Effects on Brain Excitability?

Ketones: Laboratory studies with ketones (BHB, acetoacetate, acetone) have generally been consistent with the view that these molecules affect brain excitability. However, the site and/or mode of their action(s) remain unclear. These ketones may simply represent an early step in the metabolic processes that ultimately influence brain excitability.

Fatty acids: Investigators have just begun to explore the possibility that significant changes in fatty acids, resulting from KD, contribute to decreased brain excitability.

Energy metabolites: An early and influential hypothesis regarding mechanisms of KD anticonvulsant action focused on alterations in energy metabolites (ATP, ADP, creatine, creatine phosphate). Current research has again begun to explore these changes, assisted by modern imaging technology (MR spectroscopy).

Neurotransmitters: A considerable amount of research has focused on KD effects on amino acid metabolism, particularly the possibility that KD increases GABA synthesis and/or release. More recent studies suggest that neuromodulatory agents such as norepinephrine might be affected by the KD, and produce relevant antiepileptic effects.

Hormones and neuroactive peptides: As indicated above, hormonal changes associated with altered glucose status need to be examined, particularly since it is clear that insulin can affect the synthesis of products that can increase or decrease neuroexcitability. Among those products are neuroactive peptides, such as neuropeptide Y (NPY) and galanin, that are known to decrease seizure sensitivity.

What Are the Basic Mechanisms of KD Anticonvulsant Activity?

Increased GABA-receptor-mediated inhibition: There has been much interest in the possibility that KD causes increased inhibition, presumably through action on the GABA system. Whether there is a direct effect of a KD-induced product (e.g., ketones) on the $GABA_A$ receptor, or whether the effect is "indirect" (i.e., enhancement of GABA synthesis/release) remains unclear. Experimental data do support the hypothesis, however, that some forms of inhibition are enhanced in the KD-fed rat.

Increased (or decreased) energy availability: Experimental studies also support the view that KD alters the balance of energy metabolites, providing a greater amount of high-energy molecules (e.g., ATP) than seen on a normal diet. How such changes may be translated into altered brain excitability is a matter of current speculation. Possibilities include effects on membrane "pumps" and on ATP-sensitive ion channels (e.g., the K_{ATP} channel).

Action at glia/blood–brain barrier: There is increasing attention to the possible effects of KD on mechanisms that mediate the exchange of metabolites from the brain to the vascular system, i.e., at the blood–brain barrier. Studies have suggested, for example, that the KD may affect glucose transport.

Does KD Exert Antiepileptogenic As Well As Anticonvulsant Activity (and If So, How)?

Neuroprotective function: Some preliminary data suggest that KD may, in fact, protect neurons from the damaging (neurotoxic) effects of seizures. If seizures do "beget seizures" via the neuropathological consequences of seizure activity, then neuroprotection might indeed prevent the exacerbation of seizure phenomenology (i.e., antiepileptogenesis). This protection might also provide beneficial consequences for cognitive functions that are often compromised, not only in early epilepsy, but also in other neuropathological conditions (e.g., hypoxia, stroke).

Interaction with features of the developing brain: It is widely accepted that the immature brain is more seizure-prone than the adult brain, owing to the relatively slow maturation of a large number of important "control" mechanisms (e.g., inhibition, membrane pumps, and transporters). Because KD seems to be particularly effective in pediatric epilepsies, it is possible that the diet helps the brain mature faster, and/or provides some missing or weak element characteristic of the immature central nervous system. Alternatively, it is possible that the KD interacts with salient developmental processes, e.g., brain "plasticity," that are "pro-epileptogenic." In either case, the KD may not only provide seizure-related protection, but also influence other brain functions that depend on maturational mechanisms.

Clearly, the apparent simplicity of the KD—a straightforward dietary approach to a significant clinical problem—masks a very complex set of potential avenues and mechanisms of action. For the clinical or laboratory investigator, this complexity offers an almost irresistible challenge. It also presents a problem that invites, and requires, a collaborative effort between basic scientists and clinicians. Successful explanations of the "Clinical Research Issues" listed above will undoubtedly involve input from the laboratory; unraveling the "Basic Research Issues" will likewise involve support from clinical analyses. Like solving any good mystery, elucidating the means through which KD provides anticonvulsant efficacy depends on the efficiency and coordination of our detective-work—identifying the clues, and working together to interpret them within an integrative framework (i.e., hypothesis testing). Given the sophistication of our current investigative techniques, solving this mystery seems well within our grasp.

The long list of questions, hypotheses, and possibilities presented above perhaps belies the fact that we do, in fact, know more about the KD today than even a few years ago. Although the current volume reflects the accumulated knowledge in the field, it is especially valuable for those insights obtained during the past 4 or 5 years (see earlier reviews about the KD and underlying mechanisms [1–3]). The editors have gathered an outstanding group of experts—clinical investigators and basic scientists—to provide up-to-date reviews of key issues. These descriptions and analyses should provide information valuable not only for the practicing clinicians, but also for those investigators intent on using insights from KD efficacy to develop better treatments for medically intractable epilepsy —or for other disorders that may respond to an overlapping set of mechanisms.

Philip A. Schwartzkroin, PhD
University of California, Davis, CA

REFERENCES

1. Nordli DR, DeVivo DC. The ketogenic diet revisited: back to the future. Epilepsia, 1997;38:743–749.
2. Swink TD, Vining EPG, Freeman JM. The ketogenic diet: 1997, Adv Pediatr 1997;44:297–329.
3. Schwartzkroin PA, Rho JM, eds. The ketogenic diet: mechanisms and models. Epilepsy Res 1999;37(3).

PREFACE

The ketogenic diet (KD) is a high-fat, low-carbohydrate, adequate-protein diet that has been used for more than 80 years for the treatment of medically intractable epilepsy. Effective in both children and adults, the KD provides an alternative to standard anticonvulsant drugs. The diet is now an indispensable part of our armamentarium of epilepsy treatments.

The KD was originally formulated to produce the biochemical changes ordinarily associated with fasting, a condition known since antiquity to reduce seizure activity. Despite the diet's use for so many years, fundamental questions remain about how the KD works, how to formulate and administer the diet for optimal success, and how to choose which patients will respond best to its implementation. The KD is designed to mimic the fasting state, in which the brain switches from oxidation of carbohydrates to fats as its primary energy source. Somehow, this metabolic transition is associated with improved seizure control. Laboratory efforts are currently seeking to understand how this transition occurs.

At present, there is no published text that addresses both the clinical and basic aspects of the KD in a comprehensive, up-to-date manner. With the resurgence of interest in the use of the KD over the past decade, both in the United States and worldwide, such an authoritative volume is long overdue. The principal goals of this book are to provide scientists, physicians, dietitians, and other health care professionals with detailed information about the KD, and to challenge investigators with innovative and thought provoking ideas for future research into the mechanism of the KD.

Epilepsy and the Ketogenic Diet strives to present a balance between clinical and basic science topics. We begin with an introductory discussion about epilepsy, including both clinical aspects and basic mechanisms, for those unfamiliar with the field. Clinical aspects of KD formulation, administration, and clinical usage are then described in detail. Topics include the history of how the KD originated, instructions on how to calculate and plan a KD individually tailored to the needs of each patient, how to monitor KD effectiveness, potential pitfalls and complications, and challenges for future clinical applications.

From the basic science perspective, despite the heightened interest in the KD over the past 10 years, its mechanism of action is still a mystery. Much remains to be learned about how the brain synthesizes and regulates ketone bodies, the manner in which ketones modulate neuronal excitability, and what mechanisms modify KD effectiveness at the molecular, cellular, and neuronal network levels. However, as will be seen in the chapters that follow, clinicians and basic scientists are actively pursuing an enhanced understanding of KD mechanisms, with the goal of improving the diet's effectiveness in children and adults with medically refractory epilepsy.

Epilepsy and the Ketogenic Diet should be viewed as a work in progress. We hope that its contents provoke thought and discussion about this unusual but highly effective epilepsy therapy.

Carl E. Stafstrom, MD, PhD
Jong M. Rho, MD

CONTENTS

CONTRIBUTORS

JIM ABRAHAMS • *The Charlie Foundation to Help Cure Pediatric Epilepsy, Santa Monica, CA*

KAREN R. BALLABAN-GIL, MD • *Departments of Neurology and Pediatrics, Albert Einstein College of Medicine, Montefiore Medical Center, Bronx, NY*

ANNA GUNHILD CHRISTINA BERGQVIST, MD • *Department of Neurology, Children's Hospital of Philadelphia, University of Pennsylvania , Philadelphia, PA*

KRISTOPHER J. BOUGH, PhD • *Department of Pharmacology, Emory University, Atlanta, GA*

W. MCINTYRE BURNHAM, PhD • *Department of Pharmacology, Bloorview Epilepsy Research Program, University of Toronto, Toronto, Ontario, Canada*

LIONEL CARMANT, MD • *Department of Pediatrics, Hopital Ste. Justine, Montreal, Quebec, Canada*

TIM E. CULLINGFORD, PhD • *Department of Clinical and Molecular Pharmacokinetics/ Pharmacodynamics, Showa University, Tokyo, Japan*

STEPHEN C. CUNNANE, PhD • *Department of Nutritional Sciences, University of Toronto, Toronto, Ontario, Canada*

YEVGENY DAIKHIN, MD, PhD • *Department of Pediatrics, Children's Hospital of Philadelphia, University of Pennsylvania, Philadelphia, PA*

DARRYL C. DE VIVO, MD • *Department of Neurology, Columbia University College of Physicians and Surgeons, New York, NY*

DOUGLAS A. EAGLES, PhD • *Department of Biology, Georgetown University, Washington, District of Columbia*

RIF S. EL-MALLAKH, MD • *Department of Psychiatry and Behavioral Sciences, University of Louisville, Louisville, KY*

JOHN M. FREEMAN, MD • *Pediatric Epilepsy Unit, Johns Hopkins Hospital, Baltimore, MD*

AMANDA E. GREENE • *Department of Biology, Boston College, Chestnut Hill, MA*

GREGORY L. HOLMES, MD • *Section of Neurology, Dartmouth-Hitchcock Medical Center, Lebanon, NH*

GEORGE KARVELAS, MD • *Department of Pediatrics, Hopital Ste. Justine, Montreal, Quebec, Canada*

ERIC H. KOSSOFF, MD • *Pediatric Epilepsy Unit, Johns Hopkins Hospital, Baltimore, MD*

DENIS LEBEL, BPharm, MSc • *Department of Pediatrics, Hopital Ste. Justine, Montreal, Quebec, Canada*

SERGEI LIKHODII, PhD • *Department of Pharmacology, Bloorview Epilepsy Research Program, University of Toronto, Toronto, Ontario, Canada*

DANINE MELE-HAYES, RD • *The Epilepsy and Brain Mapping Program, Pasadena, CA*

KATHY MUSA-VELOSO, PhD • *Department of Nutritional Sciences, University of Toronto, Toronto, Ontario, Canada*

MAROMI NEI, MD • *Department of Neurology, Jefferson Medical College, Philadelphia, PA*

JERI E. NICHOLS SUTHERLING, BSN, RN, PHN • *The Epilepsy and Brain Mapping Program, Pasadena, CA*

ILANA NISSIM • *Department of Pediatrics, Children's Hospital of Philadelphia, University of Pennsylvania, Philadelphia, PA*

ITZHAK NISSIM, PhD • *Department of Pediatrics, Children's Hospital of Philadelphia, University of Pennsylvania, Philadelphia, PA*

DOUGLAS NORDLI, JR., MD • *Department of Neurology, Children's Memorial Hospital, Chicago, IL*

JULLIE W. PAN, MD, PhD • *Department of Neurology and Gruss Magnetic Resonance Research Center, Albert Einstein College of Medicine, Bronx, NY*

JONG M. RHO, MD • *The Barrow Neurological Institute and St. Joseph's Hospital and Medical Center, Phoenix, AZ*

JAMES E. RUBENSTEIN, MD • *Pediatric Epilepsy Unit, Johns Hopkins Hospital, Baltimore, MD*

PHILIP A. SCHWARTZKROIN, PhD • *Department of Neurological Surgery, University of California Davis, Davis, CA*

THOMAS N. SEYFRIED, PhD • *Department of Biology, Boston College, Chestnut Hill, MA*

MICHAEL R. SPERLING, MD • *Department of Neurology, Jefferson Medical College, Philadelphia, PA*

CARL E. STAFSTROM, MD, PhD • *Department of Neurology, University of Wisconsin, Madison, WI*

PATRICIA SZOT, PhD • *Department of Psychiatry and Behavioral Sciences, University of Washington and VA Puget Sound Health Care System, Seattle, WA*

MARIANA T. TODOROVA, PhD • *Department of Biology, Boston College, Chestnut Hill, MA*

EILEEN P. G. VINING, MD • *Pediatric Epilepsy Unit, Johns Hopkins Hospital, Baltimore, MD*

DAVID WEINSHENKER, PhD • *Department of Human Genetics, Emory University, Atlanta, GA*

RHONDA ROELL WERNER, RN, BSN, MS • *Children's Hospital of Wisconsin, Milwaukee, WI*

JAMES W. WHELESS, MD • *Texas Comprehensive Epilepsy Program, University of Texas Houston, Houston, TX*

MARC YUDKOFF, MD • *Department of Pediatrics, Children's Hospital of Philadelphia, University of Pennsylvania, Philadelphia, PA*

MARY L. ZUPANC, MD • *Department of Pediatric Neurology, Medical College of Wisconsin, Children's Hospital of Wisconsin, Milwaukee, WI*

BETH ZUPEC-KANIA, RD, CD • *Children's Hospital of Wisconsin, Milwaukee, WI*

I BACKGROUND

1

An Introduction to Seizures and Epilepsy
Cellular Mechanisms Underlying Classification and Treatment

Carl E. Stafstrom

1. INTRODUCTION

Epilepsy is one of the most common neurologic disorders, affecting as many as 5% of individuals during their lifetime. Epilepsy is defined as the condition of unprovoked, recurrent seizures. The clinical manifestations of epilepsy are heterogeneous, varying from a subtle interruption of awareness and responsiveness to a full-blown convulsion of the entire body. Causes of seizures are extremely varied, ranging from acquired ("symptomatic") insults such as meningitis, traumatic brain injury, and hypoxia–ischemia to metabolic, congenital, and idiopathic, i.e., genetic, etiologies. Children are particularly susceptible to seizures, and most forms of epilepsy begin in childhood.

Despite the availability of many antiepileptic drugs (AEDs), seizures can be particularly challenging to treat. Fortunately, over the past 10 yr, there has been a flurry of new AEDs and nonpharmacologic therapies to treat epilepsy. Some of the new drugs are designed to address specific pathophysiologic defects in the sequence of events leading to seizure generation or spread. Other novel treatments that have been developed or renewed over the past decade include electrical stimulation devices, e.g., the vagus nerve stimulator, and dietary interventions, e.g., the ketogenic diet.

This chapter reviews the principles of cellular neurophysiology as a foundation for understanding how normal neuronal function goes awry in epilepsy. For health professionals who deal with epilepsy, it is important to understand some of the basic pathophysiologic mechanisms that underlie epileptic seizures. For physicians, this background will enable a rational choice of the most appropriate medication for a given seizure type or epilepsy syndrome in a particular clinical setting. For other health-care professionals, such as nurses, social workers, and dieticians, a biological foundation will allow a better understanding of the challenges in providing comprehensive medical and psychosocial care to patients with epilepsy. The background provided in this chapter will facilitate an understanding of the more technical chapters that follow.

First, seizures and epilepsy are defined and the modern classification system is explained. Second, elements contributing to normal synaptic transmission and neuronal firing are summarized. Next, the pathophysiology of acute and chronic seizures is dis-

From: *Epilepsy and the Ketogenic Diet*
Edited by: C. E. Stafstrom and J. M. Rho © Humana Press Inc., Totowa, NJ

cussed. Finally, mechanisms are considered by which AEDs and other epilepsy treatments control the hyperexcitability that underlies epilepsy. Literature citations are limited to reviews and monographs; the interested reader is encouraged to consult these reviews for primary sources.

2. SEIZURES AND EPILEPSY

2.1. Definitions

First, it is necessary to review some basic definitions. A *seizure* is a temporary disruption of brain function owing to the hypersynchronous, excessive discharge of cortical neurons. Sometimes, the term *epileptic seizure* is used to distinguish this event from a nonepileptic seizure such as a psychogenic ("pseudo") seizure, which involves abnormal clinical behavior but is not caused by hypersynchronous neuronal firing. The clinical manifestations of a seizure depend on the specific region and extent of brain involved and may include alteration in motor function, sensation, alertness, perception, autonomic function, or some combination of these. Anyone might experience a seizure in the appropriate clinical setting, e.g., meningitis, hypoglycemia, or toxin ingestion, attesting to the innate capacity of even a "normal" brain to support hypersynchronous discharges under specific circumstances.

Epilepsy is the condition of *recurrent,* unprovoked seizures, i.e., two or more seizures. Epilepsy usually occurs when a person is predisposed to seizures because of a chronic pathological state, e.g., brain tumor, cerebral dysgenesis, posttraumatic scar, a genetic susceptibility, or perhaps a combination of these. Approximately 1% of the population suffers from epilepsy, making it the second most common neurologic disorder (after stroke), affecting more than 2 million persons in the United States.

The term *epileptic syndrome* refers to a group of clinical characteristics that occur together consistently, with seizures as a primary manifestation. Such features might include similarities in seizure type, age of onset, electroencephalogram (EEG) findings, precipitating factors, etiology, inheritance pattern, natural history, prognosis, and response to AEDs. Examples of epileptic syndromes in childhood are infantile spasms, Lennox–Gastaut syndrome, febrile seizures, childhood absence epilepsy, benign rolandic epilepsy (BRE), and juvenile myoclonic epilepsy. The clinical classification of seizures and epilepsy syndromes is discussed more fully in Section 2.2.

Finally, *epileptogenesis* refers to the events by which the normal brain becomes capable of producing epileptic seizures, i.e., the process by which neural circuits are converted from normal excitability to hyperexcitability. This process may take months or years, and its mechanisms are poorly understood. The available AEDs do not have robust antiepileptogenic effects; i.e., existing drugs can suppress seizures but none prevents the formation of epileptic neuronal circuitry. Clearly, the development of an antiepileptogenic treatment is a high research priority.

2.2. Classification of Seizures and Epilepsy

The International League Against Epilepsy (ILAE) has derived two classification schemes, one for epileptic seizures *(1)* and another for epileptic syndromes *(2)*. The seizure classification scheme uses clinical criteria only: what the event looked like to an observer and the interictal (and sometimes ictal) EEG pattern. Seizures are divided into those that begin focally (partial seizures) and those that simultaneously begin in both cerebral hemispheres (generalized seizures). The epilepsy syndrome classification utilizes additional information to permit a two-tiered categorization. First, as with the seizure classification, the seizures within a syndrome are divided into generalized or localization-related, i.e., focal onset, events. Second, the syndromes are organized into those that have a known etiology (symptomatic or secondary) and those that are idiopathic (primary) or cryptogenic. The reader is referred to refs. *1* and *2* for further details. These classifications allow the clinician to choose appropriate therapy, tailored to the specific seizure type or epilepsy. Some seizure/epilepsy types respond better to one form of therapy or another. However, these schemes are not definitive and will require ongoing revision as more knowledge is gained about epilepsy genetics and pathophysiology. The ILAE is currently working on another revised classification that takes into consideration recent advances in our understanding of epilepsy, its causes, and its manifestations *(3)*.

Figure 1 utilizes this broad classification of seizures as *partial (focal)* or *generalized,* to illustrate the site of origin and spread of seizure activity. Partial seizures originate in a localized area of brain, with clinical manifestations based on the area of brain involved and how extensively discharges spread from this "focus" (Fig. 1A). For example, discharges from a focus in the left motor cortex may cause jerking of the right hand and arm. If the discharges spread to the motor area controlling the face and mouth, additional clinical ictal features would include facial twitching, drooling, and perhaps speech arrest. This pattern of clinical and electrographic seizure is typically seen in BRE, in which epileptic discharges are seen over the central–temporal area around the rolandic fissure.

On the other hand, generalized seizures begin with abnormal electrical discharges occurring in both hemispheres simultaneously. The EEG signature of a primary generalized seizure is "bilaterally synchronous spike-wave discharges" recorded over the entire brain at once. These generalized discharges reflect reciprocal excitation between the cortex and the thalamus (Fig. 1B). Generalized seizures can also spread and synchronize via the corpus callosum. A generalized seizure can manifest as anything from brief impairment of consciousness (as in an absence seizure) to rhythmic jerking of all extremities with loss of posture and consciousness (a generalized tonic–clonic [GTC] convulsion). A seizure that starts focally, then spreads widely throughout the brain is referred to as *secondarily generalized* (Fig. 1A, far right panel). For example, in BRE, seizures sometimes begin focally in face/hand motor cortex, then secondarily generalize to cause a GTC convulsion. Similarly, in a seizure of temporal lobe epilepsy (TLE), the first ictal symptom may be an aura, e.g., unusual taste or smell, motor automatism, e.g., repetitive picking at the clothes, or affective change, e.g., fear, distortion of time, déjà vu, or depersonalization, accompanied by discharges originating in the hippocampus or other temporal lobe structure; such seizures commonly generalize, resulting in a GTC convulsion. Some partial seizures secondarily generalize so quickly that they appear, both clinically and electrographically, to be generalized from the onset.

Although the mechanisms underlying partial seizures, partial seizures with secondary generalization, and primary generalized seizures differ somewhat *(4)*, it is useful to think about any seizure as *a disruption in the normal balance between excitation and inhibition* in part or all of the brain. A seizure can occur when excitation increases, inhibition decreases, or both. Hyperexcitability can occur at one or more levels of brain function, such as a network of interconnected neurons, the neuronal *membrane*

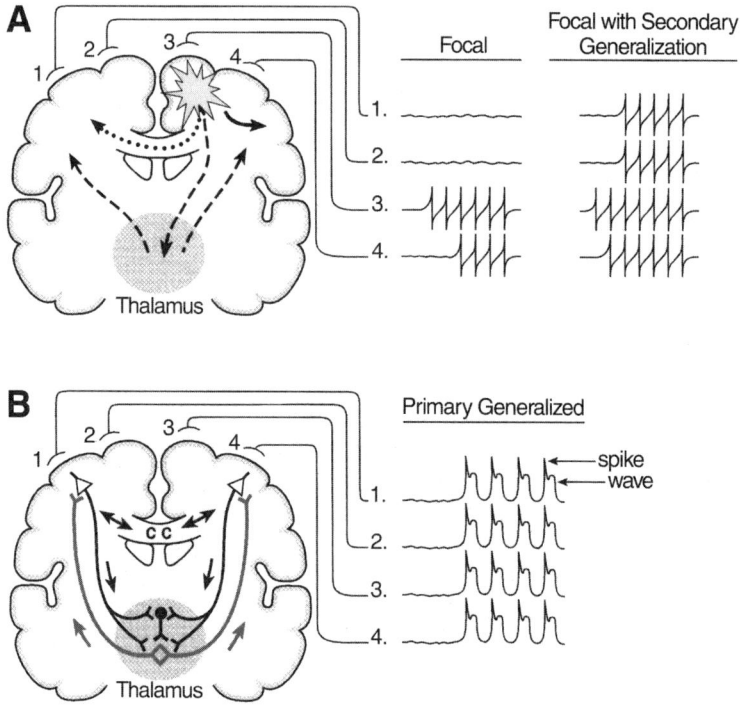

Fig. 1. Coronal brain sections depicting seizure types and potential routes of seizure spread. **(A)** Focal area of hyperexcitability (star) and spread to nearby neocortex (solid arrow), via corpus callosum or other commissures to the contralateral cerebral hemisphere (dotted arrow), or via subcortical pathways, e.g., thalamus, brainstem (downward dashed arrow), resulting in secondary generalization (upward dashed arrows). Accompanying EEGs show brain electrical activity under numbered electrodes. Focal epileptiform activity (spikes) is maximal at electrode 3 and is also seen nearby at electrode 4 (left traces). If a seizure secondarily generalizes, spike activity may be seen synchronously at all electrodes, after a delay (right-most traces). **(B)** A primary generalized seizure begins simultaneously in both hemispheres. The characteristic bilateral synchronous "spike-wave" pattern on EEG is generated by interactions between cortex and thalamus, with rapid spread via corpus callosum (CC) contributing to the rapid bilateral synchrony. One type of thalamic neuron (solid circle) is a GABAergic inhibitory cell with intrinsic oscillatory properties; this neuron has a specific type of calcium channel, which enables it to fire in bursts of action potentials, allowing the GABAergic cells to modulate ongoing excitatory corticothalamic activity. Cortical neurons send impulses to both inhibitory thalamic neurons (solid circle) and excitatory thalamic relay neurons (diamond), setting up oscillations of excitatory and inhibitory activity, which in turn give rise to the rhythmic spike waves on EEG. (Modified with permission of the American Academy of Pediatrics from ref. *58.*)

with its ionic channels, *neurotransmitters* and their receptors, or intracellular *second-messenger cascades,* and so on. Examples of specific pathophysiologic defects occurring at different sites within the nervous system are listed in Table 1 and are discussed more fully in subsequent sections. It is likely that specific genes modulate the excitability at each of these sites *(5).* Similarly, in addition to intrinsic factors, *acquired* disorders can express altered excitability at any of these levels. Just as epilepsy is not "one disease" but a broad spectrum of conditions associated with hyperexcitable neuronal function, there is no "one mechanism" of epilepsy; rather, several factors interact to create and sustain the hyperexcitable state.

Table 1
Examples of Specific Pathophysiologic Defects Leading to Epilepsy

Level of brain function	Condition	Pathophysiologic mechanism
Neuronal network	Cerebral dysgenesis, posttraumatic scar, mesial temporal sclerosis (in TLE)	Altered neuronal circuits: formation of aberrant excitatory connections ("sprouting")
Neuron structure	Downs syndrome and possibly other syndromes with mental retardation and seizures	Abnormal structure of dendrites and dendritic spines: altered current flow in neuron
Neurotransmitter synthesis	Pyridoxine (vitamin B_6) dependency	Decreased GABA synthesis: B_6, a cofactor of GAD
Neurotransmitter receptors: inhibitory	Angelman syndrome	Abnormal GABA receptor subunits
Neurotransmitter receptors: excitatory	Nonketotic hyperglycinemia	Excess glycine leads to of NMDA receptors
Synapse development	Neonatal seizures	Many possible mechanisms, including the depolarizing action of GABA early in development
Ionic channels	Benign familial neonatal convulsions	Potassium channel mutations: impaired repolarization

TLE, temporal lobe epilepsy; NMDA, *N*-methyl-D-aspartate; GABA, γ-aminobutyric acid; GAD, glutamic acid decarboxylase.

2.3. Evaluation of Seizures and Epilepsy

The EEG is our primary tool for recording the electrical activity of the human brain. Small disk electrodes are attached to the scalp at specified locations. When sufficiently amplified, voltage changes generated in neocortical neurons are recorded on the EEG as waveforms of various frequency, amplitude, and morphology. EEG patterns vary according to the patient's age, state of alertness, and genetic predisposition. The EEG may also record pathologic waveforms such spikes and sharp waves (representing the summated activity of many neurons firing synchronously) or focal slow waves (reflecting localized brain dysfunction). These abnormalities may be recorded in a given region (focal) or over the entire cortical surface (generalized). Because, however, the EEG records activity from near the brain's surface, mainly from neocortex, electrical activity emanating deep within the brain, e.g., brainstem, thalamus, and temporal lobe structures such as hippocampus, may not be recorded reliably by routine EEG. If surface recording is inadequate, special recording techniques may be required, such as electrodes surgically placed directly on the brain, e.g., subdural electrodes, or implanted into it, e.g., depth electrodes.

A variety of neuroimaging techniques continue to advance our understanding of epilepsy *(6)*. Magnetic resonance imaging (MRI) allows detection of minute developmental aberrations in brain structure, areas of brain that often comprise a seizure focus.

Techniques are now available to directly correlate MRI abnormalities with EEG activity. Positron emission tomography (PET) images the brain's regional utilization of glucose, with asymmetries in glucose utilization, suggesting interictal or ictal areas of abnormality *(7)*. Single photon emission computed tomography (SPECT) compares local blood flow discrepancies, a type of finding that is most informative when recorded during an actual seizure. Another promising new technique is magnetoencephalography (MEG), which assesses the brain's dynamic electromagnetic fields and can localize abnormally functioning areas *(8)*. Finally, a wide array of metabolic aberrations can lead to seizures and epilepsy, with the specific evaluation depending on the patient's clinical presentation *(9)*.

2.4. Refractory Epilepsy

About 70% of epilepsy patients respond favorably to AED monotherapy. However, the remaining 30% of patients respond poorly to AEDs and comprise the group whose condition is known as "refractory epilepsy." There is no uniformly accepted definition of refractory epilepsy; most commonly, epilepsy is considered to be refractory to medical treatment when there is lack of seizure control after two or three AEDs, within a defined period (usually 1–2 yr in adults; in children, this time frame is excessive for reasonable drug trial durations). In a study of 470 patients with newly diagnosed epilepsy, 61% were controlled on monotherapy (either the first or second drug chosen), and an additional 3% responded to therapy with two concurrent AEDs *(10)*. However, none of the patients who were not controlled on two AEDs together achieved seizure control when a third AED was added. Therefore, the remaining 36% of the patients would be considered to be refractory. This figure coincides closely to the wider literature, which estimates that 30–40% of patients with epilepsy are refractory to medical treatments. Depending on the epilepsy syndrome and etiology, some such patients would then be considered to be candidates for epilepsy surgery, implantable devices such as the vagus nerve stimulator, and other alternative therapies such as the ketogenic diet.

The foregoing definition of refractoriness assumes that the AEDs are chosen appropriately for the seizure type or epilepsy. Any consideration of an epilepsy as "refractory" also needs to take into account the possibility that the epilepsy itself is progressing *(11)* and that genetic drug-resistance factors may be present *(12)*. A major thrust of epilepsy research should be an attempt to identify early markers for medical refractoriness, to allow earlier, more aggressive therapeutic approaches. In particular, there are no data about whether earlier initiation of the ketogenic diet would enhance its effectiveness and prevent some of the medical and psychosocial sequelae of chronic epilepsy. Given the tendency of many childhood epilepsies to progress and become refractory, this issue is extremely timely.

3. NORMAL SYNAPTIC FUNCTION AND NEURONAL FIRING

As a preface to consideration of the abnormal firing seen in epilepsy, a review of normal synaptic transmission and neuronal firing is required. Neurons generally are one of two basic types, excitatory or inhibitory, depending on the neurotransmitter released from the neuron's terminals (Fig. 2). When a neuron is activated, it releases a transmitter from prepackaged vesicles in presynaptic terminals, a process that requires presy-

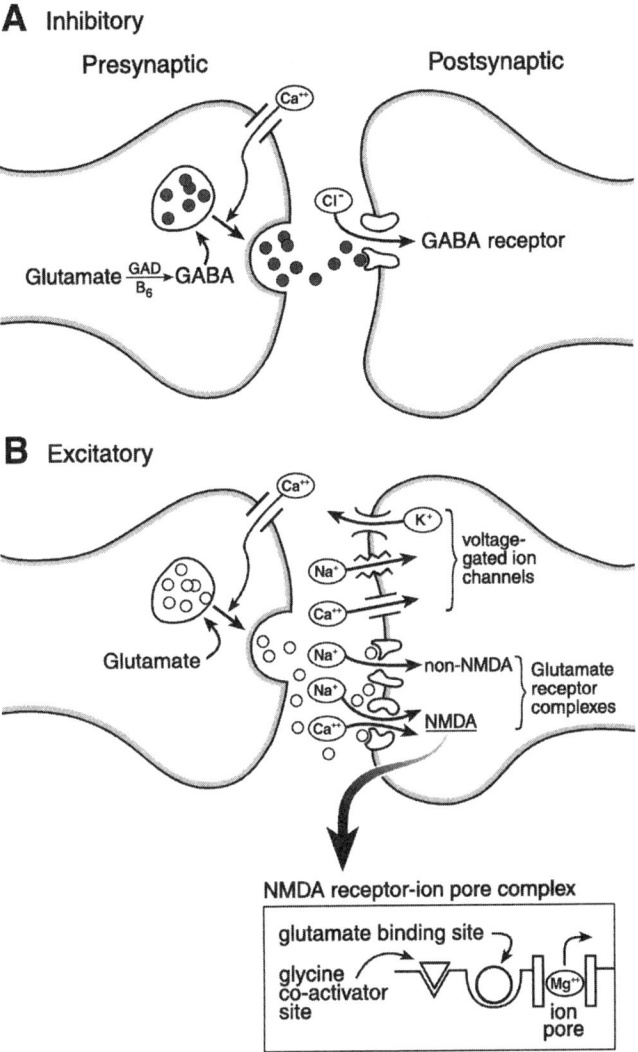

Fig. 2. Normal synaptic transmission showing representative inhibitory and excitatory presynaptic terminals and postsynaptic neurons. **(A)** Inhibitory synapse. GABA (solid circles) binding to its postsynaptic $GABA_A$ receptors allows influx of Cl^- ions, hyperpolarizing the postsynaptic neuron (IPSP; *see* text). GABA is synthesized from glutamate in a reaction catalyzed by glutamic acid decarboxylase (GAD), using pyridoxine (vitamin B_6) as a cofactor. **(B)** Excitatory synapse. Glutamate (open circles) released from the terminal crosses synaptic cleft and binds to one of several glutamate receptor subtypes (NMDA or non-NMDA; *see* text). Binding to non-NMDA receptors causes a fast EPSP; binding to NMDA receptors produces a longer, slow EPSP. If the postsynaptic neuron is sufficiently depolarized to reach firing threshold, an action potential will occur. Inset (box) shows details of the NMDA receptor–ion pore complex. For the NMDA ion pore to open, several events must occur: glutamate (open circle) must bind to the receptor, glycine (triangle) must bind to its own receptor site on the NMDA receptor complex, and when the cell is sufficiently depolarized, Mg^{2+} must leave the channel pore. Only then can Na^+ and Ca^{2+} flow into the neuron and produce a prolonged NMDA-mediated EPSP. (Modified with permission of the American Academy of Pediatrics from ref. *58*.)

naptic calcium influx. Vesicle fusion with the presynaptic terminal membrane allows release of the neurotransmitter, which then diffuses across the synaptic cleft and binds to its specific receptor on the postsynaptic membrane. Binding of a neurotransmitter to its receptor activates a cascade of events, involving ion fluxes through the receptor and a subsequent change in excitability of the postsynaptic cell (depolarization or hyperpolarization—that is, movement of the membrane potential closer to or further away from the threshold voltage for action potential generation, respectively). Since some neurotransmitters (ligands) causes the opening of ion channels, they are referred to as *ligand-gated channels.* Alternatively, ion channels may opened by voltage *(voltage-gated channels),* as discussed later.

3.1. Inhibitory Neurotransmission

The main inhibitory transmitter in the brain is γ-aminobutyric acid (GABA). GABA is synthesized from glutamate in the presynaptic terminal by action of the enzyme glutamic acid decarboxylase (GAD), which requires pyridoxine (vitamin B_6) as a cofactor (Fig. 2A). Influx of calcium ions (Ca^{2+}) caused by depolarization of the terminal of the inhibitory neuron causes vesicles to release GABA into the synaptic cleft. GABA diffuses across the cleft and binds to its receptors ($GABA_A$), and this sequence opens a pore or channel through which chloride ions (Cl^-) enter the neuron. This Cl^- influx increases the negative charge inside the postsynaptic neuron, hyperpolarizing it. The resultant change in membrane potential is called an *inhibitory postsynaptic potential* (IPSP) (Fig. 3). An IPSP reduces firing of the postsynaptic neuron by temporarily keeping the membrane potential away from its firing threshold.

Another type of GABA receptor ($GABA_B$) also exists. $GABA_B$ receptors are located both presynaptically and postsynaptically. Activation of presynaptic $GABA_B$ receptors reduces transmitter release, which could have an anti- or proepileptic effect, depending on whether the neuron is excitatory or inhibitory. Activation of postsynaptic $GABA_B$ receptors elicits a long-lasting IPSP mediated by a G protein that opens a potassium ion (K^+) channel. The role of $GABA_B$ receptors in epilepsy is being explored *(13).*

After GABA is released, it is rapidly taken up by the presynaptic neuron and degraded by the action of the catabolic enzyme GABA transaminase. Obviously, a reduction of any component of GABA synthesis, release, or binding would favor excitation and predispose to epileptic firing. Conversely, enhancing GABA function or decreasing its degradation would be a logical approach to restraining neuronal hyperexcitability. Several AEDs act on various aspects of the GABA system (*see* Section 8.).

Like all neurotransmitter receptors, GABA receptors are composed of many different subunits, each of which is under distinct genetic control. This allows for a wide diversity of GABA receptor types, which may differ from each other only in one or two subunits. Nevertheless, this subunit multiplicity creates a huge functional diversity in inhibitory control; different subunit combinations may confer differential functions and degrees of pharmacologic sensitivity on the receptor. In addition, the subunit composition may change during development. At different stages of brain maturation, GABA can mediate depolarization, hyperpolarization, or trophic (growth-regulating) actions *(14).* Obviously, this wide diversity could mediate function-specific pharmacologic modulation, which could play a significant role in seizure suppression at different ages or in different regions of the brain.

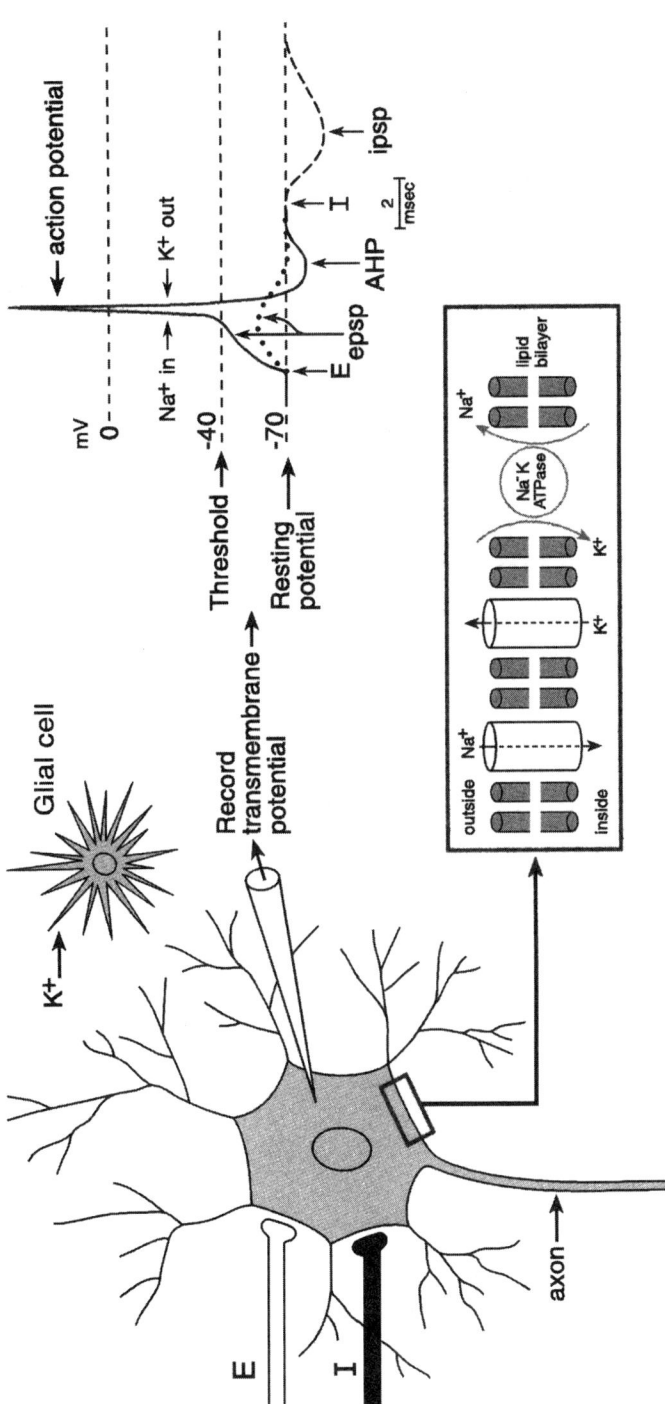

Fig. 3. Normal neuronal firing: left, schematic of neuron with one excitatory (E, open) and one inhibitory (I, solid) input; right, membrane potential, beginning at resting potential (−70 mV). Activation of E leads to graded EPSPs: a small one (dotted curve), and a larger one (solid line) that reaches threshold (approx −40 mV) for an action potential. The action potential is followed by an afterhyperpolarization (AHP), the magnitude and duration of which determine when the next action potential can occur. Activation of the inhibitory input (I) causes an IPSP (dashed curve). Inset magnified portion of the neuronal membrane as a lipid bilayer with interposed voltage-gated Na^+ and K^+ channels; the direction of ion fluxes during excitatory activation is shown. After firing, the membrane bound sodium–potassium pump (Na^+, K^+-ATPase) and star-shaped astroglial cells help to restore ionic balance. (Modified with permission of the American Academy of Pediatrics from ref. 58.)

11

3.2. Excitatory Neurotransmission and Action Potentials

3.2.1. EXCITATORY CHEMICAL NEUROTRANSMISSION

Excitatory neurotransmission in the brain is mediated largely by the excitatory amino acid, glutamate (Fig. 2B). Glutamate released from presynaptic terminals may bind to any of several glutamate receptor subtypes; for simplicity here, these are denoted as NMDA (*N*-methyl-D-aspartate) and non-NMDA (kainate and amino-3-hydroxy-5-methyl-isoxasole propionic acid [AMPA]). This confusing nomenclature arose because, experimentally, NMDA is a very selective agonist for one main subtype of glutamate receptor (therefore termed NMDA receptors), whereas AMPA and kainate prefer another type of glutamate receptor (therefore named non-NMDA receptors). However, in real life, glutamate (not NMDA, AMPA, or kainate) is the naturally occurring neurotransmitter; it is a flexible molecule that can bind to both NMDA and non-NMDA receptors, with different physiological consequences in each case. These receptor subtypes must be discussed because of their pivotal importance in the generation and maintenance of epileptic firing.

Non-NMDA receptors mediate the "fast" excitatory neurotransmission ordinarily associated with an *excitatory postsynaptic potential* (EPSP) (Fig. 3). Binding of glutamate to non-NMDA receptors causes influx of sodium ions (Na^+) through the receptor's pore, producing a "fast EPSP" (duration approx 5 ms), followed by an action potential if threshold is reached.

On the other hand, glutamate binding to NMDA receptors sets into motion a somewhat different set of physiological events. For activation of the NMDA receptor, the following must occur: (1) glutamate must bind to the NMDA receptor; (2) glycine, an essential coagonist, must bind at another, nearby site on the NMDA receptor complex; and (3) magnesium ion (Mg^{2+}) block of the channel pore must be removed (Fig. 2B, inset). Mg^{2+} ions play a unique role in the operation of the NMDA receptor. At resting potential, a Mg^{2+} ion sits in the pore, preventing influx of any other ions. Once the membrane potential is depolarized by 10–20 mV (by a non-NMDA-mediated fast EPSP), the Mg^{2+} is expelled from the pore into the extracellular space, allowing Na^+ and Ca^{2+} to flow into the neuron. This gives rise to a prolonged, NMDA-mediated EPSP. Much of the importance of NMDA receptors lies in their ability to allow Ca^{2+} influx; once inside a neuron, Ca^{2+} can participate in multiple crucial second-messenger pathways. In the normal brain, NMDA receptors play important roles in learning, in memory, and in the neuronal plasticity that underlies many critical developmental processes. However, if NMDA receptors are overstimulated, the entry of excess Ca^{2+} can wreak havoc, activating destructive intracellular enzymes, e.g., endonucleases, proteases, which may even lead to cell death. The role of NMDA receptors in epileptic firing is described in Section 4.2.

Non-NMDA and NMDA glutamate receptors are referred to as "ionotropic" or ion permeable. They mediate fast and slow excitatory neurotransmission, respectively. An even slower form of glutamate-mediated excitatory neurotransmission is mediated by another receptor class: metabotropic. Metabotropic receptors operate by means of receptor-activated signal transduction involving membrane-associated G proteins. A variety of metabotropic receptors exist and may regulate neurotransmission at a very fine level. Their importance in epilepsy is just beginning to be appreciated *(15)*.

The depolarization caused by either the fast or slow EPSP also activates voltage-gated ionic channels, such as Na^+ or Ca^{2+}, in the membrane; these channels, which

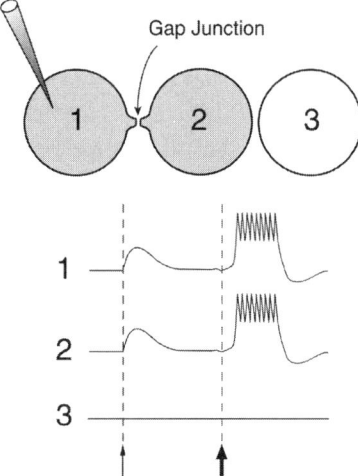

Fig. 4. Electrical synapse. Direct electrical communication via gap junctions allows rapid synchronization of electrical activity between neurons and may play a role in epileptic firing. Neurons 1 and 2 are connected via a gap junction, which allows direct passage of ionic current as well as dye (shading) between cells, when injected intracellularly into cell 1. Cell 3, which has no gap junctions, does not accumulate the dye. When an intracellular current pulse (thin arrow) is injected into cell 1, it is recorded simultaneously in cell 2. When a stronger pulse (thick arrow) is applied, an epileptic burst occurs instantaneously in cells 1 and 2. Electrical synapses provide a means for rapid synchronization of an epileptic circuit.

are distinct from those opened directly by transmitter binding, become activated and open only at certain membrane potentials. If the sum of depolarizations caused by glutamate receptor activation and by voltage-gated channels is sufficient, firing threshold may be reached, and an action potential will occur. During the longer NMDA-evoked depolarization, several action potentials may fire. Below threshold, EPSPs and IPSPs are engaged in a dynamic, electrical "tug of war," each affecting the membrane potential in the opposite direction. The final membrane potential is the sum of all excitatory and inhibitory inputs, which varies according to the magnitude and timing of each input.

3.2.2. EXCITATORY ELECTRICAL NEUROTRANSMISSION

In addition to intercellular communication via chemical synapses (excitatory or inhibitory), neurons may interact through electrical (or "electrotonic") synapses (Fig. 4). In contrast to the usual mode of chemical transmission, electrical synapses are specialized sites called gap junctions, closely apposed membranes between two cells through which electrical ionic currents can flow directly. This mode of neurotransmission, which is uniformly excitatory, does not involve the time delay that occurs at a chemical synapse; excitatory current flows directly and immediately from one neuron to its neighbor, with an action potential or even burst of action potentials occurring nearly instantaneously in the two neurons (Fig. 4). The existence of electrotonic transmission was shown in two ways: by direct cell-to-cell transmission when chemical synaptic transmission is blocked (in an environment devoid of Ca^{2+}) and by the passage of a membrane-impermeable dye from one cell to the other.

Electrotonic transmission, though rare by comparison to chemical transmission, has been identified in several parts of the brain. Obviously, if electrotonic transmission were too widespread, unbridled excitation could course through a neuronal network, leading to seizure activity (16,17). In fact, it is thought that electrical synapses mediate some aspects of epileptic synchronization, especially in the developing brain (18). The role of electrical synaptic transmission in epileptogenesis is being explored (17).

3.2.3. INTRINSIC MEMBRANE PROPERTIES

Synaptic transmission, either by chemical or electrical synapses, allows neurons to communicate with each other. A neuron's excitability (responsiveness to voltage changes) is also determined by its "intrinsic membrane properties," including membrane resistance, subthreshold voltage-dependent ionic channels, and the shape, pattern, and extent of its dendrites and other neuritic processes (collectively known as the neuron's "cable properties") (19). Some cells in the brain possess membrane properties that endow them with a "natural" hyperexcitability. For example, hippocampal CA3 neurons fire in bursts of action potentials under ordinary conditions. Therefore, these neurons may be uniquely qualified to participate in seizure generation and propagation. Intrinsic membrane properties combine with the network's synaptic characteristics to determine ultimate excitability.

3.2.4. ACTION POTENTIALS

Action potentials are "all-or-none" events; once threshold has been reached, an action potential will fire. The upstroke of the action potential is caused by a huge influx of Na^+ through voltage-gated channels, whereas the downstroke is due to efflux of K^+ out of the cell through voltage-gated K^+ channels. In one recently described epilepsy syndrome, benign familial neonatal convulsions, mutations of voltage-dependent K^+ channels were found; such mutations would prolong action potentials by reducing their repolarization rate, thus keeping the neuron depolarized longer and favoring excessive excitation (20).

At the tail end of the action potential, the membrane potential is briefly hyperpolarized beyond its original resting level; this is called the afterhyperpolarization (AHP) (Fig. 3). The AHP is mediated by another type of K^+ channel, different from the one responsible for the action potential downstroke just discussed and not dependent on voltage but rather on the intracellular Ca^{2+} level. These "Ca^{2+}-dependent K^+ channels" regulate the timing of neuronal firing by governing the neuron's refractory period, the time during which the cell is still recovering from the preceding action potential and cannot yet generate another one. Therefore, these channels can limit repetitive firing and, if they become dysfunctional, epileptic discharges may result.

3.3. Glial Cell Function and Ionic Homeostasis

Because the ionic balance inside and outside the neuron is altered after neuronal firing (especially after repetitive, epileptic discharges), a mechanism must exist to restore ionic homeostasis. After neuronal firing, there is excess Na^+ inside the cell and excess K^+ in the extracellular space. A Na^+, K^+-ATPase (an energy-dependent pump) in the neuronal membrane subserves this restorative function by pumping Na^+ back out of the cell and K^+ back into the cell (Fig. 3, inset). In addition, normalization of ionic balance is aided by nearby glial cells, which act as "ionic sponges" by soaking up excess extracellular K^+.

This role of glial cells in neuronal function is critical, because elevated extracellular K^+ can directly depolarize the membrane of the neuron and itself cause epileptic firing *(21)*.

3.4. Neuromodulators and Neurotransmitter Transporters

In addition to the standard neurotransmitters already discussed, a variety of other compounds are stored in presynaptic terminals and are released with neurotransmitters. These substances, called neuromodulators, are typically peptides that act to regulate or modify the actions of the primary neurotransmitters. Such neurosynaptic flexibility allows the brain to fine-tune excitation and inhibition in different regions, under different physiological conditions, and at different ages. For example, the excitatory neuropeptide corticotrophin-releasing hormone (CRH) is found in high concentration in neurons of seizure-prone limbic structures such as the amygdala and hippocampus *(22)*. In infant rats, exposure of the brain to a very small amount of CRH causes intense seizures, whereas the adult rat is relatively resistant to the convulsant action of CRH. This age specificity may relate to the ability of CRH antagonists to suppress seizures and could have clinical implications for the treatment of infantile spasms.

Neuropeptide Y (NPY) and somatostatin (SS) are two other peptides that have neuromodulatory roles in epilepsy; both appear to have anticonvulsant properties. NPY may act by decreasing Ca^{2+} entry into presynaptic terminals containing glutamate, thereby reducing release of this excitatory transmitter *(23,24)*. NPY and SS are colocalized in inhibitory neurons of the hippocampal dentate gyrus. Death of such neurons, as in status epilepticus, might facilitate the development of excitatory circuits. Mutant mice, deficient in NPY, develop spontaneous seizures. The modulatory role in epilepsy of these and other peptides, e.g., galanin, opioids, is under investigation *(25)*. Growth factors like brain-derived neurotrophic factor (BDNF) also modify seizure activity *(26)*.

Specific membrane-bound proteins known as neurotransmitter transporters aid in the termination of transmitter activity by transporting the neurotransmitter molecules back into neurons or glial cells *(27,28)*. These transporters play an important role in the inactivation of neurotransmitters after their release into the synaptic cleft, thus preventing their prolonged action. Obviously, extended exposure to an excitatory neurotransmitter could lead to sustained neuronal firing, and thus, defective function of the glutamate transporter could exacerbate the epileptic condition *(29,30)*. Mice with a deletion (knockout) of the gene for one glutamate transporter, GLT1, develop lethal seizures. One new anticonvulsant, tiagabine, sustains inhibitory action by blocking GABA reuptake (*see* Section 8.).

3.5. Brain Energetics and Metabolism

The brain requires a tremendous amount of energy for optimal function. Normally, the brain utilizes more than 20% of the body's basal oxygen consumption (in children, the percentage is an even higher). Much of this energy expenditure is used to operate ionic pumps and other cellular machinery. Ordinarily, the brain derives its energy from the aerobic oxidation of carbohydrate (mainly glucose), making it an "obligate" utilizer of glucose.

With both generalized and focal seizure activity, the brain's demand for energy increases markedly. Cerebral metabolic rate rises, as manifested by elevations in cerebral blood flow as well as oxygen and glucose utilization, which increase severalfold. Multiple energy metabolites increase, as summarized in Table 2 *(31)*. Glucose is

Table 2
Some Immediate-Onset Metabolic Changes Induced by Seizure Activity

Metabolic parameter	Change	Timing (persistence)
Cerebral blood flow	Increase	Sustained for duration of seizure
Oxygen consumption	Increase	Sustained for duration of seizure
Glucose uptake and metabolism	Increase	Sustained for duration of seizure
Glucose level	Decrease	Transient
Phosphocreatine	Decrease	Sustained for duration of seizure
ATP	Decrease	Transient
Lactate	Increase	Sustained for duration of seizure
pH	Decrease	Transient

depleted, phosphocreatine and ATP levels drop, and lactate accumulates, a reflection of the brain's transition to anaerobic metabolism. Other metabolites may also be altered by seizure activity, including second messengers, free fatty acids, and nucleosides, e.g., adenosine, which has inherent anticonvulsant properties *(32)*. In brief seizures, these changes are reversible, but in prolonged seizure activity (status epilepticus), permanent neuronal damage may ensue. With PET scanning, cerebral metabolism (glucose utilization) can be measured in patients. During a seizure, PET scans show a huge increase in metabolism in the brain region affected by the seizure; i.e., the region is hypermetabolic. Interictally, metabolism in the epileptic brain region is reduced below that of unaffected brain; i.e., the region is hypometabolic. Seizures also activate protein synthesis and gene expression (both immediate-early genes and longer-acting genes), which may contribute to epileptogenesis (*see* Section 5.).

If deprived of glucose, either through fasting or dietary intake predominantly of fats, e.g., ketogenic diet, the brain can shift its metabolism and utilize ketones as an energy source, rather than carbohydrates. How ketones exert an antiseizure effect is unknown; this question is addressed extensively in this volume. If the brain lacks an energy substrate, either through decreased supply, e.g., ischemia, or in prolonged seizures (status epilepticus), neuronal damage and even cell death can occur. The mechanisms by which epileptogenesis is enhanced in such situations are discussed in Section 5.

In summary, the involvement of multiple ion fluxes through a wide variety of voltage- and transmitter-dependent channels, chemical and electrical synaptic transmission, and intrinsic membrane properties (Table 3) contribute to the complexity of normal neuronal firing. This complexity also provides the opportunity for pharmacologic intervention at a diversity of sites if the system becomes pathologically hyperexcitable, i.e., in epilepsy.

4. ABNORMAL NEURONAL FIRING: EPILEPSY

4.1. Hyperexcitability and Hypersynchrony: Hallmarks of Epileptic Neurons

How is normal neuronal firing altered in epilepsy? The pathophysiology of epilepsy has two distinct but related hallmarks: *hyperexcitability* and *hypersynchrony (33,34)*. Hyperexcitability is the abnormal responsiveness of a neuron to an excitatory input; the neuron tends to fire multiple discharges instead of the usual one or two. Hypersyn-

Table 3
Roles of Channels and Receptors in Normal and Epileptic Firing

Channel or receptor	Role in normal neuronal function	Possible role in epilepsy
Voltage-gated Na^+ channel	Subthreshold EPSP; action potential upstroke	Repetitive action potential firing
Voltage-gated K^+ channel	Action potential downstroke	Abnormal action potential repolarization
Ca^{2+}-dependent K^+ channel	AHP following action potential; sets refractory period	Limits repetitive firing
Voltage-gated Ca^{2+} channel	Transmitter release; carries depolarizing charge from dendrites to soma	Excess transmitter release; activates pathologic intracellular processes
Non-NMDA receptor	Fast EPSP	Initiates paroxysmal depolarization shift (PDS)
NMDA receptor	Prolonged, slow EPSP	Maintains PDS; Ca^{2+} activates pathological intracellular processes
$GABA_A$ receptor	IPSP	Limits excitation
$GABA_B$ receptor	Prolonged IPSP	Limits excitation
Electrical synapses	Ultrafast excitatory transmission	Synchronization of neuronal firing
Na-K pump	Restores ionic balance	Prevents K^+-induced depolarization

chrony refers to the recruitment of large numbers of neighboring neurons into an abnormal firing pattern. Ultimately, epilepsy is a network phenomenon requiring participation of many neurons firing synchronously. What happens in the normally functioning brain to cause it to fire hypersynchronously, and what are possible mechanisms for excitation to increase, inhibition to diminish, or both?

Figure 5 provides a schematic overview of normal, interictal (between seizures), and ictal (during a seizure) physiological events at the level of the whole brain and in a simplified neuronal circuit. First, consider the widespread cortical networks in the top panel. Normally, excitation and inhibition in neocortex are relatively balanced. Neurons are activated when needed; otherwise they are quiescent. The EEG in the normal situation (left column) shows low-voltage "desynchronized" activity—that is, neurons in the region under the electrode are not firing synchronously. If a large number of neurons, perhaps thousands or more, begin to fire synchronously in an area of cortex, a so-called EEG spike or interictal discharge is recorded on the EEG (middle column). The larger the area of cortex involved, the greater the spread of such an interictal discharge. In Fig. 5, the largest concentration of neurons firing synchronously is under electrode 2, though electrode 1 also detects some spread of the abnormal firing, recorded as a small discharge or "sharp wave." Interictal spikes are typically 30–50 ms in duration. The third column depicts the ictal state (seizure), with a barrage of rapidly firing EEG spikes in electrodes 2 (with spread to electrode 1), which may continue for many seconds or minutes. At this point, a

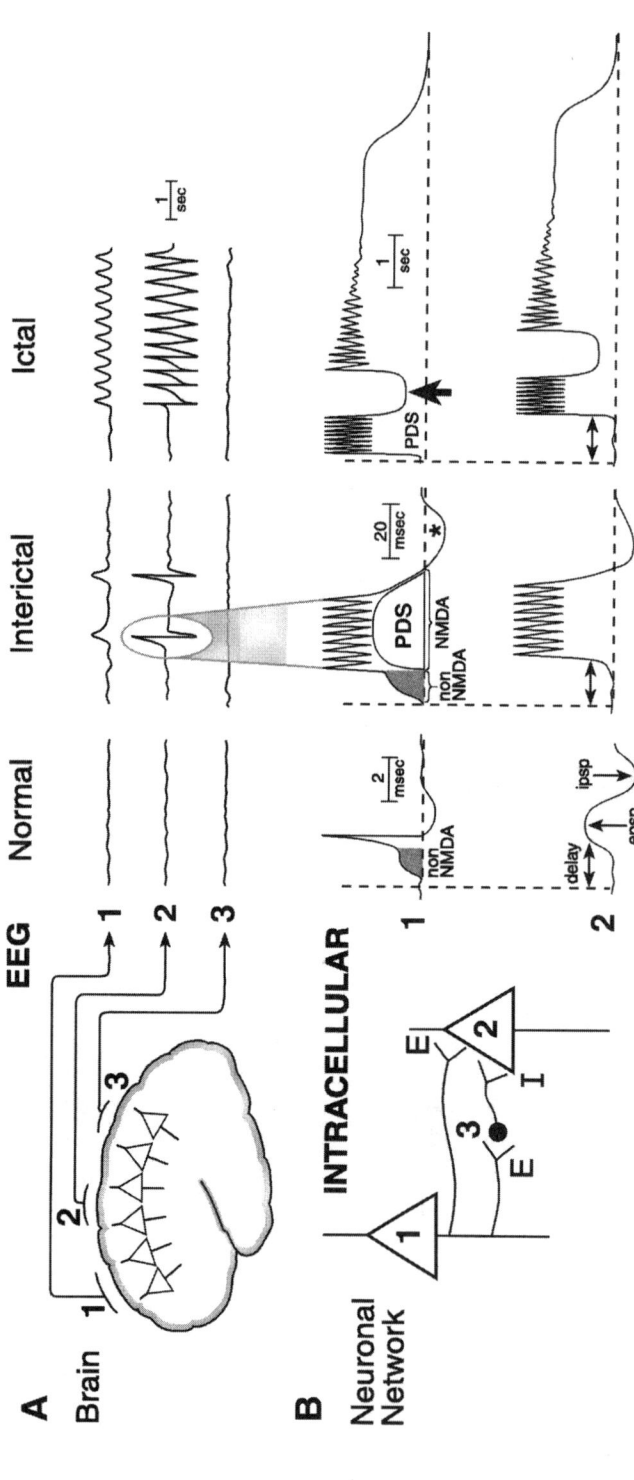

Fig. 5. Abnormal neuronal firing at the levels of (**A**) the brain and (**B**) a simplified neuronal network consisting of two excitatory neurons, 1 and 2, and an inhibitory interneuron, 3. EEG (top set of traces) and intracellular recordings (bottom set of traces) are shown for the normal (left column), interictal (middle column), and ictal conditions (right column). Numbered traces refer to like-numbered recording sites. Note time-scale differences in different traces. (A) Three EEG electrodes record activity from superficial neocortical neurons. In the normal case, activity is low voltage and "desynchronized" (neurons are not firing together in synchrony). In the interictal condition, large "spikes" are seen focally at electrode 2 (and to a lesser extent at electrode 1, where they are termed "sharp waves"), representing synchronized firing of a large population of hyperexcitable neurons (expanded in time in B). The ictal state is characterized by a long run of spikes. (B) At the neuronal network level, the intracellular correlate of the interictal EEG spike is called the paroxysmal depolarization shift (PDS). The PDS is initiated by a non-NMDA-mediated fast EPSP (shading) but is *maintained* by a longer, larger NMDA-mediated EPSP. The post-PDS hyperpolarization (asterisk) temporarily stabilizes the neuron; if this post-PDS hyperpolarization fails to restore membrane potential to the resting level (right column, thick arrow), ictal discharge can occur. The lowermost traces, recordings from neuron 2, show activity similar to that recorded in neuron 1, occurring a bit later owing to a synaptic delay (double-headed horizontal arrow). Activation of inhibitory neuron 3 by firing of neuron 1 prevents neuron 2 from generating an action potential (the IPSP counters the depolarization caused by the EPSP). But if neuron 2 does reach firing threshold, additional neurons will be recruited, leading to an entire network firing in synchrony (seizure!). (Modified with permission of the American Academy of Pediatrics from ref. 58.)

huge number of neurons is firing synchronously, the result of which would be a clinical seizure with manifestations correlating with the area of brain involved.

4.2. Pathophysiological Events in Neuronal Network

What is happening at the neuronal network level when neurons transition from their normal firing pattern to the interictal condition and then to the ictal state? Figure 5B depicts some of the physiologic features that accompany these changes. Now, rather than recording electrical activity from the surface of the brain, single electrodes are placed inside individual excitatory cortical neurons 1 and 2, thereby recording intracellular potentials. Much of our understanding of epilepsy mechanisms comes from such experiments using animal models *(35,36)*.

In the normal situation, an action potential occurs in neuron 1 when the membrane potential is depolarized to its threshold level, as previously discussed. Discharges in neuron 1 may also influence the activity of its neighbor, neuron 2. For example, with a delay of several milliseconds, an action potential in neuron 1 may give rise to an EPSP in neuron 2. If cell 3, an inhibitory interneuron, is also activated by a discharge from neuron 1, then the activity in neuron 2 will be modified by an IPSP overlapping in time with the EPSP; the recorded event will be a summed EPSP–IPSP sequence. If the IPSP occurs earlier, perhaps coincident with the EPSP, the depolarizing effect of the EPSP will be diminished. In this way, we can envision inhibition as "sculpting" or modifying ongoing excitation. If this concept is extrapolated to thousands of interconnected neurons, each influencing the activity of many neighbors, it is easy to see how an increase in excitation or decrease in inhibition in the system could lead to hypersynchronous, epileptic firing in a large area of brain. Normally, neurons fire action potentials, singly or in brief runs, and excitability is kept in check by the presence of powerful inhibitory influences (the "inhibitory surround," schematized in Fig. 6). For the activity of a small group of localized, synchronously firing neurons to spread across a wide area of cortex, the local excitation must overcome this surrounding region of strong synaptic inhibition.

The intracellular correlate of the interictal focal EEG spike is called the *paroxysmal depolarization shift* (PDS) *(37)*. It is called "paroxysmal" because it is arises suddenly from baseline activity and "depolarization shift" because the membrane potential is depolarized (less negative) for several tens of milliseconds. The PDS is actually a "giant EPSP," a prolonged depolarization causing the neuron to fire a burst of several action potentials riding on a large envelope of depolarization (Fig. 5B, middle and right columns). Importantly, the PDS is an NMDA-mediated event; experimentally, NMDA receptor blockers prevent PDSs and the transition from the interictal state to a seizure. The PDS is initiated or "kicked off" by a fast, non-NMDA-mediated EPSP and sustained by a prolonged, NMDA-mediated EPSP. Compared with the usual NMDA-mediated slow EPSP of approx 10–20 ms, the PDS is longer (30–50 ms) with many more action potentials on top of the depolarization. Note that the durations of the PDS and interictal EEG spike are similar (because they represent the same event!).

The PDS is followed by a large "post-PDS hyperpolarization" (asterisk in Fig. 5B), which serves to terminate the PDS and stop, at least temporarily, the rampant firing of action potentials. Note that a PDS in neuron 1 may activate a similar PDS in neuron 2, and so on, such that a whole network of neurons can be rapidly recruited into firing in a synchronous manner. If excitation becomes excessive or if inhibition is severely curtailed, the PDS can lead into an ictal discharge (right column). In the top trace, the post-

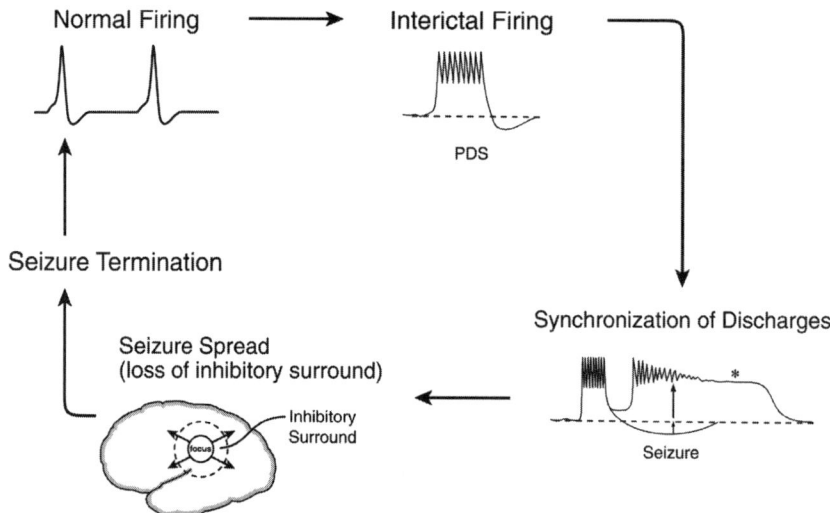

Fig. 6. Schematic diagram of the sequence of a partial seizure. Initially, neurons fire normally with single action potentials. The hallmark of interictal firing is the paroxysmal depolarizing shift (PDS). As the PDS gradually loses its post-PDS hyperpolarization (short vertical arrow), as the firing of local neurons becomes synchronized, a seizure occurs (longer vertical arrow). The ictal electrical signature of a seizure is a persistent depolarizing plateau potential (asterisk) on which are superimposed bursts of clustered spikes. Spread of the seizure beyond the local area depends on overcoming the strong inhibitory surround adjacent to the focus. Finally, the seizure stops and normal firing resumes. Separate physiologic mechanisms regulate each of these steps (*see* text).

PDS hyperpolarization is lost (thick arrow), allowing the neuron to generate a prolonged paroxysmal discharge. Such discharges in one neuron can easily spread to others, overwhelming the inhibitory control on the system and leading to an electrographic and clinical seizure. This interictal-to-ictal transition may occur because the post-PDS hyperpolarization is diminished owing to potentiation of EPSPs, decrement in IPSPs, inability to clear extracellular K^+, a large increase in intracellular calcium, or a variety of other mechanisms.

4.3. Seizure Propagation

The exact mechanisms by which seizure activity spreads from its focus of origin to distant parts of the brain are less well understood but are likely to involve similar physiologic processes *(38)*. Initially, synchronous neuronal discharges are restricted to the focus; as the post-PDS hyperpolarization shrinks (Fig. 5B), burst discharges involve successively more neurons. Eventually, excitation at the local level is sufficient to overcome the powerful inhibition surrounding the focus. As excitation propagates into this normal tissue, the inhibitory surround breaks down (at least temporarily), and hypersynchronous firing proceeds along established neural pathways to distant brain regions. For example, in neocortex, epileptic activity spreads horizontally to nearby cortical areas, as well as vertically to projection sites in brainstem, thalamus, and spinal cord. Because some areas of brain are reciprocally connected, there may be "back-propagation" to the original seizure focus as well, e.g., thalamocortical connections in Fig. 1A. The clinical manifestations of a seizure reflect the areas of brain affected, from the local circuit, e.g., "aura" of a temporal lobe seizure, to widespread brain involvement, e.g., secondarily generalized convulsion of a temporal lobe seizure.

4.4. Seizure Termination

Mechanisms by which a seizure stops are also not well delineated. Possible reasons for seizure termination include reestablishment of normal ionic gradients (with the help of glia and neuronal ion pumps), restoration of normal excitatory and inhibitory synaptic transmission and ionic currents (e.g., Ca^{2+}, Na^+, K^+), and return of metabolic homeostasis. Neuromodulators, including adenosine and many others (discussed in Section 3.4), may play a role in seizure termination as well. Clearly, to design optimal AEDs we need to understand much more about the pathophysiological factors critical for seizure termination (*see* Section 8.).

4.5. Summary

The brain can utilize its existing, normal circuitry to generate and spread seizure activity if the system is perturbed in a way that favors excitation over inhibition. Figure 6 summarizes the sequence of a partial seizure, from normal firing to interictal firing, then to synchronization and spread of neuronal activity (seizure). Finally, the seizure stops, either spontaneously or after pharmacological intervention. Distinct physiological mechanisms govern each of these steps. In the case of recurrent, unprovoked seizures (epilepsy), neuronal function is persistently abnormal. This chronic hyperexcitability can result from a number of mechanisms (Tables 1 and 3). For example, reduced inhibition can result from death or dysfunction of inhibitory neurons or from genetic conditions in which GABA synthesis is impaired or GABA receptors have an abnormal subunit composition. Lagging development, early in life, of inhibitory connections behind excitatory ones can also result in reduced inhibition. Enhanced excitation may occur if non-NMDA or NMDA receptors are overactivated owing to the presence of excessive glutamate or glycine, if excitatory connections overwhelm inhibitory ones, or if the ion channels responsible for repolarization are genetically aberrant. The transition from a single seizure to the state of chronic epilepsy will now be discussed.

5. EPILEPTOGENESIS: STRUCTURAL ALTERATIONS LEADING TO EPILEPSY

One of the great mysteries in neuroscience is how the brain becomes permanently altered to create the substrate for chronic epilepsy. Sometimes an etiology or structural cause can be determined, but often no explanation is found. One type of epilepsy, temporal lobe epilepsy or TLE, can be a consequence of structural alterations to the hippocampus, one of the most epilepsy-prone (epileptogenic) areas of the brain. Hippocampal injury, such as caused by status epilepticus (arbitrarily defined as a seizure lasting more than 30 min), may produce persistent hyperexcitability long after the end of a prolonged seizure. This chronic hyperexcitability is a result of the combined effects of several structural alterations: neuronal death, gliosis or mesial temporal sclerosis, and the growth of new, abnormal axonal connections ("sprouting"). Figure 7 depicts how such sprouting might work by producing aberrant excitatory connections. Dentate granule neurons (Fig. 7A, circles 1, 2) receive all incoming activity entering the hippocampus. Ordinarily, dentate neurons fire only single action potentials (right panel,

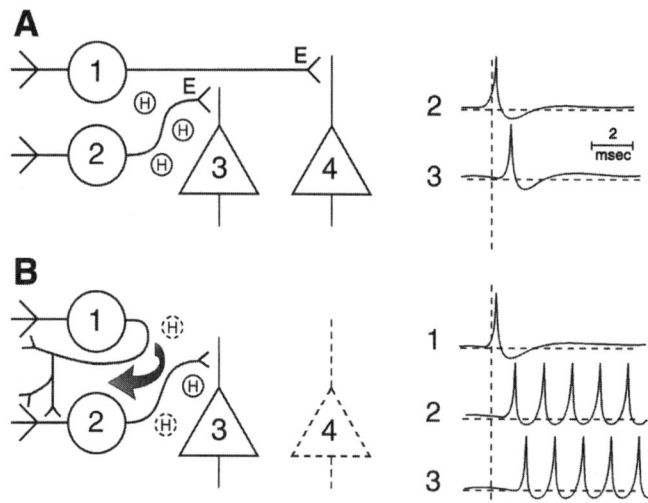

Fig. 7. Simplified depiction of sprouting in the hippocampal dentate gyrus. (**A**) Normal situation: left, Dentate granule neurons (1, 2) make excitatory synapses (E) onto dendrites of hippocampal pyramidal neurons (3, 4); right, activation of dentate neuron 2 causes single action potential in pyramidal neuron 3, after a synaptic delay. (**B**) As a consequence of status epilepticus, many pyramidal neurons die (4, dashed outline), leaving axons of dentate neuron 1 without a postsynaptic target; those axons then "sprout" and innervate the dendrites of other granule neurons (thick curved arrow), creating the substrate for a hyperexcitable circuit. Now, when neuron 1 is activated, multiple action potentials are fired in neuron 2, and therefore in neuron 3 (right traces). As described in the text, this diagram is simplified and, in fact, neurons of numerous types in the dentate hilus (labeled H) are also involved in the outcome of seizure-induced synaptic plasticity. The resultant circuit function will depend on the character (excitatory or inhibitory) and connectivity of these interneurons. (Modified with permission of the American Academy of Pediatrics from ref. *58.*)

trace 2). Dentate neurons innervate hippocampal pyramidal neurons (triangles: 3, 4), which fire single action potentials in response to dentate input (right panel, trace 3). Status epilepticus typically causes death of pyramidal cells (owing to overactivation of NMDA receptors and excessive Ca^{2+} entry, as discussed in Section 4.2.) but spares dentate neurons (Fig. 7B). Therefore, axons of dentate neuron 1 are left without a postsynaptic target, so they turn around and wind their way back to innervate their own dendrites and those of neighboring dentate neurons, forming "autoexcitatory," reverberating excitatory circuits (Fig. 7B, left). Now, dentate neuron 2 receives excessive excitatory input and fires multiple action potentials, causing surviving pyramidal neurons to do the same (trace 3). Rather than being unique to hippocampus, sprouting may comprise a more general mechanism by which brain circuits become hyperexcitable.

However, the circuit diagram in Fig. 7 is oversimplified. In fact, interspersed between the dentate granule cells and the pyramidal neurons (in the dentate "hilus," labeled H) are many other types of neuron and interneuron, some excitatory, others inhibitory. Depending on which of hilar neurons are silenced (by seizure-induced cell death) or activated by seizure activity, the physiology of the circuit could be vastly altered *(39).* This synaptic flexibility is an example of seizure-induced plasticity and can give rise to complicated circuits that can either compensate for or exacerbate the initial seizure situation.

To make matters even more complicated, seizures can induce neurogenesis in certain areas of the brain, that is, the birth of new neurons (even in the adult brain). This phenomenon is especially prominent in the dentate gyrus. Again, it can give rise to increased or decreased excitability depending on the connectivity and type of newly born neurons. The role of neurogenesis in epileptogenesis is being investigated *(40)*.

In addition to injury-induced alterations of structural neuronal networks, neural circuits can also be naturally epileptic. Children with abnormal brain development (dysgenesis) have a high predisposition to epilepsy. Aided by advances in neuroimaging, especially MRI, an ever-increasing number of dysgenetic cortical lesions is being delineated. Some of these lesions are quite subtle yet are sufficient to comprise an epileptic circuit *(41)*. Disruption at any step in the complex sequence of brain development, e.g., neuronal proliferation, migration, synaptogenesis, can lead to abnormal circuit function and epilepsy. Examination of dysgenetic cortical tissue from animals with experimentally induced abnormal brain development reveals widespread evidence of hyperexcitable circuitry *(42)*.

6. ENHANCED EXCITABILITY IN IMMATURE BRAIN

The immature brain is especially susceptible to seizures *(43,44)*. Seizure incidence is highest during the first decade and especially during the first year of life. Several physiologic features favor enhanced neuronal hyperexcitability early in life. Ca^{2+} and Na^+ channels, which mediate neuronal excitation, develop relatively early. Excitatory synapses tend to form before inhibitory ones. Excitatory NMDA receptors are transiently overexpressed early in postnatal development, when they are needed for critical developmental processes. The branching pattern of axons in the immature brain is markedly more complex than later in life, forming an exuberant network of excitatory connections *(45)*. The ability of glial cells to clear extracellular K^+ also improves with age.

GABA, perhaps paradoxically, exerts an excitatory action early in development, rather than the inhibitory effect seen later *(46)*. Early in development, chloride ion (Cl^-) concentration is greater inside the neuron than outside, and the reversal potential for Cl^- is close to action potential threshold. Therefore, early in development, when GABA binds to its receptors and opens Cl^- channels, the negatively charged chloride ions inside the neuron flow to the outside, down their electrochemical gradient. The loss of negative charge from inside the neuron depolarizes it to a membrane potential closer to the threshold for an action potential (Fig. 8). Later in development, the opposite situation occurs: Cl^+ predominates in the extracellular space as a result of the expression of a membrane protein called KCC2. KCC2 extrudes Cl^-, keeping the basal Cl^- concentration inside the neuron at about one quarter of its concentration early in life and the Cl^- reversal potential is more negative than resting membrane potential *(47,48)*. Therefore, in the mature brain, GABA receptor activation causes entry of Cl^-, thus hyperpolarizing the neuron, keeping it further away from action potential threshold.

Therefore, for many reasons, the excitatory/inhibitory balance in the brain changes dramatically over the course of development. The disadvantage of these physiological adaptations is that the brain is especially vulnerable to hyperexcitability and seizure generation during a critical window of development. Nevertheless, these neurophysiological idiosyncrasies of early brain development also provide the opportunity for producing novel, age-specific therapies.

A **Developing Brain: GABA is Depolarizing (excitatory)**

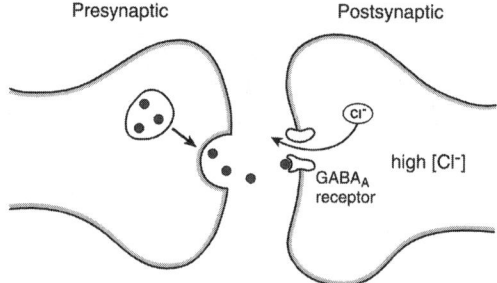

B **Mature Brain: GABA is Hyperpolarizing (inhibitory)**

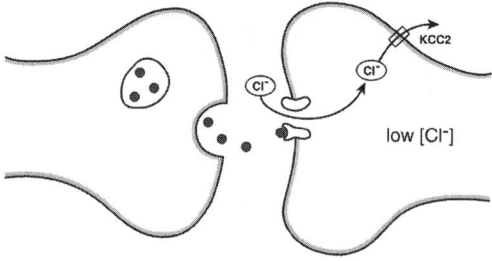

Fig. 8. Schematic diagram of the changes in GABA responsiveness over development. **(A)** In early development, activation of postsynaptic GABA$_A$ receptors causes efflux of Cl$^-$ ions because of the high intracellular Cl$^-$ concentration. This Cl$^-$ efflux causes membrane depolarization, because there is a net loss of negative charge from inside the neuron. **(B)** Later in development, the Cl$^-$ transporter KCC2 (not present early in development) reverses the Cl$^-$ gradient, such that the basal Cl$^-$ concentration is higher extracellularly. In this case, activation of GABA$_A$ receptors causes Cl$^-$ influx and hyperpolarization (net inward movement of negative charge), the usual function attributed to GABA.

7. CONSEQUENCES OF SEIZURES AND EPILEPSY

One of the most frequently asked questions in the clinical setting is, "Do seizures cause brain damage?" This question has been the subject of intense scientific scrutiny (49), yet a simple answer is not forthcoming. The outcome of epilepsy depends on many factors, including the age of the subject at the time of seizure onset, the underlying brain disorder causing the seizures, and the duration, frequency, and severity of the seizures. To address the question, the definition and methods of brain damage assessment must be taken into account (50). Brain damage can be interpreted as one or more of the following: structural damage to brain tissue, cognitive and behavioral deficits, neurologic disabilities, and subsequent seizure susceptibility. Persons with epilepsy face numerous psychosocial and medical challenges, including adjustment to the unpredictability of seizures, the need to take AEDs with their attendant side effects, and the dependence on others for certain daily functions. Therefore, the consequences of epilepsy are multiple and multifactorial.

Given this overview, it can be concluded that the longer a seizure, the more profound the consequences. For example, status epilepticus causes damage to neurons even when systemic factors, e.g., blood pressure, oxygenation, are controlled. However, even brief, recurrent seizures may lead to long-term changes in both brain structure and function, and many authorities now consider epilepsy to be a progressive disorder (11). In animal models, seizures lead to impairment of spatial memory and learning; these findings are most devastating with status epilepticus in adults, but seizures during early development also cause subtle morphologic and behavioral deficits *(51–53)*.

8. ANTIEPILEPTIC DRUG MECHANISMS

Applying the concepts developed thus far, some of the actions of various antiseizure therapies can now be examined *(54,55)* (Fig. 9). Clinical indications, pharmacokinetics, doses, and side effects are not discussed here; the reader is referred to standard textbooks for this information.

Several AEDs target aspects of the inhibitory system. Phenobarbital (PHB) and benzodiazepines (BZDs) bind to different sites on the $GABA_A$ receptor. Both drugs enhance inhibition by allowing increased Cl^- influx through the GABA receptor: PHB by increasing the duration of chloride channel openings and BZD by increasing the frequency of openings. Vigabatrin (VGB) is a new AED that is not yet available in the United States; it has shown much promise in other countries for the treatment of infantile spasms (especially in children with tuberous sclerosis) and other seizure types. VGB is an example of a "designer drug," created to target a specific pathophysiological mechanism: VGB inhibits the enzyme that degrades GABA (GABA transaminase), thereby increasing the amount of GABA available to partake in inhibitory neurotransmission. Another new AED, tiagabine (TGB), also increases GABA availability but by a different mechanism: preventing GABA reuptake into the presynaptic terminal. The mechanism of action of gabapentin (GBP), despite the presence of GABA in its name, is still unresolved; GBP may increase the rate of GABA synthesis or release.

Other AEDs affect aspects of neuronal excitation. Phenytoin and carbamazepine, and the newer AEDs lamotrigine and zonisamide, block voltage-dependent sodium channels and reduce the ability of neurons to fire repetitively. Ethosuximide, used primarily for absence seizures, blocks a unique calcium current ("T-current") present only in thalamic neurons, preventing them from firing in an oscillatory fashion and recruiting neocortical neurons into spike-wave patterns. Several of the new AEDs are believed to alter the function of NMDA receptors (lamotrigine and felbamate) or non-NMDA receptors (topiramate). The dissociative anesthetic ketamine blocks the ion pore of NMDA receptors; however, ketamine and similarly acting agents have been disappointing in clinical trials because they cause excessive sedation or behavioral activation. Much effort is being expended to design novel AEDs that selectively target other aspects of the NMDA system (Fig. 2, inset). In addition to blockage of the ion pore, antiseizure activity may be produced by antagonists of glutamate binding or blockade at other sites on the receptor complex that must be activated for the receptor complex to function (such as the glycine coagonist site). The voltage-dependent block of the NMDA receptor ion pore by Mg^{2+} may be another site for novel anticonvulsant action; in fact, magnesium sulfate has been used for years by obstetricians to control seizures in eclampsia. Topiramate, felbamate, and gabapentin, as well as the established AED valproic acid, probably have mixed excitatory and inhibitory actions. The mechanism of action of levetiracetam has not yet been clarified, but it appears to be "novel," unlike any of the other AEDs; it may block the N-subtype of calcium channels.

Mechanisms of other epilepsy treatments such as adrenocorticotrophic hormone (ACTH, used for infantile spasms) and the ketogenic diet (KD, a high-fat, low-carbohy-

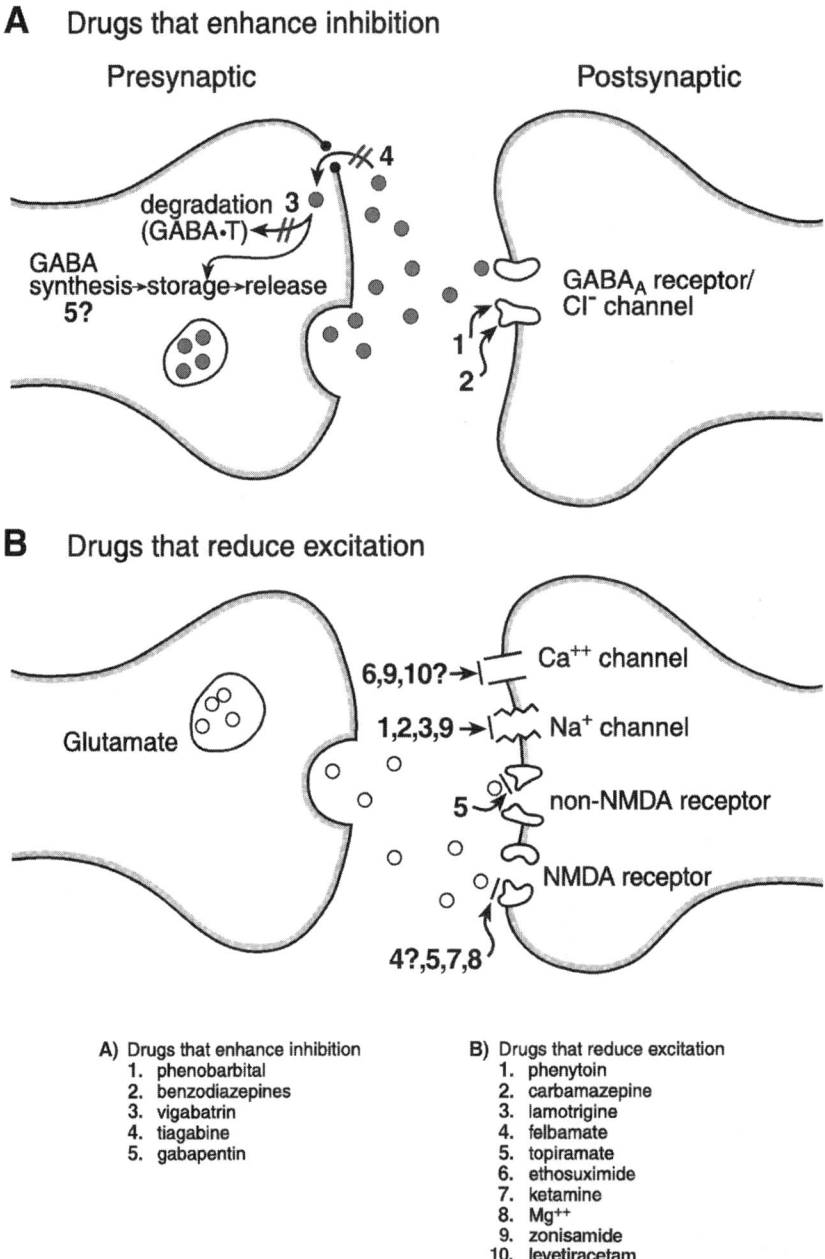

A Drugs that enhance inhibition

B Drugs that reduce excitation

A) Drugs that enhance inhibition
1. phenobarbital
2. benzodiazepines
3. vigabatrin
4. tiagabine
5. gabapentin

B) Drugs that reduce excitation
1. phenytoin
2. carbamazepine
3. lamotrigine
4. felbamate
5. topiramate
6. ethosuximide
7. ketamine
8. Mg++
9. zonisamide
10. levetiracetam

Fig. 9. Actions of antiepileptic drugs on (**A**) inhibitory and (**B**) excitatory mechanisms. Drugs in A act at both pre- and postsynaptic sites to enhance GABAergic inhibition. AEDs in B target excitation and affect mainly postsynaptic mechanisms. Ketamine and Mg^{2+} are not strictly AEDs but are shown here to illustrate their actions at a specific site (the ion pore) on the NMDA receptor. Several of the newer AEDs, e.g., gabapentin, lamotrigine, felbamate, topiramate, probably have multiple mechanisms of action. (Modified with permission of the American Academy of Pediatrics from ref. *58.*)

drate, and low-protein diet), remain largely unknown. ACTH may act in an age-specific manner to decrease the action of its excitatory precursor (corticotrophin-releasing hormone, CRH) on seizure-sensitive regions of the developing brain *(22)*. The search for mechanisms of action of the KD comprises a large portion of this volume. One could envision that the KD might alter brain energy metabolism, excitatory neurotransmission, inhibitory neurotransmission, individual ionic conductances, or several of these targets *(56,57)*. The evidence that the KD effectiveness often persists even after the diet is discontinued suggests the possibility that the KD could exert an antiepileptogenic benefit as well (*see* Chapter 22). Animal models can be used to design experiments to test each of these hypotheses.

New AEDs in the coming years are likely to increase our ability to treat seizures selectively according to specific pathophysiologic mechanisms. But to use such agents most effectively, a grasp of the underlying principles of normal and abnormal neuronal function is essential.

9. CONCLUSION

Epilepsy has many causes, both inherited and acquired. The mechanisms by which the normal brain becomes epileptic are quite diverse, ranging from the neural circuit level, to the synapse and neuronal membrane, to cascades of cellular energy production and utilization. All of these mechanisms vary over different stages of brain development. Rational treatment of epilepsy, whether with anticonvulsant medications, surgical interventions, or the ketogenic diet, requires an understanding of the age-specific physiological features that govern neuronal function.

REFERENCES

1. Commission on Classification and Terminology of the International League Against Epilepsy. Proposal for revised clinical and electroencephalographic classification of epileptic seizures. Epilepsia 1981;22:489–501.
2. Commission on Classification and Terminology of the International League Against Epilepsy. Proposal for revised classification of epilepsies and epilepsy syndromes. Epilepsia 1989;30:389–399.
3. Engel J Jr. A proposed diagnostic scheme for people with epileptic seizures and with epilepsy: report of the ILAE task force on classification and terminology. Epilepsia 2001;42:796–803.
4. Avoli M, Rogawski MA, Avanzini G. Generalized epileptic disorders: an update. Epilepsia 2001;42:445–457.
5. Stafstrom CE, Tempel BL. Epilepsy genes: the link between molecular dysfunction and pathophysiology. Ment Retard Dev Disabil Res Rev 2000;6:281–292.
6. Kuzniecky RI, Knowlton RC. Neuroimaging of epilepsy. Semin Neurol 2002;22:279–288.
7. Henry TR, Van Heertum RL. Positron emission tomography and single photon emission computed tomography in epilepsy care. Semin Nucl Med 2003;33:88–104.
8. Otsubo H, Snead OC III. Magnetoencephalography and magnetic source imaging in children. J Child Neurol 2001;16:227–235.
9. Nordli DR, DeVivo DC. Classification of infantile seizures: implications for identification and treatment of inborn errors of metabolism. J Child Neurol 2002;17 (Suppl 3):3S15–3S23.
10. Kwan P, Brodie MJ. Early identification of refractory epilepsy. N Engl J Med 2000;342:314–319.
11. Pitkanen A, Sutula TP. Is epilepsy a progressive disorder? Prospects for new therapeutic approaches in temporal lobe epilepsy. Lancet Neurol 2002;1:173–181.
12. Arroyo S, Brodie MJ, Avanzini G, Baumgartner C, Chiron C, Dulac O, French JA, Serratosa JM. Is refractory epilepsy preventable? Epilepsia 2002;43:437–444.
13. Treiman DM. GABAergic mechanisms in epilepsy. Epilepsia 2001;42 (Suppl 3):8–12.

14. Owens DF, Kriegstein AR. Is there more to GABA than synaptic inhibition? Nat Rev Neurosci 2002;3:715–727.
15. Wong RKS, Bianchi R, Taylor GW, Merlin LR. Role of metabotropic glutamate receptors in epilepsy. Adv Neurol 1999;79:685–698.
16. Dudek FE, Patrylo PR, Wuarin J-P. Mechanisms of neuronal synchronization during epileptiform activity. Adv Neurol 1999;79:699–708.
17. Velazquez JLP, Carlen PL. Gap junctions, synchrony, and seizures. Trends Neurosci 2000;23:68–74.
18. Johnston MV. Developmental aspects of epileptogenesis. Epilepsia 1996;37 (Suppl 1):S2–S9.
19. Schwindt PC, Crill WE. Membrane properties and epilepsy. Adv Neurol 1999;79:493–498.
20. Ptacek LJ, Fu YH. Channelopathies: episodic disorders of the nervous system. Epilepsia 2001;42 (Suppl 5):S35–S43.
21. Heinemann U, Gabriel S, Schuchmann S, Eder C. Contribution of astrocytes to seizure activity. Adv Neurol 1999;79:583–590.
22. Baram TZ, Hatalski CG. Neuropeptide-mediated excitability: a key triggering mechanism in the developing brain. Trends Neurosci 1998;21:471–476.
23. Vezzani A, Sperk G, Colmers WF. Neuropeptide Y: emerging evidence for a functional role in seizure modulation. Trends Neurosci 1999;22:25–30.
24. Colmers WF, Bahh BE. Neuropeptide Y and epilepsy. Epilepsy Curr 2003;3:53–58.
25. Wasterlain CG, Mazarati AM. Neuromodulators and second messengers. In: Engel J, Pedley TA (eds.). Epilepsy: A Comprehensive Textbook. Lippincott-Raven, Philadelphia, PA, 1997, pp. 277–289.
26. Binder DK, Croll SD, Gall CM, Scharfman HE. BDNF and epilepsy: too much of a good thing? Trends Neurosci 2001;24:47–53.
27. Maragakis NJ, Rothstein JD. Glutamate transporters in neurologic disease. Arch Neurol 2001;58:365–370.
28. Raiteri L, Raiteri M, Bonanno G. Coexistence and function of different neurotransmitter transporters in the plasma membrane of CNS neurons. Prog Neurobiol 2002;68:87–309.
29. Roettger VR, Amara SG. GABA and glutamate transporters: therapeutic and etiologic implications for epilepsy. Adv Neurol 1999;79:551–560.
30. Chapman AG. Glutamate and epilepsy. J Nutr 2000;130:1043S–1045S.
31. Meldrum B, Chapman A. Epileptic seizures and epilepsy. In: Siegel GJ, Agranoff BW, Albers RW, Molinoff PB (eds.). Basic Neurochemistry: Molecular, Cellular, and Medical Aspects. Lippincott-Raven, Philadelphia, PA, 1999, pp. 755–768.
32. Dunwiddie TV, Masino SA. The role and regulation of adenosine in the central nervous system. Annu Rev Neurosci 2001;24:31–55.
33. Schwartzkroin PA. Basic mechanisms of epileptogenesis. In: Wyllie E (ed.) The Treatment of Epilepsy: Principles and Practice. Lea & Fibiger, Philadelphia, 1993, pp. 83–98.
34. McCormick DA, Contreras D. On the cellular and network bases of epileptic seizures. Annu Rev Physiol 2001;63:815–846.
35. Clark S, Wilson WA. Mechanisms of epileptogenesis. Adv Neurol 1999;79:607–630.
36. Sarkisian MR. Overview of the current animal models for human seizure and epileptic disorders. Epilepsy Behav 2001;2:201–216.
37. Prince DA. Physiological mechanisms of focal epileptogenesis. Epilepsia 1985;26 (Suppl 1):S3–S14.
38. Connors BW, Pinto DJ, Telfeian AE. Local pathways of seizure propagation in neocortex. Int Rev Neurobiol 2001;45:527–546.
39. Scharfman HE. Epilepsy as an example of neural plasticity. Neuroscientist 2002;8:155–174.
40. Parent JM. The role of seizure-induced neurogenesis in epileptogenesis and brain repair. Epilepsy Res 2002;50:179–189.
41. Porter BE, Brooks-Kayal A, Golden JA. Disorders of cortical development and epilepsy. Arch Neurol 2002;59:361–365.
42. Chevassus-au-Louis N, Baraban SC, Gaiarsa J-L, Ben-Ari Y. Cortical malformations and epilepsy: new insights from animal models. Epilepsia 1999;40:811–821.
43. Holmes GL. Epilepsy in the developing brain: lessons from then laboratory and clinic. Epilepsia 1997;38:12–30.
44. Sanchez RM, Jensen FE. Maturational aspects of epilepsy mechanisms and consequences for the immature brain. Epilepsia 2001;42:577–585.

45. Swann JW, Hablitz JJ. Cellular abnormalities and synaptic plasticity in seizure disorders of the immature nervous system. Ment Retard Dev Disabil Res Rev 2000;6:258–267.
46. Ben-Ari Y. Excitatory actions of GABA during development: the nature of the nurture. Nat Rev Neurosci 2002;3:728–739.
47. Miles R. A homeostatic switch. Nature 1999;397:215–216.
48. Staley K, Smith R. A new form of feedback at the GABA-A receptor. Nat Neurosci 2001;4:674–676.
49. Sutula TP, Pitkanen A (eds.). Do Seizures Damage the Brain? Prog Brain Res 2002;135.
50. Stafstrom CE. Assessing the behavioral and cognitive effects of seizures on the developing brain. Prog Brain Res 2002;135:377–390.
51. Stafstrom CE, Lynch M, Sutula TP. Consequences of epilepsy in the developing brain: implications for surgical management. Semin Pediatr Neurol 2000;7:147–157.
52. Lado FA, Laureta EC, Moshe SL. Seizure-induced hippocampal damage in the mature and immature brain. Epileptic Disord 2002;4:83–97.
53. Holmes GL, Khazipov R, Ben-Ari Y. Seizure-induced damage in the developing brain: relevance of experimental models. Prog Brain Res 2002;135:321–334.
54. Avoli M. Molecular mechanisms of antiepileptic drugs. Sci Med 1997;4:54–63.
55. Rho JM, Sankar R. The pharmacologic basis of antiepileptic drug action. Epilepsia 1999;40:1471–1483.
56. Schwartzkroin PA. Mechanisms underlying the anti-epileptic efficacy of the ketogenic diet. Epilepsy Res 1999;37:171–180.
57. Stafstrom CE. Effects of fatty acids and ketones on neuronal excitability: implications for epilepsy and its treatment. In: Mostofsky DI, Yehuda S, Salem N (eds.). Fatty Acids—Physiological and Behavioral Functions. Humana, Totowa, NJ, 2002, pp. 273–290.
58. Stafstrom CE. The pathophysiology of epileptic seizures: a primer for pediatricians. Pediatr Rev 1998;19:335–344.

2

History and Origin
of the Ketogenic Diet

James W. Wheless

1. INTRODUCTION

In the past, many dietary "cures" for epilepsy were advocated, and such treatments included the excess or limitation of almost every substance (animal, vegetable, or mineral) *(1)*. However, fasting as a treatment for seizures was less recognized. Fasting is the only therapeutic measure against epilepsy recorded in the Hippocratic collection *(1)*. In the fifth century BC, Hippocrates reported on a man who had been seized by epileptic convulsions after having anointed himself before the fire in a bath, in winter. Complete abstinence from food and drink was prescribed, and the cure was effective.

Fasting, as a therapy for seizures, was documented in biblical times. In a quotation from the King James Version of the Bible, Mark relates the story of Jesus curing an epileptic boy *(2–4)*. When his disciples asked him privately why they had not been able to cure the boy, Jesus said "this kind can come out by nothing but prayer and fasting." Raphael's *Transfiguration of Christ,* probably the most famous painting of a person with epilepsy, is based on this passage from Mark *(5)*. This painting is divided into two parts; the upper part depicts the transfiguration of Christ, the lower part portrays the healing of the boy with epilepsy (Fig. 1).

2. FASTING (A PRECURSOR TO THE KETOGENIC DIET)

It was not until the early twentieth century that medical use of the ketogenic diet emerged as a strategy to mimic the biochemical effects of fasting (or starvation) (Fig. 2). Guelpa and Marie, both French physicians, authored the first scientific report on the value of fasting in epilepsy *(6)*. They reported that seizures were less severe during treatment, but no details were given. In the United States, contemporary accounts of fasting were also recorded early in the twentieth century (Table 1); the first was a report on a patient of an osteopathic physician, Dr. Hugh W. Conklin, of Battle Creek, Michigan, and the second concerned Bernarr Macfadden *(7,8)*. Macfadden was a physical fitness guru/cultist and publishing genius of the early part of the 20th century *(9)*. He called the medical profession an organized fraud and said that people who followed his rules could live to age 120. At age 31 (in 1899), he established his first magazine, *Phys-*

From: *Epilepsy and the Ketogenic Diet*
Edited by: C. E. Stafstrom and J. M. Rho © Humana Press Inc., Totowa, NJ

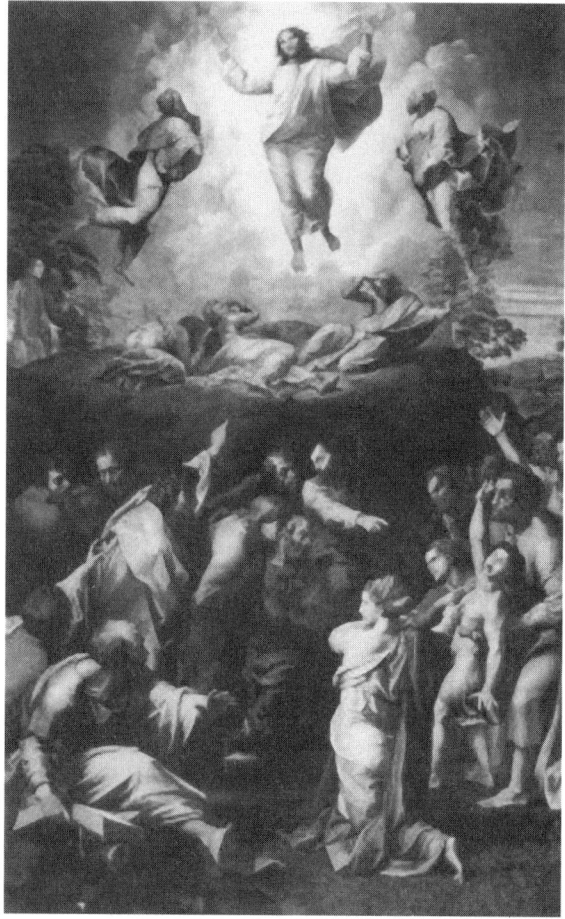

Fig. 1. Raphael's *Transfiguration of Christ.* (Reproduced with permission from ref. *5.*)

ical Culture. He advised readers how to develop themselves physically, how to maintain their health, and how to cope with illness. He illustrated it with photographs of himself lightly clad, with muscles bulging (Fig. 3A). Each issue carried articles about sickly men and women who became healthy, strong, and beautiful through proper diet and exercise. The magazine's circulation had reached 500,000 by the end of World War I. Macfadden was widely recognized, and one of his followers, Angelo Siciliano, won Macfadden's "America's Most Perfectly Developed Man" contest twice. Using the winnings, Siciliano went on to establish his own muscle-building business under the name of Charles Atlas.

Macfadden offered advice on a subject he knew very little about—coping with illness. He maintained that any disease could be cured by exercise and diet. He also emphasized fasting. His rationale was that because much of the body's energy goes into digesting food, if there is no food to digest, more energy could be applied to recovering health. Macfadden claimed that fasting for 3 d to 3 wk could alleviate and cure about any disease, including asthma, bladder disease, diabetes, prostate disease, *epilepsy,* impotence, paralysis, liver and kidney disease, and eye troubles. He had become nationally recognized, and his ideas were well known (Fig. 3B). Dr. Conklin began as an

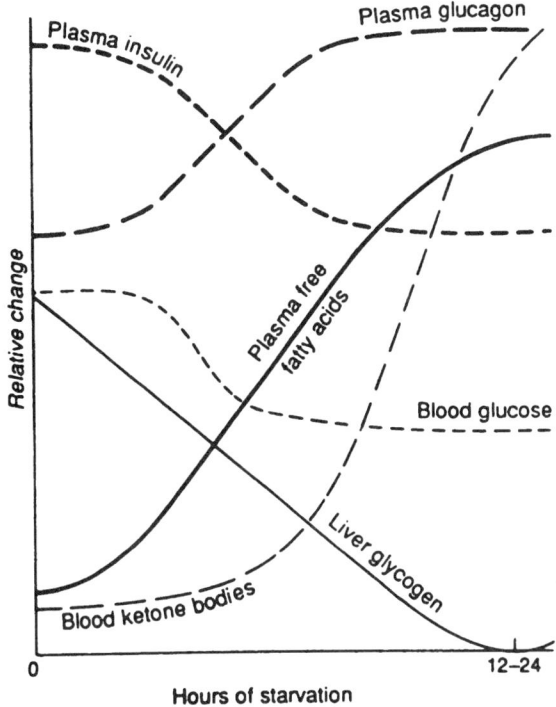

Fig. 2. Biochemical changes that occur with fasting (Reprinted with permission from ref. *94.*)

assistant to Macfadden and adopted his method of fasting to treat various ailments *(4)*. It was his practice of fasting to treat epilepsy and the results, which drew the attention of another pioneer in epilepsy studies, H. Rawle Geyelin, an endocrinologist at the New York Presbyterian Hospital.

Dr. Geyelin, a prominent physician from New York, first reported at the American Medical Association (AMA) convention in 1921 his exposure to fasting as a treatment of epilepsy *(10)*. In 1919 he had the opportunity to observe a young cousin who had epilepsy for 4 yr *(11)*. The patient's seizures were not controlled by numerous treatments that had been recommended by several neurologists. The patient also failed to respond to the conventional treatments of the day, bromides and phenobarbital. Then Dr. Conklin had the child fast four times over several months: the seizures stopped after the second day of fasting, and the boy had none in over 2 yr of follow-up. After observing two other patients who apparently had been cured of epilepsy by Dr. Conklin, Dr. Geyelin began using the same fasting treatment to see if he could confirm the results in a larger group of patients. Not knowing what the effects of the fast would be, Dr. Geyelin initially used variable periods of fasting. He finally adopted a 20-d period for the fast, although he admitted this was entirely arbitrary. Geyelin was the first to document that "when one wanted to turn a clouded mentality to a clear one it could almost always be done with fasting." This observation languished until recent times, when behavioral and developmental improvements attributed to the ketogenic diet were reported *(12)*. Dr. Geyelin documented the efficacy of fasting in 36 patients (*see* Table 1) and closed his presentation by remarking that this was a preliminary report, and further study was needed.

Table 1
Efficacy of Fasting, 1921–1928

First author	No. of patients	Age (yr) of Patients	Seizure type[a]	Diet	Success rate (%)	Comments
Geyelin R, 1921 (10)	30	3.5–35	PM, GM	Fasting	87% Seizure free	Results based on 20-d fast; no long-term follow-up
Weeks DF, 1923 (86)	64	7–61	PM, GM	Fasting	47% Seizure free during fast	Patients fasted for 3 wk; all had seizures after return to regular diet
Talbot FB, 1926 (37)	23	Children	UN	Fasting	Seizure free during fast	Seizures returned in all after fast
Lennox WG, 1928 (4)	27	13–42	UN	Fasting	50% had marked reduction in seizures during the fast	Phenobarbital stopped on admittance; fast lasted 4–21 d

[a] GM, grand mal; PM, petit mal; UN, unknown.

34

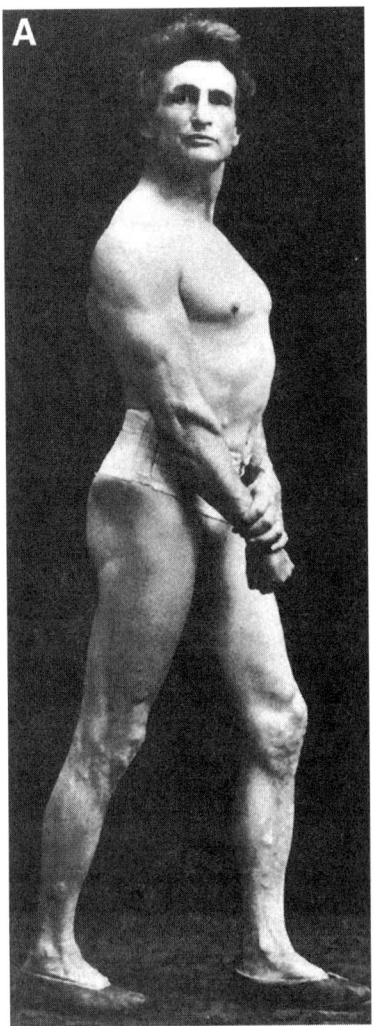

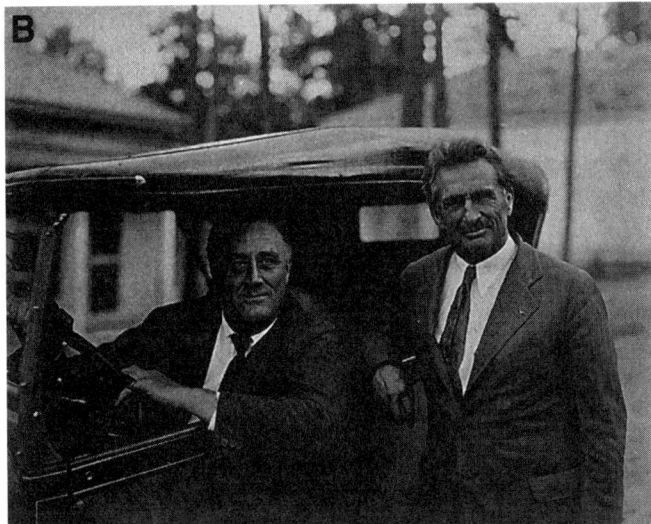

Fig. 3. Bernarr Macfadden. (**A**) As he appeared in a photograph in his magazine *Physical Culture*, illustrating his bulging muscles. (Reproduced with permission from the Qu'igley Photographic Archives, Georgetown University Library.) (**B**) With presidential candidate Franklin D. Roosevelt (in car) in 1931. Macfadden tried to ingratiate himself with Roosevelt as a part of a strategy to be appointed as the first Secretary of Health.

Dr. Stanley Cobb of Harvard was in the audience that day and commented that he had experimentally used starvation to prevent convulsions in an animal model. At that time, Cobb did not know that the father of the first child Geyelin had discussed would come to him in 1922 and ask him to explain the mechanism of action of starvation in treating epilepsy; we pick up this thread of the story again later in this section.

At this time, Dr. Conklin believed that epilepsy, which he labeled "intestinal epilepsy," had its origin in the intestines and was curable *(13)*. He thought that a toxin secreted from the Peyer's glands was taken up in the lymphatics, stored in the lymph glands and other tissues, and from time to time discharged into the bloodstream, caus-ing epileptic convulsions. He reasoned (based on influence from Macfadden) that during a fast, the tissues freely pour their poison content into the bloodstream, through which means the toxins are eliminated. In his manuscript, he outlines his treatment for epilepsy and technique for initiating and breaking the fast. Typically, he deprived the patient of all food for 18–25 d, or as long as the person was physically able to stand it. Conklin reported that his cures of epilepsy were 90% in children younger than 10 yr, 80% in adolescents 10–15 yr old, 65% in patients 15–25 yr old, and 50% between 25 and 40 yr, above age 40, the percentage was very low.

However, even before Conklin published his results with fasting, word of his successful treatment had spread to others in more conventional neurology practices *(4,14)*. Higgins, while addressing the Pennsylvania State Medical Society in 1928, commented, "About 1917 the attention of the medical world was drawn to the finding that the attacks in many cases of epilepsy were stopped, or lessened in severity and frequency, by starvation" *(14)*. Dr. Penfield, of the Montreal Neurological Institute, and his colleague Dr. Erickson, also recognized Conklin's fasting therapy in their 1941 textbook on epilepsy *(15)*. Lennox acknowledged that Conklin, by 1928, had the most experience in treating patients with epilepsy by fasting (probably hundreds of patients over approx 20 yr *[4]*).

Conklin and Macfadden's views on the origins and treatment of epilepsy were adopted by others *(4)*. This is reflected in Dr. McMurray's letter to the *New York Medical Journal* describing digestive disturbances as an impressive finding in his patients with epilepsy and the use of fasting followed by a starch- and sugar-free diet as a treatment beginning in 1912 *(16)*. Dr. A. Goldbloom, a physician at the Children's Memorial Hospital in Montreal, was more skeptical. He wrote, "A year or two ago we allowed ourselves to be startled by the news of an asserted real cure for epilepsy. A drugless healer in the middle west [Conklin] had been curing epileptics, it was said, by subjecting them to long periods of starvation" *(17)*. He then related the story of a 10-yr-old girl who had failed therapy with bromide and Luminal® (phenobarbital), was having 60–100 petit mal seizures a day, and became seizure free on the fifth day of her fast. However, after the fast was broken, the seizures gradually returned.

> Goldbloom stated, "It would seem from this case that the starvation treatment is effective only while it is continued and while the patient remains in bed, but that it has no enduring qualities. The explanation of the improvement is first that the patient is kept in bed, and secondly that the fermentative and putrefactive intestinal processes, so often the exciting causes of convulsions, even in a non-epileptic child, are reduced for the time being to a minimum. So far as children are concerned, one often sees children who have been considered epileptics in whom the epilepsy is found to be purely of intestinal origin, and who are therefore permanently cured by the application of strict dietetic measures" (17).

Lennox would later relate the relationship of Conklin's practice to the origin of the ketogenic diet *(4,18)*. In an interesting anecdote, he relates the story of HTH, the boy initially presented by Dr. Geyelin to the AMA convention.

> Lennox stated, "a New York corporation lawyer and his wife were troubled because of the daily seizures of their son. The boy's uncle (Dr. John Howland) was a professor of pediatrics, but the best medical advice and treatment of the day failed to help. In despair, the parents turned to Dr. Hugh Conklin, a disciple of Bernarr Macfadden, a physical cultist. The treatment was called, euphemistically, a water diet. This meant starvation for three or four weeks. Dramatically, the boy's seizures left him."

Around 1919, Charles Howland, the boy's father and a wealthy New York corporate lawyer, gave his brother $5000 to determine whether there was a scientific basis for the success of the starvation treatment of his son (19,20). Dr. John Howland, professor of pediatrics at Johns Hopkins and director of the newly opened Harriet Lane Home for Invalid Children was H.T.M.'s uncle. The gift from Charles Howland was used to create the first laboratory at the Harriet Lane Home. By 1937, the John Howland Memorial Fund was established at Johns Hopkins and used to support research on the ketogenic diet (21). Lennox reports that initially two physicians sought confirmation and explanation for the surprisingly favorable results of fasting. One was Dr. James Gamble. In 1915 Dr. Howland recruited Gamble, who had recently developed an interest in clinical chemistry, to the Harriett Lane staff.

By 1919, Harvey reports, "Dr. Howland had developed a deep interest in the treatment of epilepsy by the ketosis of starvation. Gamble went to work on this problem..." (22). These children were ideal subjects for the metabolic balance studies of the 1920s because their intake was limited to water, and fecal material was greatly reduced. Gamble and his colleagues initially reported the study of the acid–base balance of two fasting children (23). This report produced little information regarding the mechanism of action of fasting on epilepsy, but it was the beginning of a 30-yr study by Gamble of factors affecting the water balance in children. His report formed a pattern for clinical research and created the basis for the fields of pediatric electrolyte physiology and nephrology. He also was the first to note increased calcium excretion on the ketogenic diet, with a resulting need for calcium supplementation (24).

The other doctor recruited by Howland was H. Rawle Geyelin, who had reported his results at the 1921 AMA convention in Boston. Urinary acid excretion had been highest in patients whose seizures were best controlled. At that time, W. G. Lennox was studying cardiology under Dr. Francis Peabody at Boston's Peter Bent Brigham Hospital. Lennox reported that he was "Thrilled by Geyelin's demonstration and having a compelling interest in epilepsy and its treatment, my missionary zeal was abruptly transferred from Chinese to the epileptic" (18). Geyelin's extensive clinical and laboratory data were never published, but he later told Lennox that long-term freedom from seizures occurred in 15 of 79 children treated (19%), but in only 1 of 200 adults (0.5%) (4,11). Lennox's personal review of Conklin's short case records of 127 patients with epilepsy indicated that 20% achieved seizure freedom, and some improvement occurred in 50% (4).

In 1922 the parents of H.T.H. asked Dr. Stanley Cobb, associate professor of neuropathology at Harvard Medical School, to explain why starvation worked as a treatment for epilepsy (18). Cobb enlisted the assistance of a young colleague, W. G. Lennox. Lennox and Cobb reported on a selected group of five patients during a 2-wk period of fasting (24). Lennox himself served as a control during one fast period of 14 d and several shorter ones. Chemical assays of the blood and urine were performed in the subjects and controls. All showed an increase in serum uric acid and acidosis, which was excreted in the urine if the fast was broken with carbohydrate or by a purine-free protein diet, but not if broken by the intake of 40% cream. Also, they noted the increase in serum uric acid and acidosis typically developed after 2 or 3 d and was accompanied by a decrease in seizures.

Lennox stated, "Initiation of the use of bromides in 1857 and of phenobarbital in 1912 had demonstrated that the chemical action of these sedative drugs could lessen seizures. The third decade of the twentieth century witnessed a measure of control through a change of body metabolism. Simple absence of food or dearth of carbohydrate in the body forced the body to burn acid-forming fat" *(18)*. The efficacy of fasting led to a flurry of clinical and research activity. Theories arose to explain the success of starvation. Dehydration *(23,26)*, ketosis *(24,27–29)*, and acidosis *(25,30,31)* were all advanced as mechanisms to explain the efficacy of fasting. Metabolic balance studies had been used by many investigators of this era to understand the interrelationships of fat, protein, and carbohydrate metabolism to the ketoacidosis and disturbed glucose utilization that occurs in diabetes.

3. THE KETOGENIC DIET

At about the same time as the study of Cobb and Lennox, in 1921, a review article about diet adjustments and diabetes by Woodyatt stated "acetone, acetic acid, and beta-hydroxybutyric acid appear … in a normal subject by starvation, or a diet containing too low a proportion of carbohydrate and too high a proportion of fat. It [ketoacidosis] appears to be the immediate result of the oxidation of certain fatty acids in the absence of a sufficient proportion of 'oxidizing' glucose" *(32)*.

Concurrently, Dr. Wilder at the Mayo Clinic proposed, probably based on the work summarized by Woodyatt, "that the benefits of … fasting … could be obtained if ketonemia was produced by other means. The ketone bodies … are formed from fat and protein whenever a disproportion exists between the amount of fatty acid and the amount of sugar actually burning in the tissues. In any case, as has long been known, it is possible to provoke ketogenesis by feeding diets which are very rich in fat and low in carbohydrate. It is proposed therefore, to try the effects of such ketogenic diets on a series of epileptics" *(27)*. Wilder suggested that a ketogenic diet should be as effective as fasting and could be maintained for a much longer period, compensating for the obvious disadvantages of a prolonged fast.

In a report issued the following day, he described the dramatic improvement in seizure control of three patients with epilepsy who had been admitted to the Mayo Clinic for initiation of the ketogenic diet *(33)*. He concluded, "It is impossible to draw conclusions from the results of these few patients treated with high fat diets, but we have here a method of observing the effect of ketosis on the epileptic. If this is the mechanism responsible for the beneficial effect of fasting, it may be possible to substitute for that rather brutal procedure a dietary therapy which the patient can follow with little inconvenience and continue at home as long as seems necessary" *(33)*. It was Wilder who coined the term *ketogenic diet*.

Peterman and other pediatricians eagerly acted on Wilder's suggestion *(34,35)*. Peterman first reported the calculation and effectiveness of the ketogenic diet from the Mayo Clinic in 1924 *(35)*. Peterman's ketogenic diet, composed of one gram of protein per kilogram of body weight in children, 10–15 g of carbohydrate per day, and the remainder of the calories in fat, is identical to the ketogenic diet that is used today. Peterman documented the importance of teaching the caregivers management of the diet before discharge, individualization of the diet, close follow-up, and the potential for further adjustments at home. He also made the early observation that excess ketosis could lead to nausea and vomiting, symptoms that were quickly relieved by orange juice *(34)*. This clinical caveat is still useful to know and is employed as needed during initiation of the ketogenic diet *(36)*.

Peterman also noted improvements in behavior and cognitive effects that accompanied the ketogenic diet.

"The mental development has been normal in all patients, and exceptionally good in seven of the twenty who are now free from attacks. In all the children treated with the ketogenic diet there was a marked change in character, concomitant with the ketosis, a decrease in irritability, and an increased interest and alertness; the children slept better and were more easily disciplined. This action of the diet warrants further study" (34).

This last comment is as true today as it was in 1925! M. B. Pulsifer and others, 75 yr later, performed the first prospective study of the effects of the ketogenic diet on development and behavior *(12)*. She concluded, "At follow-up, mean developmental quotient showed statistically significant improvement ($p < 0.05$), with significant behavioral improvements in attention and social functioning," verifying Peterman's earlier observation.

These initial reports were rapidly followed by reports from Talbot and colleagues (Harvard) *(28,37–39)* and from McQuarrie and Keith (Mayo Clinic) *(40)* in 1926 and 1927. Talbot introduced the first report as follows: "In 1921, the children's medical service of the Massachusetts General Hospital (MGH) initiated a study of the treatment of idiopathic epilepsy. The first method of attack was by the fasting method recommended by Conklin of Battle Creek" *(37)*. This statement verifies the impact Macfadden ultimately had, even on such prestigious institutions as MGH.

Talbot noticed some seizure freedom in all 21 children during the fast, but the seizures returned after the fast was broken. As a result, in 1924 MGH adopted the ketogenic diet as performed by the Mayo Clinic (Dr. Peterman). Talbot also noted that the diet was well tolerated, "without causing any untoward symptoms in the patients. On the contrary, they seem to be more alert and less nervous" *(37)*. Talbot also acknowledged the critical role of the dietician and noted that "a clever dietician works out various little tricks to get in fat" *(37)*. Talbot's 1930 textbook on the treatment of epilepsy included tables with complete discussion and instructions for the ketogenic diet *(41)*. The current Johns Hopkins Hospital protocol *(see* ref. *42)* for calculating and initiating the ketogenic diet after a period of fasting to hasten the production of ketosis, and gradually increasing the amount dietary fat introduced over several days, was well discussed by Talbot in 1926 *(38)*.

By 1928, Talbot had experience with differing compositions of ketogenic diets and wrote that "the best therapeutic results in epilepsy are not obtained until the ratio has approached 4:1..." *(24)*, which is now recognized as the most common composition for the ketogenic diet. McQuarrie and Keith, while studying the biochemistry of children on the ketogenic diet in 1927, made the initial observation that the proportion of acetone bodies in the blood runs parallel to that in the urine *(40)*, a finding validated 62 yr later by Schwartz et al. *(43)*. The Mayo Clinic investigators also were the first to note variations during the day in the intensity of ketosis, with a maximum in the late afternoon and the nadir in the early morning hours.

McQuarrie and Keith were aware of the recently rerecognized tendency of children to have seizures early in the morning, when ketosis is minimal, and they suggested the addition of a midnight snack to maintain early ketosis. They also recognized that the degree of ketosis to prevent seizures may vary across individuals, and as a result adjusting the diet for the individual patient was necessary to ensure optimal ketosis. Such adjustments are routinely made in multidisciplinary epilepsy clinics today.

By 1927 Helmholz at the Mayo Clinic was aware that if the child did not have definite improvement in seizure control after 2 mo of the ketogenic diet, it was fair to say that a therapeutic failure had occurred and appropriate to abandon the diet (29). In 1927 the Section on Pediatrics and Nutrition at the Mayo Clinic prepared a pamphlet that describes in detail meal plans and recipes for a ketogenic diet (44). This was done in response to the demand for this type of practical information.

The use of the ketogenic diet was recorded in almost every comprehensive textbook on epilepsy in childhood that appeared between 1941 and 1980 (3,15,18,45–51). Most of these texts had full chapters describing the diet, telling how to initiate it and how to calculate meal plans. Extensive tables listed the nutritional composition of foods and discussed meal planning.

Throughout the 1920s and 1930s, the ketogenic diet was widely used (see next section). When Merritt and Putnam discovered diphenylhydantoin in 1938, the attention of physicians and researchers shifted focus from the mechanism of action and efficacy of the ketogenic diet to new antiepileptic drugs (AEDs) (see ref. 52). A new era of medical therapy for epilepsy had begun, and the ketogenic diet fell by the wayside. Medications were easier to administer and new chemical compounds were always on the horizon. As early as 1937, Ford, in a pediatric neurology text, found the ketogenic diet difficult, rigid, and expensive (53).

In an effort to make the classic ketogenic diet more palatable, Huttenlocher et al., in 1971, introduced a medium-chain triglyceride (MCT) oil diet that was more ketogenic per calorie, allowing less restriction of other foods (54). This 1971 report from Yale University documented a therapeutically significant anticonvulsant effect in 6 of 12 children with daily myoclonic and astatic seizures. As a result, other centers adopted the MCT diet in place of the classic ketogenic diet and reported it as the "ketogenic diet" (55–60). Almost 20 yr went by before Schwartz and colleagues conducted the only comparative trial of the MCT diet and the classic ketogenic diet (see Section 3.2.) (43,61). This report documented more side effects and less palatability of the MCT diet.

As new AEDs became available, the ketogenic diet was used less and less. After the introduction of sodium valproate, it was believed that this branched-chain fatty acid would treat children previously placed on the diet to treat the seizures of Lennox–Gastaut syndrome and that the diet could no longer be justified (62). Pediatric neurologists and epileptologists were led to believe that better understanding of central nervous system neurotransmitters and rationally designed AEDs were the hope for the future. Fewer children were placed on the ketogenic diet, resulting in fewer dieticians who were trained in the initiation and maintenance of the diet. As Lennox stated in 1960, "Though interest in fasting (or the ketogenic diet) as a treatment has almost vanished, doubtless much scientific gold remains in 'them thar hills'" (18).

3.1. Ketogenic Diet in the 1990s

Use of the ketogenic diet decreased greatly until it received national media attention in October 1994, when NBC-TV's *Dateline* aired a program on the treatment (7,8,42,63–66). This television program was based on the true story of Charlie, a 2-yr-old with intractable myoclonic, generalized tonic, and tonic–clonic seizures (Fig. 4). A videotape presentation made later summarizes Charlie's condition in 1994: "Thousands

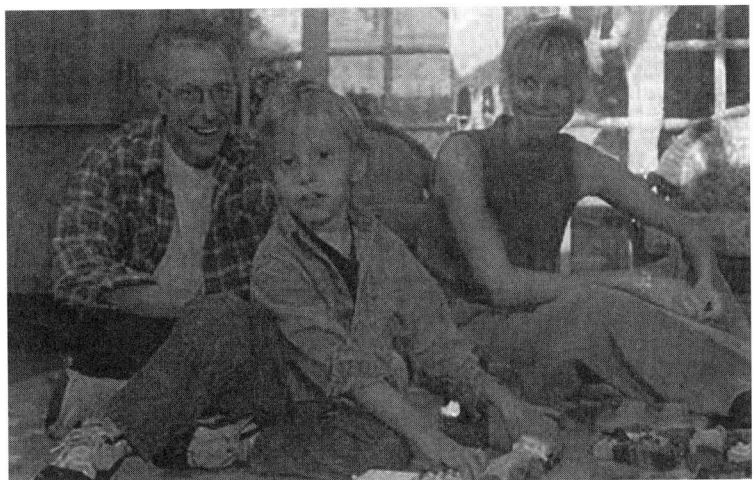

Fig. 4. Charlie Abrahams, age 4, with his parents Jim and Nancy, as they appeared in 1997 in a story on Charlie and the ketogenic diet published in the *New York Times* (Reproduced with permission from Bart Bartholomew.)

of seizures and countless medications later, after five pediatric neurologists, two homeopathic physicians, one faith healer, and one fruitless surgery, Charlie's seizures remained unchecked and his prognosis was for continued seizures and progressive retardation" *(65)*.

While researching treatments for epilepsy on his own, Charlie's father found a reference to the ketogenic diet and Johns Hopkins *(67)*. Charlie was brought to Johns Hopkins for initiation of the diet. There the diet continued to be used in the epilepsy center, under the discretion of Ms. Millicent Kelly, an experienced dietician. Charlie initiated the diet, became seizure-free, and soon posted developmental progress. Charlie's father was disturbed that no one had told him about the diet. He reviewed the references of the success rate (*see* Section 3.2.) and was determined that the information should be available so that other parents could become aware of the ketogenic diet. He created the Charlie Foundation and made videos for parents about the diet, as well as one directed at physicians and another, an instructional video, for dieticians. The foundation has distributed over 50,000 of these videotapes gratis.

The Charlie Foundation also funded the initial publication of *The Epilepsy Diet Treatment: An Introduction to the Ketogenic Diet (8)* and underwrote conferences to train physicians and dieticians from epilepsy centers nationwide. The first conference attendees were responsible for developing the first multicenter prospective report on the efficacy of the ketogenic diet *(68)*. In 1995 Wheless concluded that the ketogenic diet compares favorably with other new treatments for epilepsy in children and should be available at every pediatric epilepsy center *(69)*. This echoed a comment made by Dr. Geyelin at a presentation to the American College of Physicians in New Orleans on March, 7, 1928: "The results of fasting and the ketogenic diet are apparently the best that are obtained by any therapeutic procedure that we have to offer epileptics in childhood today" (*see* ref. *11*).

The ketogenic diet has experienced a significant reemergence in recent years, and modern clinical studies have established the treatment as significantly effective (*see* next section). This is reflected by the dramatic increase in scientific articles regarding this treatment. Between January 1965 and December 1995, PubMed recorded 93 publications pertaining to the with ketogenic diet; however, from January 1996 to January 2003, a website of the National Institutes of Health recorded 172 publications (www.ncbi.nih.gov/entrez/query.fcgi). This documents the increased interest in the diet in the scientific community over the last 5–10 yr, and the timeliness of this book.

3.2. Early Efficacy of the Ketogenic Diet

In the 1920s and 1930s, initial reports documented the efficacy of the ketogenic diet (Table 2) *(14,29,70–78)*. These were all retrospective reports. Some included a small number of patients and provided few clinical details or specifications of epilepsy syndrome or seizure type. The studies clearly showed some patients had improved seizure control on the ketogenic diet. Over the next 60–70 yr, many more clinical reports appeared on the ketogenic diet (Tables 2 and 3) *(79)*. Meta-analysis of the published data is not possible, given differences in study design and sparse clinical detail; additionally, it is often not clear what is meant by "good" or "partial" response to the ketogenic diet. Despite these limitations from older studies, however, the literature supports the consensus view that the ketogenic diet improves seizure control in some children. Overall, one-third to one-half of children have an excellent response to the ketogenic diet, defined by marked cessation of seizures or reduction in seizure severity. Younger children are more likely to have a favorable response than older children.

Few early studies evaluated the ketogenic diet treatment in adults (Table 4). Reports from the Mayo Clinic experience in 100 adults treated during the 1920s found that seizures were controlled in 12 patients and that an additional 44 benefited *(80,81)*. Another early report of 20 institutionalized adult patients with epilepsy and mental impairment found an increase in seizure frequency upon initiation of the diet *(82)*. However, all antiepileptic drugs have been stopped before diet initiation. In 1999, over 70 yr after the initial Mayo Clinic report, Sirven and colleagues, performed a modern, prospective study evaluating the efficacy and safety of the ketogenic diet as a treatment for adults with intractable, symptomatic partial, or generalized epilepsy *(83)*. These patients had failed an average of 5.4 AEDs and had weekly to daily seizures. At 8 mo of follow-up, 54.5% (6 of 11) had a greater than 50% reduction in seizure frequency, and 4 patients discontinued the diet. All seizure types responded to the diet, and most patients tolerated the diet.

Some modern studies have looked more critically at the ketogenic diet and have provided good clinical details of the clinic population. Hopkins and Lynch reported on the first group of children in Australia *(84)*. They followed 34 children who had not responded to adequate drug therapy, and this group experienced an overall success rate of 29%. Improvement was dramatic in some patients who had been earlier regarded as hopeless.

Schwartz et al. reported on the results of 24-h metabolic profiles performed on epileptic children receiving normal diets, the classic (4:1) ketogenic diet, the MCT diet, and the modified MCT diet (Radcliffe diet, which incorporates both long-chain and medium-chain fatty acids) *(43)*. The authors hoped the study would establish relative efficacy of the various forms of the diet. They evaluated 59 patients who were fasted for 18 h and then placed on one of the three diets. Patients continued on the diet with recording of seizures and then were readmitted for a follow-up metabolic profile.

Several biochemical parameters were analyzed, but specifically, blood samples were assayed for the measurements of ketone bodies (acetoacetate, β-hydroxybutyrate), serum glucose, pyruvate, and lactate. The studies showed that all three therapeutic diets produced a significant increase in total ketone body levels, but this effect was most marked on the classic ketogenic diet. In addition, the work documented that ketone body concentrations elevated during the day, reached a maximum in the afternoon, and often were lower in the morning. Measured urinary ketones reflected changes noted in the serum. This led to the adoption of urine ketone body measurement as a standard method for determining the degree of ketosis on the ketogenic diet.

The study by Schwartz et al. documented that all three therapeutic diets resulted in seizure control and that one was not superior to another in this brief period; however, it also documented that the classic ketogenic diet, using the Johns Hopkins Hospital's protocol, induced the greatest degree of ketosis. Additionally, Schwartz et al. analyzed short-term clinical efficacy of the ketogenic diet in the treatment of epilepsy *(61)*. They again used the three dietary therapies that were used in the 1980s: the classic (4:1) diet as administered at the Johns Hopkins Hospital, the MCT diet, and the modified MCT diet. They evaluated 59 patients who were followed for at least 6 wk and reported a very high (81%) responder rate (defined as >50% reduction in seizures). They noted that drowsiness, a frequent side effect during initiation of the diet resolved as the children obtained the full diet. They documented the efficacy of all forms of the ketogenic diet, but they also showed that there were more side effects associated with the MCT diet, including diarrhea and vomiting. In addition, the MCT diet was less palatable.

In 1992 a report updated the efficacy of the ketogenic diet in the modern era of antiepileptic drug therapy *(85)*. The authors reviewed the results of 58 consecutive patients who were placed on the ketogenic diet at Johns Hopkins Hospital in the 1980s. All the children treated had severe, intractable epilepsy: 80% had multiple seizure types, and 88% were on multiple AEDs. Despite this high morbidity, improved seizure control occurred in 67% of the patients on the ketogenic diet, 64% were able to reduce their antiepileptic drugs, 36% became more alert, and 23% had better behavior. These findings are remarkable because they were reported in a group of patients with refractory epilepsy who also had mental retardation (84%), microcephaly (15%), and cerebral palsy (45%). In this study, seizure type did not predict success with the ketogenic diet. Additionally, 75% of the improved patients continued the diet for at least 18 mo, confirming the efficacy and palatability of the diet and patient willingness to continue with it. This study confirmed the earlier work by Livingston on a large number of patients at the same institution, demonstrating that 52% had complete control and an additional 27% had improved control *(3)*.

The first multicenter study of the efficacy of the ketogenic diet was completed in 1998 *(68)*. Seven comprehensive epilepsy centers prospectively entered 51 children into this study of the efficacy of the classic ketogenic diet. The parents recorded baseline seizure frequency for one month prior to initiation of the diet. These children had intractable epilepsy and an average of 230 seizures per month. Their seizure frequency was evaluated at 3, 6, and 12 mo on the ketogenic diet. Ten percent of the patients were seizure free at one year, and 54, 53, and 40% achieved greater than 50% decrease in seizure frequency at 3, 6, and 12 mo of follow-up on the diet. In addition, using an intention-to-treat analysis, 47% remained on the diet at one year. This study again showed that the patient's age, seizure type, and electroencephalographic results are not

Table 2

Efficacy of the Ketogenic Diet (KD), 1921–1976

First author	No. of patients	Age (yr) of Patients	Seizure type[a]	Diet	Success rate (%)	Comments
Peterman MG, 1925 (34)	37	2.25–14.5	PM, GM	KD	60% Seizure free, 34.5% improved, 5.5% not improved	All idiopathic etiology; follow-up 0.33–2.5 yr; only 2 on phenobarbital
Talbot FB, 1926 (37)	12	Children	PM, GM	KD	50% Seizure free, 33% improved, 17% no change	Follow-up period 3–6 mo; all idiopathic etiology
Cooder HR, 1933 (87)	38	≤12	GM, PT	KD	50% Seizure free, 34% improved, 16% not improved	>3 mo follow-up
Helmholz HF, 1937 (88)	501	Children	UN	KD	Idiopathic etiology	92 had symptomatic epilepsy and 142 could not maintain diet. All children had > 1 yr follow-up. Results from children treated between 1922 and 1936; 1 child developed pellagra.
Wilkins L, 1937 (21)	30	3–14	GM, PT, MM	KD	27% Seizure free, 50% no benefit	Idiopathic etiology, follow-up >1.5 yr; all seizure-free patients resumed a normal diet
Keith HM, 1963 (49)	729	Unknown	UN	KD	Of 530 idiopathic patients, 31% seizure free, 24% improved, 39% no benefit	Patients treated between 1922 and 1944, follow-up 1–30 yr (some included in ref. 88). Excluded 84 with symptomatic epilepsy; 115 unable to follow diet
Hopkins IJ, 1970 (84)	34	1–13	GM, MM	KD	29% Successful (seizure free or much reduced), 32% unsuccessful, 26% inadequate trial	No deaths from diet. 1 Renal calculus
Livingston S, 1972 (3)	1001	Unknown	UN	KD	52% Seizures controlled, 27% seizures marked improvement, 21% no improvement	
Dodson WE, 1976 (89)	50	5–38	UN	KD	50% Seizure free, 20–30% seizures improved considerably	

[a] GM, grand mal; MM, minor motor; ; PM, petit mal; UN, unknown; KD, classic ketogenic diet.

Table 3
Efficacy of the Ketogenic Diet, 1989–1999

First author	No. of patients	Age (yr) of patients	Seizure type[a]	Diet	Success rate (%)	Comments
Schwartz RH, 1989 (61)	59	<5–54	M, A, IS, GTC, AB, SP, CP	KD-24 MCT-22 Modifield MCT-13	81% had a >50% reduction of seizures	MCT diet more unpalatable; prospective series
Kinsman SL, 1992 (85)	58	1–20	80% multiple seizure types	KD	29% seizure controlled 38% had >50% seizure reduction, 29%	All had severe neurology handicaps: mental retardation (84%), cerebral palsy (45%), micrecphaly (15%); 3 renal nodes
Swink T, 1997 (90)	18	6.5–1.75	934 seizures/mo average	KD	At 6 months: 50% seizure free; 42% have ≥50 seizure reductions, only 1 discontinued diet.	Prospective, all children <2 yr at enrollment
Vining EPG, 1998 (68)	51	1–8	230 seizures/mo average (IS, SP, GTC, AB, CP, A, M)	KD	At 1 year 53% off diet (half poor seizure control, half poor tolerance), 40% of original group had ≥50% decrease in seizure frequency and 10% are seizure free	Prospective, multi center; failed average of 7 drugs previously
Freeman JM, 1998 (91)	150	0.34–16	410 seizures/mo average (multiple types)	KD	At 1 yr 55% on diet 27% had 90% decrease in seizure frequency; 7% were seizure free	Prospective; 70% had IQ <69, prior trials 6.24 AEDs on average
Hassan AM, 1999 (92)	52	Mean = 5.5	81% Mixed seizure types	KD-49 MCT-3	67% have > 50% decrease in seizures 11.5% seizure-free (no duration given)	Retrospective; no duration of follow-up given. 60% stopped diet in ≤ 3 mo.

M, myoclonic; A, atonic; IS, infantile spasms; GTC, generalized tonic-clonic; AB, absence; SP, simple partial; CP, complex partial; KD, classic ketogenic diet; MCT, medium-chain triglyceride diet; modified MCT, modified MCT diet; AEDs, antiepileptic drugs.

Table 4
Efficacy of the Ketogenic Diet in Adults

Author	No. of patients	Age (yr) of patients	Seizure type*	Diet*	Success rate (%)	Comments
Barborka CJ, 1928 (80)	49	17–42	GM, PM	KD	25% seizure free; 34% improved; 41% not benefited; 17 did not cooperate and stay on diet.	Idiopathic epilepsy in all. Only 5 on an AED (PB)*
Barborka CJ, 1930 (81)	100	16–51	GM, PM	KD	12% seizure free; 44% not benefited.	Idiopathic epilepsy in all.
Bastible C, 1931 (93)	45	19–51	GM, PM	KD	Of those staying on diet 7% seizure free; 69% improved; 21% seizures increased. 16/45 unable to maintain diet.	All females, diagnosed with eplieptic insanity, all idiopathic etiology. 6-mo follow up. Best response seen in those with least mental disorder.
Notkin J, 1934 (82)	20	22–47	GM	KD	No improvement in any, 90% had an increase in seizure number.	All institutionalized patients And off AEDs, cryptogenic Etiology. Average time on the diet 11 mo.
Sirven J, 1999 (83)	11	19–4	CP, SGTC, GTC, Atonic Absence	KD	6/11 had >50% seizure decrease. None seizure free.	All symptomatic epilepsy. All seizure types responded. 8-mo follow-up.

GM, grand mal; PM, petit mal; GTC, generalized tonic-clonic; SGTC, secondary GTC; AED, antiepileptic drug; PB, phenobarbitol.

related to outcome. Reasons that patients discontinued the ketogenic diet included insufficient seizure control, inability to medically tolerate the diet, concurrent medical illnesses, and inability to tolerate the nature of the dietary regimen. This study demonstrated that the ketogenic diet is effective in different epilepsy centers with different support staff. Children and families comply with the diet if it is effective, and results are similar to those obtained over the past seven decades.

Almost a century has passed since the ketogenic diet was initially used, and many more therapies are now available for children with epilepsy. The ketogenic diet continues to compare favorably with other new treatments that have been introduced to treat epilepsy in children. The renewed interest in the ketogenic diet has once again raised several research questions that, if answered, have the potential to improve our understanding of the neurochemistry of epilepsy and would allow better treatment of all patients with epilepsy. The ketogenic diet, a therapy that started at the beginning of the twentieth century, appears to have a definite role in the treatment of childhood epilepsy well into, and perhaps beyond, the twenty-first century.

4. CONCLUSION

Fasting, the precursor to the ketogenic diet, has been used to treat a spectrum of human maladies for centuries. The ketogenic diet emerged about 100 yr ago as a viable alternative, allowing the biochemical effects of fasting to persist, while providing fuel for the body. The ketogenic diet has a rich history in the United States and continues to be utilized to treat refractory childhood epilepsies. Its use has increased the last 10 yr, and now it is available at all major children's hospitals. Our understanding of the scientific underpinnings of this unique therapy has evolved dramatically, culminating in this medical textbook, the first ever devoted to the ketogenic diet. A better understanding of the scientific basis of this unique dietary therapy will continue to emerge with this renewed scientific interest, resulting in improved epilepsy care for all children. This will be a fitting legacy for the ketogenic diet.

REFERENCES

1. Temkin O. The Falling Sickness, 2nd ed. Johns Hopkins University Press, Baltimore, 1971, pp. 66–67.
2. Mark 9:14–29. (New King James Version.) Guideposts, Carmel, NY, 1982.
3. Livingston S. Comprehensive Management of Epilepsy in Infancy, Childhood, and Adolescence. Charles C Thomas, Springfield, IL, 1972, pp. 378–405.
4. Lennox WG, Cobb S. Studies in epilepsy. VIII: The clinical effect of fasting. Arch Neurol Psychiatr 1928;20:771–779.
5. www.epilepsiemuseum.de/alt/raffaelen.html. Site accessed January 5, 2003.
6. Guelpa G, Marie A. La lutte contre l'épilepsie par la désintoxication et par la rééducation alimentaire. Rev Ther Medico–Chirurgicale 1911;78:8–13.
7. Hendricks M. High fat and seizure free. Johns Hopkins Mag April 1995, 14–20.
8. Freeman JM, Kelly MT, Freeman JB. The Epilepsy Diet Treatment: An Introduction to the Ketogenic Diet, 1st ed. Demos, New York, 1994.
9. Wilkinson JF. Look at me. Smithsonian 1997;28(9):136–151.
10. Geyelin HR. Fasting as a method for treating epilepsy. Med Rec 1921;99:1037–1039.
11. Geyelin HR. The relation of chemical influences, including diet and endocrine disturbances, to epilepsy. Ann Intern Med 1929;2:678–681.
12. Pulsifer MB, Gordon JM, Brandt J, Vinig EPG, Freeman JM. Effects of the ketogenic diet on development and behavior: preliminary report of a prospective study. Dev Med Child Neurol 2001;43:301–306.

13. Conklin HW. Cause and treatment of epilepsy. J Am Osteopath 1922;22(1):11–14.
14. Higgins HL. Some physiological and clinical effects of high fat feeding. N Engl J Med 1930;203(4):145–150.
15. Penfield W, Erickson TC. Epilepsy and Cerebral Localization. A Study of the Mechanism, Treatment, and Prevention of Epileptic Seizures. Charles C Thomas, Baltimore, 1941, pp. 504–509.
16. McMurray TE. Epilepsy. N Y Med J 1916;109:934.
17. Goldbloom A. Some observations on the starvation treatment of epilepsy. Can Med Assoc J 1922;12:539–540.
18. Lennox WG, Lennox MA. Epilepsy and Related Disorders, Vol. 2. Little, Brown, Boston, 1960, pp. 735–739.
19. Welch HW, Goodnow FJ, Flexner S, et al. Memorial meeting for Dr. John Howland. Bull Johns Hopkins Hosp 1927;41:311–321.
20. Swink TD, Vining EPG, Freeman JM. The ketogenic diet: 1997. Adv Pediatr 1997;44:297–329.
21. Wilkins L. Epilepsy in childhood: III. Results with the ketogenic diet. J Pediatr 1937;10:341–357.
22. Harvey AM. The First Fulltime Academic Department of Pediatrics: The Story of the Harriet Lane Home. Johns Hopkins University Press, Baltimore, 1976, p. 198.
23. Gamble JL, Ross GS, Tisdall FF. The metabolism of fixed base during fasting. J Biol Chem 1923;57:633–695.
24. Talbot FB. The ketogenic diet in epilepsy. Bull N Y Acad Med 1928;4:401–408.
25. Lennox WG, Cobb S. Epilepsy from the standpoint of physiology and treatment. Medicine 1928;7:105–290.
26. McQuarrie I. Epilepsy in children: the relationship of water balance to the occurrence of seizures. Am J Dis Child 1929;38:451–467.
27. Wilder RM. The effect on ketonemia on the course of epilepsy. Mayo Clin Bull 1921;2:307.
28. Talbot FB, Metcalf KM, Moriarty ME. Epilepsy: chemical investigations of rational treatment by production of ketosis. Am J Dis Child 1927;33:218–225.
29. Helmholz HF. The treatment of epilepsy in childhood: five years' experience with the ketogenic diet. JAMA 1927;88(26):2028–2032.
30. Bridge EM, Iob LV. The mechanism of the ketogenic diet in epilepsy. Bull Johns Hopkins Hosp 1931;48:373–389.
31. Lennox WG. Ketogenic diet in the treatment of epilepsy. N Engl J Med 1928;199(2):74–75.
32. Woodyatt RT. Objects and method of diet adjustment in diabetics. Arch Intern Med 1921;28:125–141.
33. Wilder RM. High fat diets in epilepsy. Mayo Clin Bull 1921;2:308.
34. Peterman MG. The ketogenic diet in epilepsy. JAMA 1925;84(26):1979–1983.
35. Peterman MG. The ketogenic diet in the treatment of epilepsy: a preliminary report. Am J Dis Child 1924;28:28–33.
36. Wheless JW. The ketogenic diet: an effective medical therapy with side effects. J Child Neurol 2001;16(9):633–635.
37. Talbot FB, Metcalf K, Moriarty M. The ketogenic diet in the treatment of idiopathic epilepsy. Am J Dis Child 1926;32:316–318.
38. Talbot FB, Metcalf KM, Moriarty ME. A clinical study of epileptic children treated by the ketogenic diet. Boston Med Surg J 1926;196(3):89–96.
39. Talbot FB. The treatment of epilepsy of childhood by the ketogenic diet. R I Med J 1927;10(11):159–162.
40. McQuarrie I, Keith HM. Epilepsy in children: relationships of variations in the degree of ketonuria to occurrence of convulsions in epileptic children on ketogenic diets. Am J Dis Child 1927;34:1013–1029.
41. Talbot FB. Treatment of Epilepsy. Macmillan Co, New York, 1930.
42. Freeman JM, Freeman JB, Kelly MT. The Ketogenic Diet, 3rd ed. Demos, New York, 2000.
43. Schwartz RM, Boyes S, Aynsley-Green A. Metabolic effects of three ketogenic diets in the treatment of severe epilepsy. Dev Med Child Neurol 1989;31:152–160.
44. Section on Nutrition and Pediatrics, Mayo Clinic. Arranging the ketogenic diet in cases of epilepsy. Dietary administration and therapy, 1927;5:245–260.
45. Bridge EM. Epilepsy and Convulsive Disorders in Children. McGraw-Hill, New York, 1949, pp. 386–414.

46. Lennox WG. Science and Seizures: New Light on Epilepsy and Migraine. Harper & Row, New York, 1941, pp. 141–144.

47. Livingston S. The Diagnosis and Treatment of Convulsive Disorders in Children. Charles C Thomas, Springfield, IL, 1954, pp. 213–235.

48. Livingston S. Living with Epileptic Seizures. Charles C Thomas, Springfield, IL, 1963, pp. 143–163.

49. Keith HM. Convulsive Disorders in Children: With Reference to Treatment with Ketogenic Diet. Little, Brown, Boston, 1963, pp. 146–183.

50. Withrow CD. Antiepileptic drugs, the ketogenic diet: mechanism of anticonvulsant action. In: Glaser GH, Penry JK, Woodbury DM (eds.). Antiepileptic Drugs: Mechanism of Action. Raven, New York, 1980, pp. 635–642.

51. Bower BD. Epilepsy in childhood and adolescence. In: Tyrer JG (ed.). Current Status of Modern Therapy: The Treatment of Epilepsy, Vol. 5. JB Lippincott, Philadelphia, 1980, pp. 251–273.

52. Livingston S, Pauli LL. Ketogenic diet and epilepsy. Dev Med Child Neurol 1975;17:818–819.

53. Ford F. The Epilepsies and Paroxysmal Disorders of the Nervous System. Charles C Thomas, Springfield, IL, 1937, p. 888.

54. Huttenlocher PR, Wilbourn AJ, Signore JM. Medium-chain triglycerides as a therapy for intractable childhood epilepsy. Neurology 1971;21:1097–1103.

55. Gordon N. Medium-chain triglycerides in a ketogenic diet. Dev Med Child Neurol 1977;19:535–544.

56. Signore JM. Ketogenic diet containing medium-chain triglycerides. Perspectives in practice. J Am Diet Assoc 1973;62:285–290.

57. Ross DL, Swaiman KF, Torres K, Hansen J. Early biochemical and EEG correlates of the ketogenic diet in children with atypical absence epilepsy. Pediatr Neurol 1985;1(2):104–108.

58. Trauner DA. Medium-chain triglyceride (MCT) diet in intractable seizure disorders. Neurology 1985;35(2):237–238.

59. Woody RC, Brodie M, Hampton DK, Fiser RH. Corn oil ketogenic diet for children with intractable seizures. J Child Neurol 1988;3(1):21–24.

60. Sills MA, Forsythe WI, Haidukewych D, MacDonald A, Robinson M. The medium-chain triglyceride diet and intractable epilepsy. Arch Disease Child 1986;61:1168–1172.

61. Schwartz RH, Eaton J, Bower BD, Aynsley-Green A. Ketogenic diets in the treatment of epilepsy: short term clinical effects. Dev Med Child Neurol 1989;31:145–151.

62. Aicadi J. The International Review of Child Neurology. Epilepsy in Children, 2nd ed. Raven, New York, 1994, pp. 426–427.

63. *NBC Dateline.* The ketogenic diet. October 26, 1994.

64. Schneider KS, Wagner J. Recipe for hope. People, April 17, 1995, pp. 54–57.

65. Charlie Foundation to Help Cure Pediatric Epilepsy. An Introduction to the Ketogenic Diet—A Treatment for Pediatric Epilepsy. Videotape. Charlie Foundation, Santa Monica, CA, 1994.

66. Freeman JM, Kelly MT, Freeman MT. The Epilepsy Diet Treatment, 2nd ed. Demos, New York, 1996.

67. Freeman J, Vining EPG, Pillas DJ. Seizures and Epilepsy in Childhood: A Guide for Parents. Johns Hopkins Unversity Press, Baltimore, 1990, pp. 151–155.

68. Vining EPG, Freeman JM, Ballaban-Gil K, et al. and the Ketogenic Diet Multi-Center Study Group. A multi-center study of the efficacy of the ketogenic diet. Arch Neurol 1998;55:1433–1437.

69. Wheless J. The ketogenic diet: fa(c)t or fiction. J Child Neurol 1995;10:419–423.

70. Barborka CJ. The ketogenic diet. Proc Meet Mayo Clin 1928;3(36):273–275.

71. Smith WA. The ketogenic diet in the treatment of epilepsy. Ann Intern Med 1929;2:1300–1308.

72. Keeton RW, MacKenzie H. The principles underlying the calculation of flexible diabetic and ketogenic diets. Ann Intern Med 1929;3:546–556.

73. Barborka CJ. The ketogenic diet and its use. Med Clin North Am 1929;12(6):1639–1653.

74. Helmholz HF, Keith HM. Eight years' experience with the ketogenic diet in the treatment of epilepsy. JAMA 1930;95(10):707–709.

75. Helmholz HF, Keith HM. Ten years experience in the treatment of epilepsy with the ketogenic diet. Proc Meet Mayo Clin 1932;7(28):406–408.

76. Pulford DS. The present status of the ketogenic diet. Ann Intern Med 1932;6:795–801.

77. Wilder RM, Pollack H. Ketosis and the ketogenic diet: their application to treatment of epilepsy and infections of the urinary tract. Int Clin 1935;1(45th Ser):1–12.

78. Fischer L. Epilepsy: its treatment by the use of the ketogenic diet versus drugs. Arch Pediatr 1935;52(1):131–136.
79. Keith HM. Results of treatment of recurring convulsive attacks of epilepsy. Am J Dis Child 1942;74:140–146.
80. Barborka CJ. Ketogenic diet treatment of epilepsy in adults. JAMA 1928;91(2):73–78.
81. Barborka CJ. Epilepsy in adults: results of treatment by ketogenic diet in one hundred cases. Arch Neurol Psychiatr 1930;23:904–914.
82. Notkin J. Epilepsy: treatment of institutionalized adult patients with a ketogenic diet. Arch Neurol 1934;31:787–793.
83. Sirven J, Whedon B, Caplan D, et al. The ketogenic diet for intractable epilepsy in adults: preliminary results. Epilepsia 1999;40:1721–1726.
84. Hopkins IJ, Lynch BC. Use of ketogenic diet in epilepsy in childhood. Aust Pediatr J 1970;6:25–29.
85. Kinsman SL, Vining EPG, Quaskey SA, et al. Efficacy of the ketogenic diet for intractable seizure disorders: review of 58 cases. Epilepsia 1992;33(6):1132–1136.
86. Weeks DF, Renner DS, Allen FM, Wishart MB. Observations on fasting and diets in the treatment of epilepsy. J Metab Res 1923;3:317–364.
87. Cooder HR. Epilepsy in children: with particular reference to the ketogenic diet. Calif West Med 1933;39:169–173.
88. Helmholz HF, Goldstein M. Results of fifteen years experience with the ketogenic diet in the treatment of epilepsy in children. Proc Mayo Clin 1937;12(28):433–436.
89. Dodson WE, Prensky AL, DeVivo DC, et al. Management of seizure disorders: selected aspects. Part II. J Pediatr 1976;89(5):695–703.
90. Swink TD, Vining EPG, Casey JC, et al. Efficacy of the ketogenic diet in children under 2 years of age. Epilepsia 1997;18 (Suppl 3):26.
91. Freeman JM, Vining EPG, Pillas DJ, et al. The efficacy of the ketogenic diet 1998: a prospective evaluation of intervention in 150 children. Pediatrics 1998;102:1358–1363.
92. Hassan AM, Keene DL, Whiting SE et al. Ketogenic diet in the treatment of refractory epilepsy in childhood. Pediatr Neurol 1999;21:548–552.
93. Bastible C. The ketogenic treatment of epilepsy. Ir J Med Sci 1931;2:506–519.
94. Murray RK, Granner DK, Mayes PA, Rodwell VW (eds.). Harper's Biochemistry, 24th ed., Vol. 29. Appleton & Lange, Norwalk, CT, 1996, p. 288.

II   CLINICAL ASPECTS

3

The Ketogenic Diet

The Physician's Perspective

Eric H. Kossoff and John M. Freeman

1. INTRODUCTION

Children with medically refractory epilepsy, i.e., those with seizures that are not controlled by the first two antiepileptic drugs (AEDs) used appropriately, are likely to experience not only continuing seizures but concomitant morbidities associated with the epileptic condition. Why would any rational pediatric neurologist use the ketogenic diet (KD) when new AEDs are being rapidly introduced to treat children with difficult-to-control seizures? Each of these new medications claims efficacy equal to prior medications, but with fewer side effects. It is possible to use each of these medications, pushed to efficacy or toxicity, in individual or multiple combinations with older drugs. Done slowly and properly, this can take many years. Vagus nerve stimulation may also be helpful for some who do not respond to medications. Patients with localization-related epilepsies may benefit from surgery. So why would a physician choose the KD, a difficult therapy that involves meticulous weighing of foods and calorie restriction?

There has been increasing literature on the efficacy of the KD for even the most intractable of epileptic patients *(1–3)*. The ability to reduce medications and avoid their side effects provides an obvious additional benefit *(4)*. Use of the KD is associated with relatively few problems in comparison to most AEDs, used either alone or in combination *(5)*. Physicians are now more aware of the diet and are more open minded about using it. Our most recent survey *(6)* found that since 1994, increasing numbers of pediatric neurologists have used the diet for their patients. The major impediment to its use is the lack of adequately trained dieticians.

In general, the KD has historically been used as a therapy of desperation for many parents and physicians, when there has been failure of multiple medications, and when there is not a surgically remediable lesion. If the diet is effective when most other therapies have failed, why is it reserved for last?

2. CHOOSING PATIENTS

The KD appears to work well against seizures of all types and in children of all ages. Our reported experience with 150 children who had failed an average of more than six

From: *Epilepsy and the Ketogenic Diet*
Edited by: C. E. Stafstrom and J. M. Rho © Humana Press Inc., Totowa, NJ

medications indicated that no specific epilepsy syndrome had a higher response rate to the ketogenic diet *(2)*. In one trial, there was no difference in outcome between seizure types, although a small diminished efficacy was seen for children with multifocal spikes on electroencephalograms (EEGs) at 3 mo ($p = 0.04$) *(3)*. However, our impression is that children with the highest frequency of seizures, and those who are most refractory to medications, are most likely to respond. Children with the Lennox–Gastaut syndrome and atonic and tonic seizures seem to have the best clinical response. As demonstrated in our retrospective experience with 23 infants, infantile spasms may also show similar benefit from the KD *(7)*.

There is a misconception that the diet cannot, or should not, be used in children under 2 yr of age, or in adolescents. However, our data indicate that children as young as 4 mo and even teenagers may benefit from the KD *(7,8)*. In addition, limited data suggest that the diet may be effective in adults *(9)*.

Profoundly retarded children with intractable epilepsy may be good candidates for the diet because their eating habits can be more easily modified. However, ambulatory children with normal intelligence can stick with the diet and remember to refuse nondiet foods, especially if the diet controls their seizures and relieves them of the sedative effects of AEDs. We have frequently heard young children, when faced with cookies, say, "I can't have that—it's not on my special diet." Adolescents (and perhaps adults) have more difficulty with the rigorous compliance issues of the diet and should attempt the diet only when they are highly motivated and when their seizures, or medications, are clearly interfering with their quality of life.

In a child with a gastrostomy tube, compliance is not an issue, especially with the widespread use of ketogenic formulas. The commercially prepared ketogenic formulas can be provided enterally via a gastrostomy tube with significant ease of preparation *(10)*. Although infants with an increased risk of growth retardation will need careful electrolyte maintenance, the benefits of the KD in this age group can be considerable *(7,11,12)*. Bottle-fed infants readily accept the diet in place of their formula.

The KD, like surgery, should be considered for every patient with seizures. It, like surgery, should rarely be used as the first treatment, because 70% of seizures will be controlled by the initial AED when appropriately used *(13)*. Clearly, monotherapy is easier than the diet—when it works, and when it does not produce too many unacceptable side effects. When a second medication has not brought the seizures under control, the diet should be seriously considered. In our estimation, the diet should *not* be saved for the last desperate attempt at seizure control.

3. PREDIET REFERRAL AND EVALUATION

Patients evaluated at the Pediatric Epilepsy Center at Johns Hopkins are often self-referred. They have heard about our successes from a friend or through the Internet. They may be seeking alternatives to drugs because they are afraid of the side effects of these medications. They often want a more "natural" way of controlling seizures. The KD is not natural, however, and it may not be the best choice for that child or that family at that time and at that stage of the epilepsy. So how do we address all these issues?

All patient inquiries about the diet (except patients already under our care) are screened over the phone by our coordinator, Ms. Diana Pillas. Ms. Pillas has a wealth of experience in dealing with families of children with epilepsy and discusses the risks

Table 1
Studies to Obtain Prior to Ketogenic Diet Initiation

Urine organic acids
Plasma amino acids
Complete blood count with differential and platelets
Lactate
Electrolytes
Electroencephalogram
Magnetic resonance imaging of brain
Cerebrospinal fluid (if a history of neurologic degeneration)

and benefits of the diet with them at length. She will determine the type and frequency of the seizures, the medications previously tried, and the reason the parent wishes to try the diet. If the diet represents a reasonable option, Ms. Pillas will often refer the patient to a KD center closer to the family's home. She will instruct those coming to Johns Hopkins to obtain medical records so that we can prescreen for structural or metabolic conditions.

Parents are asked to send a letter to accompany the records that describes their child, his or her epilepsy, and the family's goals and expectations. Occasionally these goals are surprising, such as "reduce the larger seizures by 50%, but the daily staring ones can stay the same." These goals will later provide a benchmark against which to measure the success of the diet. This exercise is quite valuable because it forces the parents to think about their expectations for the child and for the seizures. The letter further enables us to understand the child's role in the family.

Many of our patients come from great distances, and we will communicate with their local physician about the diet, the medications that may be used, and the partnership we hope to establish. If families are coming to Hopkins for initiation of the diet, we request that they read our book, *The Ketogenic Diet: A Treatment for Epilepsy,* and that if possible they view the video made by the Charlie Foundation *(14,15).* Our dietician will contact them by phone prior to admission to assess the child's usual dietary intake, food preferences, and weight and height.

Because most of our patients are referred from other centers, one of our major tasks is to ensure the validity of their histories and the completeness of prior evaluations. The laboratory studies we either obtain, or ensure that they were done accurately elsewhere, are listed in Table 1. The condition of children with underlying metabolic disorders or certain mitochondrial syndromes may be worsened by the KD *(5).* Children with pyruvate carboxylase deficiency, fatty acid oxidation defects, and other syndromes in which energy metabolism is compromised could experience increased seizures on the diet and/or metabolic decompensation, especially during periods of illness. For that reason, we ensure that all children have had a urine and plasma metabolic screen and a serum lactate prior to admission. Children become acidotic on the diet, and baseline acidosis may indicate a metabolic problem that might worsen with the diet. We have not seen the bruising on the ketogenic diet reported by others, although obtaining a baseline complete blood count, including platelets, is reasonable. We do not routinely check carnitine levels, platelet aggregation function, electrocardiograms, mineral (zinc, selenium) levels, or pancreatic function *(16–20).*

Table 2
Timeline of Ketogenic Diet Initiation

Before diet
    Less carbohydrates for 1–2 d
    Fasting starts the night before admission
Day 1
    Admitted to the hospital
    Fasting continues
    Fluids restricted to 60–75 mL/kg
    Blood glucose monitored every 6 h
    Use carbohydrate-free medication
Day 2
    Dinner given as one-third of calculated diet meal as eggnog
    Blood glucose checks discontinued after dinner
Day 3
    Breakfast and lunch given as one-third of diet
    Dinner increased to two-thirds (still eggnog)
Day 4
    Breakfast and lunch given as two-thirds of diet allowance
    Dinner is first full ketogenic meal (not eggnog)
Day 5
    Full ketogenic diet breakfast given
    Child discharged to home

In cases of central nervous system degeneration, we recommend studies of the cerebrospinal fluid, especially for glucose, to check for a glucose transport defect. Any child with partial-onset epilepsy needs to have recent EEG and magnetic resonance imaging records to enable us to investigate for a surgically resectable focus. Many families opt for the ketogenic diet as a "last resort" of medical therapy prior to surgery, and although the treatment is less successful when structural lesions are present, we have occasionally achieved seizure control in such patients.

4. DIET INITIATION

We have continued to initiate the diet in the hospital during a preapproved 4-d admission. Although others have stated that the diet can be initiated without fasting *(21)* and that it can be initiated on an outpatient basis, we have found that fasting hastens the diet initiation and development of ketosis *(22,23)*. Hospitalization also allows the child's blood sugar to be closely monitored and any fluctuations to be corrected promptly. In the inpatient setting, the occasional severe acidosis, vomiting, and sedation that may accompany diet initiation can be monitored and corrected, and during the hospital admission better teaching of the parents can take place. Over the past several years, we have adopted a standardized protocol for a 4-d diet initiation admission period (Table 2). The creation of preprinted order sheets helps streamline the entire process for the families, physicians, and nurses.

We usually admit three to five children at a time, once a month. This allows the families to bond and form small support groups, which can continue after discharge. It also permits far more efficient teaching. Many friendships have formed during the hospital admission. One potential drawback is that some children will have very different initial responses to the ketogenic diet, and families with children having less success in the first few days may become discouraged.

For first 2 d prior to admission, the family decreases the child's carbohydrate intake. The child begins to fast after the clinic visit and is admitted to the hospital the following day, after what has been an overnight fast. Occasionally, younger or smaller children will be fasted for only 24 h. The children are seen in our outpatient clinic on Tuesday afternoons, allowing us to confirm previous information, discuss last-minute issues in a quiet setting, and ensure that the child is medically stable for this elective admission. It also serves for a 2-h session in which to teach the family about the diet and to answer their questions.

On Day 1 of hospitalization, the child is admitted. Fluids are restricted to 60–75 mL per kilogram of body weight, and children often require encouragement to drink owing to thirst arising from ketosis. Blood glucose is monitored with finger sticks every 6 h unless it falls below 40 mg/dL, in which case it is checked every 2 h. If the child has symptoms of hypoglycemia or the glucose level falls below 25 mg/dL, 30 mL of orange juice is provided and the glucose is checked one hour later. Even small children tolerate the fast well, with rare symptomatic hypoglycemia. Urine ketones are checked daily as well. Ketosis can begin during the fasting period, and the resultant nausea and vomiting can occasionally require intravenous hydration using fluids containing no dextrose.

AEDs are continued during the fasting period at their previous doses. The only exception is phenobarbital, a drug whose blood level can increase with ketosis (and we will routinely reduce the dose by 30% during admission to compensate for this interaction). All medications are carefully examined for carbohydrate content and formulations changed when necessary.

On day 2, fasting continues until dinner, when one-third of the calculated diet is provided as an "eggnog," which looks and tastes like a milkshake and can be sipped, frozen as ice cream, or cooked as scrambled eggs. Excess ketosis at this time that causes nausea and vomiting can be relieved with a small amount (30 mL) of orange juice. Once the child begins eating, serum glucose checks are no longer necessary and are thus discontinued.

Breakfast and lunch remain at one-third of the calculated calories as eggnog on day 3, but dinner increases to two-thirds of the usual allowance (still eggnog). On day 4, breakfast and lunch are also increased to two-thirds of allowance, and dinner is then given as the first full KD meal (with actual foods provided). On the fifth hospital day, the child receives a full ketogenic breakfast and is discharged to home. All children are sent home with prescriptions for urine ketosticks, additional calcium, and a sugar-free, fat-soluble vitamin and mineral supplement. Medications are left unchanged unless side effects are problematic, it is always better to use tablets or a carbohydrate-free solution whenever possible. Follow-up is arranged.

Throughout the 5-d hospital stay, classes are held with physicians, nurses, and dieticians to teach the family about the rationale of the ketogenic diet, calculation of meals, nutrition label reading, and management of their children during illnesses. This is just as important in achieving a favorable outcome as the actual logistics of diet initiation. Even families that do not speak English can be trained by using videotapes (which can be paused and reviewed multiple times), written handouts, and translators. We encourage both parents to be present for classes, to prepare for the likely future event of having to make meals and handle problems individually. Older children are also asked to participate in classes as cognitively appropriate.

After discharge, parents are instructed to check urine ketones daily, and the diet is individually adjusted after consultation by telephone to maximize seizure control. Serum glucose or electrolytes are not routinely monitored after discharge. Weight is monitored by the parents, and any significant change is reported. We strongly advocate the care of these children by only one primary medical center. Problems arise when different providers make medication changes. Parents need to have a consistent plan and a single contact person for this very serious therapy.

5. MEDICAL FOLLOW-UP

Children are followed by phone by our dietician, quite frequently at first, until parents become more secure. The dieticians have estimated that as much as 30 h of telephone support per patient may be necessary. For our many patients who live far from Johns Hopkins, we have instituted a full-day KD clinic day each month. Children return for follow-up 3, 6, and 12 mo after diet initiation. Laboratory results (urine calcium/creatinine, serum lipid profile, electrolytes, AED levels) are obtained prior to these clinic visits to monitor for side effects.

During the visit, our dietician evaluates the dietary history and laboratory values and makes recommendations for meal or calorie changes based on this assessment. A physician discusses these recommendations and assesses the child for seizure control, adjusting AEDs as appropriate. Finally, our epilepsy counselor will meet with the family and child to discuss home and school issues. After the large amount of work needed to institute the diet, the pleasure of seeing these children return with significantly improved seizure control can make a busy clinic day quite enjoyable.

6. MEDICATIONS

A common goal of parents with children with intractable epilepsy is to reduce their medications. The side effects of sedation, irritability, and mood changes that can be seen with AEDs are much less commonly seen with the ketogenic diet. Even when the diet does not completely control the seizures, children will remain on the diet if medications can be eliminated. However, we encourage patience. In general, no changes are made in medications during the diet initiation period or for the first few weeks afterward. There is often a need to titrate each individual patient's diet before seizure reduction is achieved. Therefore, medication changes would considerably complicate the assessment of efficacy and are hence discouraged.

We have not found any AEDs to be particularly beneficial or detrimental when used in combination with the KD. Valproate has been reported to increase potential liver abnormalities when used with the KD, but this has never been conclusively proven (16). Traditionally, carbonic anhydrase inhibitors (acetazolamide, zonisamide, topiramate) have been discouraged in combination with the KD because of the common side effect of kidney stones. A retrospective study of our cohort did not find any increased risk of nephrolithiasis when these drugs were used in combination with the KD (24). In a study by Takeoka et al., topiramate did not worsen acidosis (25). As stated earlier, phenobarbital levels tend to rise slightly with ketosis; therefore we decrease the dose by approximately one-third in all patients to prevent this.

Carnitine levels have been shown to decrease initially on the KD and then stabilize, without clinical symptoms *(26)*. We have not seen liver problems owing to carnitine insufficiency in our population. Children on the diet who complain of fatigue or weakness have been given carnitine for a one-month trial, but this has only rarely made a difference.

7. HANDLING INCREASED SEIZURES

Seizures are predicted to decrease after initiation of the diet, and often they do. However, some patients derive marked benefit from the diet but later have an increase in seizures again. When a child who had been doing well once more experiences seizures, the question is always "Why?" In searching for an answer, we immediately ask whether the child has an infection. As with any epilepsy, the threshold for seizures is lower during an infection and will return to a higher level when the infection disappears. It is always prudent to look for sore throats, ear infections, or urinary tract infection, as well as common viruses.

It is also important to ascertain whether new medications or different foods have been introduced. In some children, the diet is so carefully titrated for seizure control that even small amounts of carbohydrate can induce seizures. One child had an increase in seizures when the family changed to a different luncheon meat. Several others experienced increased seizures after using suntan lotion, which may contain so much sorbitol that some is absorbed through the skin. Hair gels, lotions, and ointments also often contain enough sorbitol to negate ketosis and cause seizures in susceptible patients. Many food additives described as "sugar free" contain carbohydrate-containing chemicals such as maltodextrin, sorbitol, starch, and fructose. Seven macadamia nuts rather than the three allowed in one child's diet caused a recurrence of seizures.

It is important that the family check urine ketones routinely to ensure adequate ketosis. If ketones are not greater than 4, the child can be fasted with clear liquids for 24 h to improve ketosis rapidly. Periodic oral or rectal benzodiazepines can be useful for seizure exacerbations.

Kidney stones may be subtle and can exacerbate seizures *(27)*. The seizures will again abate when the stone is dissolved with citrates and increased fluids. Although the stress of surgery can cause increased seizure activity, a recent review of patients undergoing general anesthesia did not find any worsening with close observation *(28)*. Most, but not all, children whose seizures have had a marked decrease with the diet will be brought back under control when a diligent search has uncovered the cause of the recurrence.

8. DISCONTINUATION OF THE DIET

The KD, if successful, is traditionally continued for 2 yr. The origins of this tradition are unknown. An outcome study of 150 children, questioned 3–6 yr after starting the diet, revealed that only 10% were still on the KD after more than 4 yr *(1)*. Discontinuation during the first year of therapy was often secondary to perceived ineffectiveness or restrictiveness. After 1 yr, significantly fewer children were discontinued for these reasons, and comparatively more had the diet stopped because they were seizure free (often >2 yr) or had an intercurrent illness. Of those remaining on the diet at 1 yr, 36% (30 of 83) became medication free.

As with AEDs, the KD is traditionally tapered slowly over 3–6 mo by gradually lowering the ratio of fat to protein and carbohydrate, then relaxing the weighing of ingredients, and finally adding new carbohydrate foods over weeks while keeping calories constant. An alternative method that appears to work, although it has never been rigorously tested, is to substitute whole milk for heavy cream while maintaining the remainder of the diet. After 2 wk we gradually switch to 2% and then to 1% milk.

If this protocol does not cause seizures to recur, it is followed by the relaxation of calorie restriction, then gradual introduction of carbohydrate-containing foods. The advantage of this approach is that it is far faster and, if seizures recur, it is easy to return to cream without fasting again and retraining the child. If the child is having significant difficulty with the KD or in the event of a severe intercurrent illness, the diet can be discontinued immediately, often without a dramatic increase in seizures.

9. CONCLUSION

The ketogenic diet can be very effective when patients are carefully selected and potentially negative predisposing conditions are excluded. The protocol for diet initiation at our center has made the entire admission process much less difficult for the patients and their families, while maximizing diet efficacy and education. After admission, we use a team approach to strictly monitor medication changes, laboratory results, dietary changes, and nondiet medical issues. Despite the difficulty in maintaining the diet, the care of these children can be vastly rewarding, not only for the pediatric neurologist, nurse, and dietician, but more importantly for the patients and their family members.

REFERENCES

1. Hemingway C, Freeman JM, Pillas DJ, Pyzik PL. The ketogenic diet: a 3 to 6 year follow-up of 150 children enrolled prospectively. Pediatrics 2001;108:898–905.
2. Freeman JM, Vining EPG, Pillas DJ, Pyzik PL, Casey JC, Kelly MT. The efficacy of the ketogenic diet—1998: a prospective evaluation of intervention in 150 children. Pediatrics 1998;102:1358–1363.
3. Vining EPG, Freeman JM, Ballaban-Gil K, et al. A multicenter study of the efficacy of the ketogenic diet. Arch Neurol 1998;55:1433–1437.
4. Gilbert DL, Pyzik PL, Vining EP, Freeman JM. Medication cost reduction in children on the ketogenic diet: data from a prospective study. J Child Neurol 1999;14:469–471.
5. Wheless JW. The ketogenic diet: an effective medical therapy with side effects. J Child Neurol 2001;16:633–635.
6. Hemingway C, Pyzik PL, Freeman JM. Changing physician attitudes toward the ketogenic diet: a parent-centered approach to physician education about a medication alternative. Epilepsy Behav 2001;2:574–578.
7. Kossoff EH, Pyzik PL, McGrogan JR, Vining EPG, Freeman JM. Efficacy of the ketogenic diet for infantile spasms. Pediatrics 2002;109:780–783.
8. Mady MA, Kossoff EH, McGregor AL, Wheless JW. The ketogenic diet: adolescents can do it, too. Epilepsia 2003;44:847–851.
9. Sirven JI, Liporace JD, O'Dwyer JL, et. al. A prospective trial of the ketogenic diet as add-on therapy in adults: preliminary results (abstr). Epilepsia 1998;39:195.
10. La Vega-Talbott M, Solomon GE, Mast J, Green NS, Hosain SA. Ketogenic diet in pediatric epilepsy patients with gastrostomy feeding (abst). Ann Neurol 2001;50(3 Suppl 1):S102.
11. Nordli DR, Jr., Kuroda MM, Carroll J, et al. Experience with the ketogenic diet in infants. Pediatrics 2001;108:129–133.
12. Vining EPG, Pyzik P, McGrogan J, et al. Growth of children on the ketogenic diet. Dev Med Child Neurol 2002;44:796–802.
13. Shinnar S, Berg AT, O'Dell C, Newstein D, Moshe SL, Hauser WA. Predictors of multiple seizures in a cohort of children prospectively followed from the time of their first unprovoked seizure. Ann Neurol 2000;48:140–147.

14. Abrahams J. An Introduction to the Ketogenic Diet: A Treatment for Pediatric Epilepsy. The Charlie Foundation, Santa Monica, CA (videotape), 1994.
15. Freeman JM, Kelly MT, Freeman JB. The Epilepsy Diet Treatment, 2nd ed. Demos, New York, 1996.
16. Ballaban-Gil K, Callahan C, O'Dell C, Pappo M, Moshe S, Shinnar S. Complications of the ketogenic diet. Epilepsia 1998;39:744–748.
17. Best TH, Franz DN, Gilbert DL, Nelson DP, Epstein MR. Cardiac complications in pediatric patients on the ketogenic diet. Neurology 2000;54:2328–2330.
18. Berry-Kravis E, Booth G, Taylor A, Valentino LA. Bruising and the ketogenic diet: evidence for diet-induced changes in platelet function. Ann Neurol 2001;49:98–103.
19. Stewart WA, Gordon K, Camfield P. Acute pancreatitis causing death in a child on the ketogenic diet. J Child Neurol 2001;16:682.
20. Hahn TJ, Halstead LR, DeVivo DC. Disordered mineral metabolism produced by ketogenic diet therapy. Calcif Tissue Int 1979;28:17–22.
21. Wirrell EC, Darwish HZ, Williams-Dyjur C, Blackman M, Lange V. Is a fast necessary when initiating the ketogenic diet? J Child Neurol 2002;17:179–182.
22. Pan JW, Rothman TL, Behar KL, Stein DT, Hetherington HP. Human brain beta-hydroxybutyrate and lactate increase in fasting-induced ketosis. J Cereb Blood Flow Metab 2000;20:1502–1507.
23. Freeman JM, Vining EPG. Seizures decrease rapidly after fasting: preliminary studies of the ketogenic diet. Arch Pediatr Adolesc Med 1999;153:946–949.
24. Kossoff EH, Pyzik PL, Furth SL, Hladky HD, Freeman JM, Vining EPG. Kidney stones, carbonic anhydrase inhibitors, and the ketogenic diet. Epilepsia 2002;43:1168–1171.
25. Takeoka M, Riviello JJ, Pfeifer H, Thiele EA. Concomitant treatment with topiramate and ketogenic diet in pediatric epilepsy. Epilepsia 2002;43:1072–1075.
26. Berry-Kravis E, Booth G, Sanchez AC, Woodbury-Kolb J. Carnitine levels and the ketogenic diet. Epilepsia 2001;42:1445–1451.
27. Furth SL, Casey JC, Pyzik PL, et al. Risk factors for urolithiasis in children on the ketogenic diet. Pediatr Nephrol 2000;15:125–128.
28. Valenica I, Pfeifer H, Thiele EA. General anesthesia and the ketogenic diet: clinical experience in nine patients. Epilepsia 2002;43:525–529.

4

Clinical Use of the Ketogenic Diet
The Dietitian's Role

Beth Zupec-Kania, Rhonda Roell Werner, and Mary L. Zupanc

1. INTRODUCTION

The ketogenic diet is a multidisciplinary therapy that requires the dedicated support of physicians, nurses, dietitians, and social workers. A registered dietitian with pediatric experience is vital to the success of a ketogenic diet program, for this person is responsible for calculating, initiating, and fine-tuning the ketogenic diet. The dietitian must assure that nutritional needs are met during the course of diet therapy. The dietitian's responsibilities include communicating medical concerns to medical team members and communicating regularly with the caregiver of the individual on the ketogenic diet. It is the responsibility of the epileptologist or neurologist and the nurse clinician to provide medical supervision of the ketogenic diet.

1.1. Planning for Ketogenic Diet Therapy

The decision to use the ketogenic diet is based on the appropriateness of this therapy to the patient's medical condition, the willingness and ability of the patient to comply with the diet, and the availability of a ketogenic diet program. When managed successfully, the ketogenic diet can provide seizure control and even seizure freedom to individuals with difficult-to-control seizures. The ketogenic diet can also provide cost savings in the overall medical budget of the family of a child who has epilepsy *(1)*.

1.2. Candidate Selection

The typical ketogenic diet candidate has failed to achieve seizure control with antiepileptic drug treatment or has suffered unwanted effects from the antiepileptic drug(s). Children with disorders of fatty acid oxidation would not be candidates for the ketogenic diet. If these disorders exist during ketogenic diet therapy, the individual would be unable to metabolize the fatty acids that constitute the majority of the calories in the diet. In the absence of this major energy source, the body would metabolize its own protein stores, leading to severe acidosis, coma, and even death if untreated. Biochemical screening prior to admission should include profiles for urine organic and amino acids, serum amino acids, lactate, pyruvate, and carnitine *(2)*.

From: *Epilepsy and the Ketogenic Diet*
Edited by: C. E. Stafstrom and J. M. Rho © Humana Press Inc., Totowa, NJ

The ketogenic diet has been used more frequently in children than adults. A 1997 survey of 30 medical centers utilizing the diet throughout the United States reported that 80% of the individuals who had been treated with the ketogenic diet were children between the ages of 1 and 10 yr, 15% between the ages of 11 and 17 yr, 3% infants, and 2% adults under the age of 40 *(3)*.

1.3. Overview of Ketogenic Diet Therapy

A suitable candidate for initiation of the ketogenic diet is hospitalized to begin the diet and then is followed by regularly scheduled outpatient visits during the course of diet therapy *(4)*. If successful in controlling or minimizing seizures, ketogenic diet therapy is usually continued for 2–3 yr. Children whose seizures fail to improve after 2–3 mo or who are unable to tolerate the diet should be discontinued from the diet early.

1.4. Pre-Ketogenic Diet Session

The rigors of ketogenic diet management should be discussed during the pre-ketogenic diet session. The process of food preparation and food weighing should be explained. The caregiver should be provided with the information for purchasing a scale that weighs in tenths of a gram (0.1 g). A description of the typical meals and beverages, and the requirement for the omission of carbohydrate-rich foods, should be clearly communicated. The caregiver should be informed about the appropriate foods and nutritional supplements that must accompany the diet. The follow-up appointments required to monitor the diet safely should be reviewed. The caregiver should understand the possible adverse effects of the diet, including constipation, kidney stones, and difficulty with compliance (particularly with older children). The expected length of ketogenic diet therapy should also be reviewed in this session.

Eating is an activity that is highly celebrated in our society with every holiday and major event. The caregiver should be aware of the impact that food restriction may have on child and family alike and should be willing to discuss alternative ways to enjoy these events. The caregiver who understands the ketogenic diet and is motivated to adjust to the demands of this therapy will find the diet a worthwhile endeavor. Disorganized or unreliable families will find the diet difficult and may jeopardize the seizure control and health of an individual if the diet is poorly managed. Single-parent households and children in childcare and institutional settings have had positive experiences with the diet; therefore, these settings should not be considered to be contraindications to utilizing the ketogenic diet.

A nutrition assessment of the candidate should be completed before the ketogenic diet is initiated. Information regarding growth history, dietary practices, and chewing or swallowing difficulties should be reviewed. Feeding difficulties such as gastrointestinal reflux may need to be resolved prior to ketogenic diet therapy.

Baseline laboratory collected to determine nutritional status and to establish a reference point for follow-up nutrition and neurologic evaluations should include a complete blood count, chemistry or endocrine panel, electrolytes, lipids, serum carnitine levels, and antiepileptic drug levels. If not previously completed, metabolic studies for disorders in fatty acid oxidation and mitochondrial function should be included at this evaluation.

A pre-ketogenic diet history intake form can assist in collecting data for the nutrition assessment and planning a safe and well-tolerated ketogenic diet (*see* Appendix 1 in this chapter). The ketogenic diet should be individualized to the special needs of the child. A growth chart should be initiated and monitored during the course of ketogenic diet therapy.

Food allergies, intolerances, and cultural and religious preferences require special consideration and may necessitate adjustments in the diet. Information regarding current medications and nutritional supplements is needed to determine appropriateness to the diet. Medications and supplements in suspension, syrup, elixirs, and chewable-tablet forms generally contain concentrated sources of carbohydrate, and alternatives should be used. A 3-d food diary is also recommended prior to ketogenic diet initiation to determine the child's dietary practices, food preferences, and method of nutritional intake. The ketogenic diet can be formulated for oral intake, enteral intake, or a combination of these methods.

2. CALCULATING THE KETOGENIC DIET PRESCRIPTION

Calculating the ketogenic diet requires the consideration of many factors. It is important to individualize the calculations to the needs of the candidate and to use outcome data such as growth parameters, level of ketosis, seizure control, and nutritional needs to fine-tune the calculations later during therapy. The hand calculations described in the section that follow are based on the traditional long-chain triglyceride ketogenic diet. Computerized diet programs are available and can save time and ensure the accuracy of diet calculations. "Ketocalculator" is one example.

2.1. Calculating Energy Requirements

The calculation of the energy requirement is aimed at achieving normal growth and development while maintaining ketosis during the course of ketogenic diet therapy. A calorie level that is too high will result in rapid weight gain. A calorie level that is too low may result in poor growth and insufficient ketosis. Experience has shown that children can grow on the ketogenic diet, but often growth occurs at a decelerated rate. The calorie level may need to be adjusted several times during the course of ketogenic diet therapy to support individual growth needs. The child's ideal weight for height is the main parameter for determining caloric needs. If the child is underweight, his or her actual weight should be used as the initial caloric goal. Overweight children should be calculated at or close to their ideal weight for height. Factors affecting energy expenditure, such as immobility (low energy expenditure) or muscle spasticity (increased energy expenditure), should be taken into account.

The thermic effect of a high-fat diet is also a factor in determining caloric needs. The thermic effect is the increase in energy expenditure resulting from the obligatory metabolic costs of processing a meal, which include nutrient digestion, absorption, transport, and storage. Since the ketogenic diet is highest in fat, the energy level of the ketogenic diet can be lower than a typical high carbohydrate diet. The initial energy level is therefore calculated at 80–90% of the Recommended Dietary Allowance (RDA) *(5)*. The final energy value is extrapolated from this range based upon activity level as described earlier. For example, the energy recommendation (RDA, 2002) for a 7-yr-old, physically active female weighing 23 kg is 1473 kg *(5)*. Then calculate 80–90% of this value [(1473 kcal × 0.8–0.9) = 1178–1326 kcal]. The final energy level chosen for the purpose of these calculations is 1300 kcal.

2.2. The Ketogenic Ratio

The ketogenic ratio represents the relationship between the grams of fat and the combined grams of protein and carbohydrate. In a 4:1 ratio, there are four times as many

Table 1
**Recommended Starting Ketogenic Ratios
of Fat: Protein + Carbohydrate**

Age	Ratio
≤ 18 mo	3:1
19 mo–12 yr	4:1
>12 yr	3:1
Obesity	3:1

Table 2
Kilocalories per Dietary Unit

Fat: Protein + carbohydrate ratio	Nutrients (kcal)		Value/dietary unit (kcal)
	Fat	Protein + carbohydrate	
2.0:1	2 g × 9 kcal = 18	1 g × 4 kcal/g = 4	22
2.5:1	2 g × 9 kcal = 22.5	1 g × 4 kcal/g = 4	26.5
3.0:1	2 g × 9 kcal = 27	1 g × 4 kcal/g = 4	31
3.5:1	2 g × 9 kcal = 31.5	1 g × 4 kcal/g = 4	35.5
4.0:1	2 g × 9 kcal = 36	1 g × 4 kcal/g = 4	40
4.5:1	2 g × 9 kcal = 40.5	1 g × 4 kcal/g = 4	44.5
5.0:1	2 g × 9 kcal = 45	1 g × 4 kcal/g = 4	49

grams of fat for every 1 g of protein and carbohydrate combined. The ratio is intended to regulate the degree of ketosis, with higher ratios theoretically stimulating greater ketosis. The higher the ratio, the lower the protein and carbohydrate content of the diet. The ratio can be manipulated during the course of ketogenic diet therapy to achieve nutritional goals and to optimize seizure control. The ratio at which the ketogenic diet should be started is outlined in Table 1. It is important to keep in mind that the degree of ketosis may vary among individuals. Two different individuals of the same age and weight may experience a completely different level of ketosis on the same ratio. This difference is tentatively attributed to individual variations in energy metabolism and expenditure. The ratio is tapered at the end of ketogenic diet therapy to gradually reduce and eliminate ketosis.

2.3. Calculating Dietary Units

Dietary units represent a caloric value based on the ratio of grams of fat to carbohydrate and protein. In a 4:1 ratio, a dietary unit has 4 g of fat for every gram of protein and carbohydrate combined. Because fat has 9 kcal/g and protein and carbohydrate has 4 kcal/g, the dietary unit in the 4:1 ratio has 40 kcal per dietary unit: (9 kcal/g × 4 g = 36 kcal) + (4 kcal/g × 1 g = 4 kcal) = 40 kcal/dietary unit.

To calculate the number of dietary units for a given diet prescription, divide the energy goal by the kilocalories per Dietary Unit for the indicated ratio (Table 2). For example,

Table 3
Protein Goals

Age group	Protein (g/kg)
Infant	1.5
1–3 yr	1.1
4–13 yr	0.95
14–18 yr	0.85
> 18 yr	0.8

From ref. 5.

1300 kcal, 4:1 diet
1300 kcal ÷ 40 kcal/dietary unit = 32.5 dietary units

2.4. Calculating the Fat

The number of grams of fat that are required to satisfy the ratio requirement is determined by multiplying the dietary units by the fat unit in the ratio. Continuing the example from Section 2.3. for a 4:1 ratio, we write

32.5 dietary units × 4 = 130 g fat daily

2.5. Calculating the Protein

The ketogenic diet calculations should allow sufficient protein for normal growth and tissue turnover. The Dietary Reference Intakes (DRIs) provide protein goals based on age and weight as shown in Table 3. For example, A 7-yr-old child weighing 23 kg requires 22 g protein daily:

23 kg × 0.95 g/kg = 22 g of protein

It is important to consider that limited energy intake may cause some of the dietary protein to be used for energy. Careful monitoring of growth and protein status (albumin and prealbumin) during ketogenic diet therapy will provide guidance in modifying the diet to preserve endogenous protein.

2.6. Calculating the Carbohydrate

To calculate the grams of carbohydrate, you must first have calculated the grams of protein as described in Section 2.5. The next step is to multiply the dietary units (determined in Section 2.3) by the unit in the ratio (which is always 1). The last step is to subtract the grams of protein from this number to achieve the grams of carbohydrate allowed daily. For example,

32.5 dietary units × 1 = 32.5
A 7-yr-old weighing 23 kg requires 22 g of protein:
32.5–22 = 10.5 g of carbohydrate

2.7. Adjusting the Carbohydrate

The carbohydrate value may need to be adjusted to account for nonfood sources of carbohydrate such as medications and supplements. If the sum total of the carbohydrate

Table 4
Sample Ketogenic Diet Prescription for a 7-yr-old Child (1300-kcal, 4:1 diet ratio)

Nutrient	Daily intake (g)	Grams per meal (3 meals/d)
Protein	22	7.3
Fat	130	43.3
Carbohydrate	10.5	3.5

Table 5
Nutrient Values of Selected Foods

Food	Amount (g)	Nutrients (g)		
		Protein	Fat	Carbohydrate
36% Cream	100	2	36	3.7
Raw mixed egg	100	12	12	0
10% Fruit	100	1	0	10
Group B vegetable	100	2	0	7
Soybean oil	100	0	100	0
Butter	100	0.8	81	0
Chicken breast, no skin	100	31.1	3.6	0

content from medications and supplements exceeds 500 mg, the excess amount of carbohydrate should be subtracted from the total dietary carbohydrate allowance. If the carbohydrate from medications and supplements together equal 1 g, the daily carbohydrate should be adjusted as follows. For example,

10.5 g carbohydrate (diet) – 0.5 g (nonfood) = 10.0 g carbohydrate

2.8. The Final Ketogenic Diet Prescription

The final calculations for the daily grams of protein, carbohydrate, and fat should be divided evenly into the number of daily meals as shown in Table 4. The diet is usually divided into three equal meals per day. It is equally effective to divide the values into smaller meals, such as four equal meals per day for a toddler.

3. COLLECTING FOOD COMPOSITION DATA

Food composition information should be collected and updated regularly for accuracy. Converting food value data to amounts per 100 g is necessary to perform the calculations described in these examples. Food labels are not reliable sources for precise nutrient values because manufacturers are not required to reveal nutrient values that are less than 1 g for the serving size listed on the label. The food manufacturer should be contacted to obtain accurate values for processed foods. The US Department of Agriculture maintains a large database of processed and unprocessed foods with detailed macro- and micronutrient information that is available on their website (www.nal.usda.gov/fnic/foodcomp). Table 5 gives some sample values.

The ketogenic diet is based on unprocessed foods such as fresh fruits and vegetables, meats, fish, and poultry, and butter and vegetable oils. Processed foods that are low in carbohydrate may be used in the diet but must be evaluated for precise food composition. Foods should be identified according to the form in which they will be consumed. For example, the nutrient values for cooked chicken breast should be used to calculate a meal, not the values for raw chicken breast.

Fruits and vegetables that are low in carbohydrate are classified into food groups based on similarity in macronutrient composition. The fruit is divided into groups that contain 10 and 15% of their weight in carbohydrate (Appendix 2). Vegetables are divided into those that are lowest in carbohydrate (group A) and those that contain twice this amount of carbohydrate (group B). Fruits and vegetables that are rich in carbohydrate, such as bananas, potatoes, peas, and corn, are omitted from the diet but may be included when liberal ketogenic ratios (e.g., 3:1 or 2:1) are used.

Heavy whipping cream, which is a component of most ketogenic meals, is identified according to butterfat content. Heavy whipping cream is most commonly available with 36% or 40% butterfat. (These percentages are arrived at by dividing the gram weight of fat by the gram weight of the serving size listed on the carton). Creams that contain additives such as polysorbate, dextrose, or other sugars should be avoided.

4. CALCULATING A MEAL

The basic ketogenic diet meals are a combination of four food items: heavy cream, a protein-rich food, a fruit or vegetable, and butter, vegetable oil, or mayonnaise. Specific amounts of these foods are calculated in sequential order starting with the cream, followed by the protein-rich food, the fruit or vegetable, and finally the butter or oil. The following examples demonstrate the calculations of a basic meal using the diet prescription shown in Table 4.

4.1. Calculating Heavy Cream

The cream is generally calculated first. No greater than half of the total meal allotment of carbohydrate should be provided by the cream. Half of the meal allotment of carbohydrate derived from our example is 1.75 g. If 100 g of cream has 3.7 g of carbohydrate, how much cream provides 1.75 g?

Step 1. $100/3.7 = x/1.75$
Step 2. $3.7x = 175$
Step 3. $x = 175/3.7 = 47.3$ rounded down to 45 g of cream for a simplified value that will be used to calculate all of the initial ketogenic meals.
Step 4. Calculate the actual protein, fat and carbohydrate values for 45 g of cream:

45 g of cream × 2 g protein/100 g cream = 0.9 g protein
45 g of cream × 36 g fat/100 g cream = 16.2 g fat
45 g of cream × 3.7 g carbohydrate/100 g cream = 1.7 g carbohydrate

Step 5. Subtract these actual values from the goal values for the meal as shown in Table 6.

4.2. Calculating Protein-Rich Food

The next step is to calculate the quantity of the protein-rich food from the remaining values of protein, fat, and carbohydrate as shown above. If 100 g of chicken breast

Table 6
Calculating the Cream

Nutrient	Protein	Fat	Carbohydrate
Goal values for a ketogenic meal	7.3	43.3	3.5
Subtract calculated values for 45 g of cream	−0.9	−16.2	−1.7
Remaining values	6.4	27.1	1.8

Table 7
Calculating the Protein-Rich Food

Nutrient	Protein (g)	Fat (g)	Carbohydrate (g)
Remaining values from previous calculation	6.4	27.1	1.8
Subtract values for 20 g of chicken breast	−5.9	−0.7	−0
Remaining values	0.5	26.4	1.8

Table 8
Calculating the Carbohydrate Food

Nutrient	Protein (g)	Fat (g)	Carbohydrate (g)
Remaining values from previous calculation	0.5	26.4	1.8
Subtract values for 20 g of group B vegetable	−0.5	−0	−1.8
Remaining value	0	26.4	0

(cooked, without skin) contains 31.1 g of protein, how much chicken breast provides the remaining value of protein calculated in Table 7?

Step 1. $100/31.1 = x/6.4$
Step 2. $31.1x = 640$
Step 3. $x = 20.5$ = rounded down to 19 g (knowing that the vegetable will also contain protein)
Step 4. Calculate the protein, fat, and carbohydrate values for 19 g of chicken breast:
    19 g of chicken × g 31.1 g protein/100 g chicken = 5.9 g protein
    19 g of chicken × 3.6 g fat/100 g chicken = 0.7 g fat
    19 g of chicken × g 0 g carbohydrate/100 g chicken = 0 g carbohydrate
Step 5. Subtract these values from the remaining values of the calculation shown in Table 6.

4.3. Calculating Carbohydrate (Fruit or Vegetable)

The next step is to calculate the quantity of fruit or vegetable that will provide the remaining carbohydrate for this meal. If 100 g of group B vegetable contains 7 g of carbohydrate, how much group B vegetable provides the value of carbohydrate remaining in the meal in Table 8?

Table 9
Calculating the Remaining Fat

Nutrient	Protein (g)	Fat (g)	Carbohydrate (g)
Remaining values from previous calculation	0	26.4	0
Subtract values for 33 g of butter	–0.26	–26.7	–0
Remaining value	–0.26	–0.3	0

Step 1. $100/7 = x/1.8$
Step 2. $7x = 180$
Step 3. $x = 25.7$ g rounded to 25 g of group B vegetable (knowing that the butter will also contain protein)
Step 4. Calculate the protein, fat, and carbohydrate values for 25 g of group B vegetable:
  25 g of group B veg × 2 g protein/100 g group B veg = 0.5 g protein
  25 g of group B veg × 0 g fat/100 g group B veg = 0 g fat
  25 g of group B veg × 7 g carbohydrate/100 g group B veg = 1.8 g carbohydrate
Step 5. Subtract these values from the remaining values of the calculation shown in Table 7.

4.4. Calculating Dietary Fat

The next step is to calculate the quantity of dietary fat that will complete the remaining fat required for this meal. If 100 g of grade A butter contains 81 g of fat, how much butter provides the value of remaining fat in the meal in Table 9?

Step 1. $100/81 = x/26.4$
Step 2. $81x = 2640$
Step 3. $x = 32.6$ g rounded to 33 g of butter
Step 4. Calculate the protein, fat, and carbohydrate values for 33 g of butter:
  33 g of butter × 0.8 g protein/100 g = 0.26 g protein
  33 g of butter × 81 g fat/100 g butter = 26.7 g fat
  33 g of butter × 0 g carbohydrate 100 g butter = 0 g carbohydrate
Step 5. Subtract these values from the remaining values of the calculation shown in Table 8.

4.5. Summarizing the Final Calculations

Upon completion of the calculations of Sections 4.1.–4.4., the final meal can be put together (*see* Table 10). The actual values are compared with the goal values. Check the meal for accuracy by multiplying the actual values by their respective caloric value to arrive at the total kilocalories. The actual meal contains 436 cal (vs the goal of 432 cal). This 1% difference in calories is sufficient for accuracy. Next, check the ratio for accuracy by calculating the actual dietary units of the meal (7.5 protein + 3.5 fat = 11) by the desired ratio (11 × 4 = 44) and compare the actual fat value, which is 43.6. This ratio is within 1% of the desired ratio and is sufficient for accuracy.

Upon completion of these calculations, you will arrive at a mathematically balanced ketogenic meal. Because all meals are mathematically identical, all meals can be used interchangeably within a given diet prescription.

Table 10
Meal Calculation for 1300-calorie, 4:1 Diet (3 meals daily)

Food	Amount (g)	Nutrients (g)		
		Protein	Fat	Carbohydrate
36% Cream	45	0.9	16.2	1.7
Chicken breast (cooked, no skin)	19	5.9	0.7	0
Group B vegetable	16	0.5	0	1.8
Butter	33	0.2	26.7	0
		Values (kcal)		
		Protein	Fat	Carbohydrate
	Actual	7.5	43.6	3.5
	Goal	7.3	43.3	3.5

4.6. Ketogenic Diet Snacks

A "free" snack may be given once daily if needed to help curtail hunger. Snacks include three small black (ripe) olives, one English walnut, two butternuts, one Brazil nut, two macadamia nuts, two pecan halves, or three filberts. These foods are high in fat and low in carbohydrate. It may become necessary to calculate a snack, i.e., 50–100 cal, into the diet if the child is always hungry at a given time each day. The snack must be ketogenically balanced, using the same ratio as the diet prescription. Typical ketogenic snacks include whipped cream with fruit or sugar-free gelatin and frozen eggnog.

4.7. Incorporating Creativity into Ketogenic Diet Meals

Several ketogenic meals should be calculated for each child initially to provide variety. A protein-rich food paired with a fruit or vegetable provides the foundation of the ketogenic meal. Cream, butter, margarine, vegetable oils, and mayonnaise complete the requirement for fat. For variations of the ketogenic meals, families can incorporate combinations of protein-rich foods such as bacon and eggs or small amounts of low-carbohydrate food items such as avocado, nuts, sugar-free gelatin, and cheese.

The child's preferences will largely determine the adjustments that are needed to improve his or her acceptance of the diet. Some children will prefer larger volumes of cream and less butter or vegetable fat. This increase in cream will however reduce the quantity of carbohydrate and protein available for the vegetable or fruit in the meal. Other children may prefer to drink vegetable oil or melted butter and consume less cream.

Creative meals can be designed to provide variety, such as tacos made with an egg-white shell, pizza made with an eggplant crust, and spaghetti squash with a tomato–meat sauce. The heavy cream can be prepared in different ways. It can be whipped and served with fruit, mixed with diet caffeine-free root beer, or thinned down with water to resemble milk. Creative ideas for ketogenic meals often come from caregivers who are eager to make the diet more interesting.

5. CALCULATING AN INFANT OR ENTERAL FORMULA

The ketogenic diet can be prepared in liquid form for bottle-fed infants or children who receive their nutrition enterally. The diet is calculated in the same fashion as

Table 11
Holiday–Segar Method for Determining Maintenance
Fluid Needs

Body weight	Water (mL/kg/d)
First 10 kg	100
Second 10 kg	50
Each additional kilogram	20

described for the oral diet except that it is calculated as one daily recipe (rather than in individual meals). Combinations of enteral and oral diets can be also be prepared. The following are examples of different types of ketogenic formulas.

- KetoCal™ (Scientific Hospital Supplies). This product comes in powder form and requires mixing with water. It is formulated at a 4:1 ratio, but the ratio can be adjusted with the addition of carbohydrate. It is fortified with vitamins and minerals. KetoCal can be used for enteral or oral consumption.
- RCF™ (Ross Pharmaceuticals). This is a carbohydrate-free formula concentrate that requires mixing with water plus fat and carbohydrate modulars to achieve the desired ratio. Although originally designed for infants, it can be utilized for older children with additional vitamin and mineral supplementation. RCF is very low in sodium.
- Blenderized formula. This can be achieved by blenderizing together foods such as commercial baby foods, water, and vegetable oil or Microlipid™ to achieve the desired ratio. Vitamin and mineral supplementation is required.

6. CALCULATING FLUID

Adequate fluid intake is necessary to maintain normal hydration during ketogenic diet therapy. Insufficient fluids can increase the risk for kidney stones and constipation. The ketogenic diet restricts fluids to noncaloric, caffeine-free beverages such as water, decaffeinated weak tea, and noncaloric caffeine-free soda. Fluid should be calculated for the maintenance needs of the individual. The Holiday–Segar Method is a fluid calculation that is based on weight alone (6) (Table 11). This formula does not account for abnormal fluid losses, for example, from excessive drooling or febrile illness. For example, a child weighing 23 kg needs 1000 mL (for first 10 kg) plus 500 (10 kg × 50 mL/kg) plus 60 mL (3 kg × 20 mL/kg) for a total of 1560 mL daily. This can be divided into six servings of 250 mL as a simple daily guide for the caregiver to manage. The child should not be allowed to drink large volumes of fluid at one time because this may upset internal fluid balance and ketosis. The caregiver should also be instructed to allow additional fluids during periods of illness or exposure to warm weather.

7. SUPPLEMENTING THE KETOGENIC DIET: VITAMINS, MINERALS, AND ESSENTIAL FATTY ACIDS

The ketogenic diet is deficient in several vitamins and minerals owing to its high fat component and consequently low volume of carbohydrate- and protein-rich foods. The restriction of these foods limits the intake of many vitamins and minerals particularly B vitamins, vitamin D, calcium, phosphorus, potassium, iron, selenium, magnesium, and zinc *(7,8)*. A computerized nutrient analysis of an individual's ketogenic diet selections over an extended period is helpful to identify the actual micronutrients absent from the diet.

Vitamin and mineral supplementation is essential for all ketogenic diet candidates in efforts to provide optimal nutrition and to prevent micronutrient deficiencies. Supplements should be in sugar-free form. The Recommended Dietary Intakes published by the Food and Nutrition Board (2002) provide a guide for daily level of intakes of vitamins, minerals, and trace minerals based on age *(5)*. A typical supplementation profile for a child on the oral ketogenic diet includes a multivitamin with minerals supplement plus a calcium and a phosphorus and potassium supplement. A multivitamin-with-minerals supplement and individual mineral supplements should be given to the child at separate times throughout the day for optimal absorption.

The ketogenic diet can be low in essential fatty acids if animal sources of the fatty and protein-rich foods are the only sources of fat in the diet. Fresh or canned tuna, salmon, sardines, and herring are good sources of essential fatty acids. Vegetable oils such as walnut and soybean oils and mayonnaise (made with soybean oil) are also excellent sources and can easily be incorporated into the ketogenic diet. The DRI of essential fatty acids ranges between 4.4 and 17 g daily, based on age *(5)*.

8. INITIATION OF THE KETOGENIC DIET

During the initiation of the diet, the child is at risk for hypoglycemia, dehydration, acidosis, and antiepileptic drug toxicity. Therefore, initiation is recommended in a hospital setting under the guidance of the ketogenic diet team. Initiation of the diet has been managed in the home setting when 24-h nursing care is present. Methods of ketogenic diet initiation vary among medical centers, from fasting prior to initiating the diet to initiating the diet without any fasting period at all. Initiating the diet gradually (with or without a fast) is the usual practice among medical centers.

8.1. Initiating the Oral Ketogenic Diet

The process of initiating the diet gradually is usually achieved by providing one-third of the ketogenic diet (calories) on the first day, two-thirds of the ketogenic diet on the second day, and the full ketogenic diet on the third and subsequent days. The deprivation of calories incurred by this stepwise increment in calories stimulates hunger and encourages the child to consume all the diet. Ketogenic eggnog, a combination of heavy cream and pasteurized raw eggs, is often used for the first 2 d of this method because it is a ketogenically balanced liquid that is easily prepared and accepted favorably by most children. It can be sweetened with saccharine to the child's liking and flavored with vanilla extract and consumed in small portions throughout the day. For variation, the eggnog can be cooked to a custard consistency or frozen like ice cream.

8.2. Initiating the Infant or Enteral Ketogenic Diet

Children with enteral feeding tubes and bottle-fed infants can be safely acclimated to the ketogenic diet with a gradual transition from the home formula to the ketogenic diet formula by combining the two formulas in a systematic fashion. Two-thirds of the home formula can be mixed with one-third of the ketogenic formula for the first day of the diet initiation, then gradually increased by thirds each day while reducing the home formula by equal volume, until the third day, when full ketogenic formula is reached. This transition method allows a gentle adjustment to the ketogenic formula and serves to stimulate ketosis in a nonfasting manner.

8.3. Monitoring Complications

During ketogenic diet initiation children are routinely monitored for complications that may arise. Blood glucose levels are checked every 2 h for infants and 4 h for children over the age of one year then reduced to every 4–6 h, respectively, once a child is stable and the diet is being well tolerated. Symptoms of hypoglycemia include dizziness, fatigue, and nausea. If the blood glucose level drops below 50 mg/dL, the child is treated with 15–30 cc of apple juice and rechecked in 30–60 min. If the child is unable or refuses to consume the juice orally or enterally, an iv bolus of glucose (0.25 g/kg) may be given. Theoretically, children who are very active, very young, or very thin have minimal glycogen stores and thus become hypoglycemic more easily than children who are at or above their ideal weight or who are inactive. Untreated hypoglycemia may result in excessive ketosis.

Ketosis is measured with urine test strips upon each urine void that the child produces. Ketone levels usually appear in the urine when glucose levels fall below 70 mg/dL. If the child is monitored appropriately for hypoglycemia, it is unlikely that excessive ketosis will occur (unless there is an underlying metabolic disorder). Symptoms of excessive ketosis include lethargy, nausea, vomiting, and rapid shallow breathing (Kussmaul respirations). The condition can progress to coma and even death if untreated. Excessive ketosis can be remedied with glucose administration as described in the paragraph above. The caregiver needs to be instructed on how to remedy hypoglycemia and excessive ketosis, should these symptoms develop at home.

During ketogenic diet initiation it is important to monitor the hydration status of the individual. A urine specific gravity test performed at bedside can quickly determine urine concentration. A fluid "schedule" should be outlined with reasonable quantities of calorie-free, caffeine-free fluids to be consumed daily based on the child's maintenance fluid goals. If the child is unable to meet these goals and the urine specific gravity is overconcentrated, i.e., >1.020 on a Bayer Multistix 10SG, a bolus of iv fluids without dextrose should be given. Continuous intravenous administration may discourage the child from drinking fluids and should be avoided.

The child's vital signs should be checked every 8 h during ketogenic diet initiation, until they are stable and the child is tolerating the full diet. The child's weight should be measured daily in the hospital and weekly at home. Children often experience weight loss during the initial stages of the diet as a result of the diets diuretic effect. However, the weight should stabilize and return to baseline in a few weeks.

9. KETOGENIC DIET EDUCATION

While the child is becoming acclimated to the ketogenic diet, the dietitian and the nurse can begin to train the caregiver on the management of the ketogenic diet at home.

9.1. Diet Preparation

The family can be taught to manage the fluid schedule that will be continued for home use. Ketogenic diet food weighing can be taught on the day after admission so that the parents can prepare the meals that are consumed in the hospital and for the first few meals at home. Access to a small kitchen on or near the inpatient unit is ideal for accommodating this process. Simple ketogenic meals should be taught initially to minimize food preparation and to facilitate learning. Ketogenic diet education should also include a session on appropriate vitamin and mineral supplementation and a list of carbohydrate-free health care products such as toothpastes, pain relievers, and cold remedies.

9.2. Constipation

Guidelines for constipation management should be discussed with the caregiver, with the emphasis focused on prevention. Adequate fluid intake and the inclusion of vegetables into daily meals may be enough to prevent constipation for many children. Adding up to 25 g of iceberg lettuce as a "free food" to the diet may also help. Calculating 10–20 g of avocado into a meal for daily consumption may also promote regularity. Some children will need further dietary manipulation such as the calculation of medium-chain triglycerides (MCT) oil into meals. Pharmacologic intervention with a carbohydrate-free stool softener may also help to prevent constipation.

Constipation may be treated with use of carbohydrate-free laxatives such as Milk of Magnesia™, a glycerin suppository, or an enema. In children on the ketogenic diet, a bowel movement should be expected every 2–4 d, and treatment should be instituted otherwise.

9.3. Sick Days

The caregiver must also receive counseling on management of intercurrent illnesses ("sick days"). If the child is vomiting or has diarrhea, ketogenic meals should be temporarily stopped and the emphasis should be on maintaining hydration with fluids. Diluted broth, noncaloric caffeine-free soda and sugar-free gelatin can be offered. If vomiting and/or diarrhea persists, an oral rehydration solution may be given at half-strength. Easy-to-digest ketogenic meals such as ketogenic eggnog or chicken salad with applesauce can be restarted in half portions when the child is ready to begin eating. The signs and symptoms of hypoglycemia and excessive ketosis should be taught during the hospitalization, and the method of treatment should be outlined for home use. A visit to the pediatrician or emergency room may be necessary if symptoms persist after treatment. Caregivers should be assured that these problems are unlikely to occur once the child has begun to consume the full diet. Close contact with the ketogenic diet team will also help the caregiver to feel comfortable managing illnesses.

9.4. Hunger Behavior

Caregivers often feel that they are "starving their child" because of the limited volume of food that the diet provides. Some children will become upset that they are not allowed additional servings of food when their meal is completed. The caregiver should be taught to maximize the quantity of foods by using the higher volume vegetables (group A) and fruit (10% fruit). A small spatula should be used at each meal to ensure that every morsel of fat and cream (which tends to adhere to dishes) is consumed. A free-food snack can be provided daily to lessen hunger between meals. Chewing on ice chips or drinking allowed fluids may also delay appetite. Feeding the child his or her meals at evenly spaced intervals throughout the day will assist with hunger management. If hunger behavior persists, the caregiver should discern between true hunger and manipulative behavior. One approach is to remove the child from the eating area as soon as he or she completes a meal and offer the distraction of other activities. The ketosis effect of the diet suppresses appetite, and children usually adapt to the smaller quantity of food without difficulty. If true hunger persists, a ketogenic snack can be calculated by the dietitian. The dietitian can also reevaluate the child's energy needs and increase the diet accordingly.

10. KETOGENIC DIET THERAPY FOLLOW-UP PROGRAM

Management of the ketogenic diet is best achieved through phone calls and regularly scheduled follow-up appointments with the ketogenic diet team. Phone calls at least weekly with the dietitian during the early weeks of this therapy are vital to the success of this therapy. A 1-mo visit after ketogenic diet initiation followed by a visit every 3 mo is commonly practiced. At each visit the child's seizures, growth, and neurological and nutritional status are evaluated. The initial laboratory studies are repeated at each visit to monitor metabolic responses. Caregivers are asked to keep a journal of seizure activity and ketone readings to facilitate objective decisions regarding therapy adjustments.

10.1. Fine-Tuning the Ketogenic Diet

The goal of ketogenic diet therapy is to find and maintain a state of ketosis that serves to abate seizures. After a few weeks of ketogenic diet therapy, a defining pattern of ketosis will emerge. Ketosis is monitored at home by the caregiver with a urine ketone testing kit. Ketosis is usually lower in the morning and higher in the afternoon and evening. Urine ketone levels are a crude estimate of serum ketone levels and can be sufficient for determining level of ketosis on a daily basis. β-Hydroxybutryate is the serum ketone that is thought to impact seizure control and can be measured quantitatively by blood analysis. A β-hydroxybutryate level may be helpful when attempts to fine-tune the diet by means of urine ketone levels are inadequate. Diet manipulation can alter ketosis and effect seizure control. Several factors should be considered before deciding how to adjust the ketogenic diet. The initial goal is to ensure that 100% of the ketogenic diet is being consumed. This may take a few weeks for children who are learning to adjust to this high-fat regimen. Offering new and creative meals may improve diet acceptance. Once the child has adjusted to the diet, is consistently eating all the foods, and has been taking the required supplements and fluids for at least a month, it is time to evaluate the history of ketosis. Urine ketones should be at least moderate to large or large consistently. If ketosis is below these levels, a dietary adjustment may be warranted. There are exceptions to this rule, however, and certain children will achieve excellent seizure control with lower ketosis. Also, some children may become too ketotic and require lower ratios.

Fine-tuning the diet should be discussed with the ketogenic diet team. It is important to make only one change at a time to ascertain the effect of each change. Each diet or medication change should be tried for at least 6 wk prior to initiating a new change. As the team develops experience in managing children successfully on the ketogenic diet, these decisions will become second nature.

Breakthrough seizure activity after a period of control can be triggered by many factors. If the cause of the breakthrough can be determined and remedied, there may be no need to make any changes. Possible causes of a temporary breakthrough in seizures may include the stressors that have triggered the child's seizures in the past, such as sleep deprivation or illness. Seizures may result from disruptions in the ketogenic diet such as a mistake made in the preparation or weighing of the food, eating or drinking the wrong brand of food, or the introduction of a new medication (even if it is carbohydrate free).

Fine-tuning of the ketogenic diet should be pursued if the seizure breakthrough persists. The following diet adjustments may improve seizure control:

- Recalculate the diet with specific fruits and vegetables instead of using the exchange groups.
- Adjust the carbohydrate content of the diet to account for the carbohydrate supplied by medications and or supplements.
- Reassess energy needs and recalculate the diet accordingly; i.e., reduce the diet by 50 or 100 kcal to effect stronger ketosis.
- Increase the ratio by half-step increments to effect stronger ketosis.
- Introduce MCT oil into the diet in substitution for some of the fat to effect stronger ketosis.
- Assess carnitine status and supplement if low.
- Redistribute calories to provide a meal or snack before bedtime.

11. DECIDING TO TERMINATE KETOGENIC DIET THERAPY

If there is no improvement in seizure control after 2–3 mo of ketogenic diet therapy, the diet should be discontinued. Reasons for early termination of the diet may include the following:

- The individual refuses to comply with the diet despite multiple attempts to provide acceptable meals in a positive atmosphere.
- Seizures worsen.
- Caregivers find the diet too difficult and want to discontinue it.
- The patient experiences an adverse effect of the diet that cannot be corrected without discontinuation of the diet.

11.1. Early Termination

The process for early termination of the diet is individualized and may be done gradually over a week or longer. The following are suggestions for tapering the diet.

- Reduce the ratio every 3 d: i.e., if on a 4:1 diet, use a 3:1 diet for 3 d, then a 2:1 diet for 3 d, then add a small portion of carbohydrate-rich food into each meal for 3 d, increasing daily until child is out of ketosis.
- Reduce the ratio by doubling the carbohydrate portion of the meal, i.e., fruit or vegetable. Then after 2–3 d, introduce a small carbohydrate-rich food with each meal such as rice, potatoes, peas, pasta, pudding, or milk, while at the same time reducing the cream by half.

11.2. Tapering the Diet After Successful Therapy

Tapering of the ketogenic diet should occur after 1–2 yr of successful seizure control. Reduction in the ratio is used to gradually reduce ketosis and taper off the diet. Ketone levels should be checked after each reduction in the ketogenic diet ratio. Children usually remain on the 4:1 ratio (or the ratio that has enabled them to produce large ketones consistently) for up to 2 yr. The ratio can be gradually tapered to 3:1 for 6 mo then 2:1 for another 6 mo. Carbohydrate can be gradually added to the diet in the form of bread, pasta, rice, cereal, crackers, and dairy products to eliminate the remaining ketosis. Milk may not be tolerated initially because after a long period on the ketogenic diet, there may be no lactase stimulation in the gut.

11.3. Deciding Not to Terminate

Some families may request to continue ketogenic diet therapy because of the marked improvement in their child's quality of life, which they fear will be lost if the diet is terminated. Continued surveillance of these children is necessary to ensure safety in continued therapy. Lowering the ratio to 3:1 or 2:1 can improve the nutritional quality of the diet and reduce possible adverse effects.

12. CONCLUSION

Ketogenic diet therapy is a unique therapy that requires the expertise of a mutltidisciplinary medical team. The expertise of the dietitian is an essential part of the ketogenic diet team. The dietitian writes diet prescriptions, calculates meal plans, determines nutritional supplementation, and provides the majority of education to the family during ketogenic diet therapy. The dietitian also tracks growth and laboratory data relevant to nutritional status and diet therapy. A successful ketogenic diet program allows for the allocation of time and resources to this endeavor.

REFERENCES

1. Mandel A, Ballew M, Pina-Garza J, Stalmasek V, Eck Clements L. Medical costs are reduced in children with severe epilepsy who are successfully maintained on a ketogenic diet. Future Dimens Clin Nutr Manage 1998;17:12–13.
2. Wheless JW. The ketogenic diet: An effective medical therapy with side effects. J Child Neurol 2001;16:633–635.
3. Zupec-Kania BA. Summary of ketogenic diet survey of practitioners. Building Block for Life (a publication of the Pediatric Nutrition Practice Group) 2001;24:12–14.
4. Cassilly Casey J, McGrogan J, Pillas D, Pyzik P, Freeman J, Vining EP. The Implementation and maintenance of the ketogenic diet in children. J Neurosci Nurs 1999;31:294–302.
5. Food and Nutrition Board. Dietary Reference Intakes for Energy, Carbohydrate, Fiber, Fat, Fatty Acids, Cholesterol, Protein and Amino Acids (Macronutrients). Institute of Medicine, Washington DC, 2002, pp. 335–432, 465–608.
6. Johns Hopkins Hospital. The Harriet Lane Handbook; A Manual for Pediatric House Officers, 14th ed. Mosby-Year Book, Chicago, 1997, pp. 216–217.
7. Ballaban-Gil K, Callahan C,O'Dell C, Pappo M, Moshe S, Shinnar S. Complications of the ketogenic diet. Epilepsia 1998;39:744–748.
8. Bettler MA. Vitamin and mineral deficiencies related to the ketogenic diet. Building Block for Life (a Publication of the Pediatric Nutrition Practice Group) 2001;24:5–9
9. Johns Hopkins Hospital, Ketogenic Meal Plan Guide. Ketogenic Diet Conference Manual. Baltimore, MD, 2002.

Appendix 1
Pre-Ketogenic Diet Intake

Name:_____ Date of birth:_____ M F

Weight:_____ Height:_____ Head circumference_____ Date measurements taken:_____

Has there been any recent change in weight? If yes, please explain:_____

_____

Current medicines:
      Name   Dose   Dose time   Manufacturer

_____   _____   _____   _____

_____   _____   _____   _____

_____   _____   _____   _____

_____   _____   _____   _____

Current vitamins/nutritional supplements:
      Name   Dose   Dose time   Manufacturer

_____   _____   _____   _____

_____   _____   _____   _____

Bowel habits: ____Normal ____Constipation ____Loose stools

Activity level: (please describe):_____

_____

Seizure type and frequency: _____

_____

Previous seizure
medicines: _____

Family history: ____Heart disease or stroke ____High lipids ____Kidney stones

Food allergies:_____ Food intolerances:_____

Chewing difficulties:_____ Swallowing difficulties:_____

Feeding route: ____Oral ____Feeding tube ____Both oral and feeding tube

Religious or cultural dietary restrictions: _____

Appendix 2
Ketogenic Diet Fruit and Vegetable Lists*

Fruit or Juice: Fresh, Frozen or Canned Without Sugar (Do Not Use Dried Fruit)

10% (use amount prescribed)	15% (use 2/3 the amount of 10% fruit)
Applesauce (unsweetened)	Apple
Apricot	Blueberries
Blackberries	Figs
Cantaloupe	Grapes-green-purple-red
Grapefruit	Mango
Guava	Pear
Honeydew melon	Pineapple
Nectarine	Plums—Damson
Orange	Kiwi
Papaya	
Peach	
Raspberries	
Strawberries	
Tangerine	
Watermelon	

Vegetables: Fresh, Canned, or Frozen; Measure Raw (R) or Cooked (C) as Specified

Group A (use twice amount of group B)		Group B (use amount prescribed)	
Asparagus–C	Radish–R	Beets–C	Kohlrabi–C
Beet greens–C	Rhubarb–R	Broccoli–C	Mushroom–R
Cabbage–C	Sauerkraut–C	Brussels sprouts–C	Mustard greens–C
Celery–C/R	Scallion–R	Cabbage–R	Okra–C
Chicory–R	Summer squash–C	Carrots–R/C	Onion–R/C
Cucumbers–R	Swiss chard–C	Cauliflower–C	Rutabaga–C
Eggplant–C	Tomato–R	Collards–C	Spinach–C
Endive–R	Turnips–C	Dandelion greens–C	Tomato–C
Green pepper–R/C	Turnip greens–C	Green beans–C	Wintersquash–C
Poke–C	Watercress–R	Kale–C	

*From ref. *10*.

5 How to Maintain and Support a Ketogenic Diet Program

A Nursing Perspective

*Jeri E. Nichols Sutherling
and Danine Mele-Hayes*

1. INTRODUCTION

This chapter describes the experience of one center (Epilepsy and Brain Mapping Program, Pasadena, CA) in starting and maintaining a ketogenic diet (KD) program. We hope that our experience will be useful to other centers contemplating starting a KD program.

Our program began in 1993, when our medical director, primary nurse, and dietitian visited the Pediatric Epilepsy Center at Johns Hopkins Hospital in Baltimore, for training in the KD. Representatives from several other centers from across the United States and Canada participated in the training sessions. In addition to group teaching, we had private teaching sessions with Millicent Kelly, R.D., one of the most experienced dietitian with expertise in the KD. These private sessions allowed us to pose specific questions about the KD. Upon our return to California, it took another 6 mo to set up KD protocols, train hospital and clinic staff, and begin administering the KD.

The diet was implemented in the hospital for all patients at that time, and we adhered strictly to Johns Hopkins protocol. Patients were fasted and stayed 4–5 d in the hospital. The parents were trained in the diet while the child was admitted for initiation of the diet. With time and experience, we have revised some of the initial protocols. We have always operated under the assumption that there are many ways to achieve the same goal with the diet.

One notable improvement has been the perception of the KD within the community. When we first started putting children on the diet, we had numerous calls from emergency room (ER) doctors reporting mothers who were abusing their children by starving them and giving them high fat. Those physicians were reassured that the diet indeed had a medical rationale and actually helped to control seizures. This lack of awareness about the KD, even among medical professionals, has largely abated at this point.

We believe that the KD is extremely beneficial for many patients if formulated and administered properly. Our outcome data support this belief. Long-term results of the

From: *Epilepsy and the Ketogenic Diet*
Edited by: C. E. Stafstrom and J. M. Rho © Humana Press Inc., Totowa, NJ

KD in our center showed that as of 2000, 63% of the patients were seizure free or had 90% reduction in seizures, and 88% had at least 50% seizure reduction *(1)*. These results are even more impressive when it is noted that most of the patients had medically intractable epilepsy.

2. PREPARATION FOR THE DIET

2.1. Candidacy for the KD

The KD is an elective procedure and is not used in emergencies. Our standard criteria are medically intractable seizures in a patient who has failed two first-line anticonvulsant drugs. We sometimes accept patients with medication toxicity. Seizure frequency must be 1–2 seizures per week to establish a pattern to assess KD efficacy.

Exceptions to the foregoing criteria have occurred. A family in which four of five children had the same epilepsy syndrome was allowed to put the remaining three epileptic children on the KD after the eldest became seizure free immediately after starting the diet. All the children had excellent results and have been seizure free since beginning the diet. All but the eldest are now off the diet and remain seizure free and medication free. We require a recent video electroencephalography (VEEG) inpatient telemetry study to rule out nonepileptic seizures in adults or older children. One 12-yr-old child was being considered for the diet but was found to have nonepileptic seizures. This emphasizes the importance of an accurate epilepsy diagnosis before starting the KD. Because most of our patients are young children, in whom nonepileptic seizures are of less concern, an outpatient EEG or VEEG is usually sufficient.

2.2. Screening

Each patient has a complete history and physical examination, and an extensive 1-h evaluation with the epilepsy nurse. The nurse explains the rigors of the diet and explores family background to determine which family members will primarily oversee the diet's preparation and administration. The family also has a consultation with the dietitian, who assesses the patient's nutritional status, eating habits, allergies, and other dietary concerns.

We inquire about a family history of hyperlipidemia, hypercholesteremia, and renal stones, as well as the child's seizure type(s) and frequency and his or her epilepsy syndrome. Laboratory studies include a comprehensive metabolic panel (liver function tests, albumin, CO_2), complete blood count, fasting lipid panel, serum pyruvate and lactate, magnesium, zinc, ammonia, uric acid, free and total carnitine, selenium, serum ketone levels, anticonvulsant levels, and a urinalysis. Computed tomographic or magnetic resonance images of the head are obtained if recent images are not available.

If the patient is on a carbonic anhydrase inhibitor, e.g., acetazolamide or topiramate, it is discontinued before diet initiation, to reduce the risks of severe serum bicarbonate deficits and acidosis. Such metabolic derangements could potentially become life threatening if status epilepticus occurred. We also check key blood test results one week after initiation of the diet to identify any unanticipated side effects. The initial and follow-up laboratory studies (with standing orders as appropriate) should be developed by the neurologist in conjunction with the dietitian.

2.3. Developing Protocols for Office and Hospital

A questionnaire for prospective patients should be developed, detailing the patient's medical and dietary history. When a patient is referred, the family is contacted by our nurse, who obtains a brief history. A "keto packet" is then sent to the family, which provides detailed information about the diet, the medical questionnaire, and a chronology of the events that will take place as the child is evaluated for the KD.

First and foremost, we expect the family to obtain and read Dr. John Freeman's book, *The Ketogenic Diet: A Treatment for Epilepsy (2)*. We feel that it is crucial for the family to take the initiative to locate and purchase the book themselves, to demonstrate their willingness to become involved in the KD process. Because so much training and energy is devoted to KD patients, we want to ensure parental commitment. When we receive the completed packet, the child goes on our "start list." It is the parents' responsibility to follow the steps and have the checklist completed before KD training begins (*see* Appendix 1 of this chapter).

2.4. Training of Nursing and Dietary Hospital Staff

It is essential that nursing and dietary staff who will be involved in the care of pediatric patients be trained fully. We provide extensive in-service teaching for nurses and dietary personnel to ensure that there is consistency in provision of the KD and care of the hospitalized children. Some of the instruction is a modified version of the parent teaching. Nursing staff is instructed in the basic principles of the KD, with emphasis on early metabolic issues during fasting and KD initiation. For the dietary staff, a 1- to 2-h class is given by our KD dietitian on basic principles, weighing techniques, and diet preparation.

2.5. Developing a Training Manual for Parents and Nursing Staff

Because we have found that similar questions arise repeatedly in our training classes, we developed our own handbook for staff and families. This manual describes the KD and includes the goals and course outline for each teaching session, authorization forms (mentioning possible complications and risks) for families to sign, and information on the purpose and background of the KD, dietary tips, the most common mistakes, how to get through the first month, how to use other medications concurrently, how to calibrate and troubleshoot the scale, 3-d food logs, fluid schedules, how to keep a home checklist of intake, and how to document concerns and problems. We instruct the family to always take the manual with them when traveling and to medical and dental appointments (*see* Appendix 2 of this chapter).

We have also found the manual to be helpful for physicians who are not familiar with the KD. It lists medications that can be used in conjunction with the KD and the carbohydrate content of each.

2.6. Training of Emergency Room Staff, School Personnel, Physicians, and Social Workers

It is vital that everyone who will be involved with the patient's care be educated about the diet at the start of a KD program. The hospital ER staff should receive in-service training on how to deal with common emergency problems. It is especially important for them to know about appropriate intravenous solutions and that dextrose-containing solutions should be avoided unless absolutely necessary. Elixirs of common medications should be avoided because of their high carbohydrate content. Most important, emergency personnel must understand that in an emergency situation, maintaining the diet becomes secondary to the child's urgent health needs. The parents must also understand this priority.

We also try to prepare a child's siblings, school, and classmates when appropriate. This effort pays off in key aspects of compliance with the diet. We have a parent make up a sample of the food "desserts" and take it into the child's classroom for everyone to try. This "treat" can provide the basis for a brief in-service session for teachers, the school nurse, and other school personnel. We have found that most children are very understanding and become diligent in helping to "patrol" the child who is on the diet. Ordinarily, both teachers and classmates are dedicated to helping the patient comply with the diet and monitor for seizures.

Another useful tool is the Charlie Foundation's videotape *Introduction to the Ketogenic Diet*. Teachers and school personnel have found this video to be very informative about the KD and the challenges facing a child on the KD. In teaching about the KD, we are also educating the community about epilepsy in general.

We require our patients' parents to have a referral from their primary physician. In our institution, the child must have a private physician who is willing to work with us and with the diet. Because many of our patients come from out of state and even from other countries, it is mandatory that a physician with familiarity with the diet be available to evaluate the child, should an acute situation arise. We also send our information packet to the local physician, providing the contact information for our physician, nurse, and dietitian. It is critical that a member of the KD team be available 24 h a day.

2.7. The Dietitian's Role

The most important member of our ketogenic diet team is the dietitian. Our dietitian is employed by our Epilepsy Center, a private clinic, rather than by the hospital, thereby assuring that she does not have conflicting responsibilities. Other centers need to utilize dietitians whose duties are shared by other clinics and by inpatient units. Based on the dietitian's workload, we have found that we can initiate and follow a maximum of one to three patients per month, also dependent on the needs of the patient and the abilities of the caregivers.

Because our dietitian works part time, we allow flexibility in her schedule. This flexibility permits her to initiate and teach new patients and to manage problems with established patients. Her extensive experience (she has been with us since the beginning of the KD program) has proven to be an invaluable asset to continuity of patient care.

Once a new patient has been seen by the dietitian, he or she is put on the initiation schedule. The dietitian then confers with the pediatric neurologist and nurse to establish when the child will be started on the KD, details of diet initiation, and follow-up plans. The dietitian must analyze the child's diet history and dietary needs, review with family the checklist for preparing the home, develop the meal plans with the food preferences and dislikes of the patient in mind, educate the patient and family, fine-tune the diet, review 3-d logs, and perform product analyses. She prepares reports and letters of explanation to schools, physicians, and insurance companies, consults by telephone with pharmacists, nurse coordinators, pediatricians, and neurologists, and attends team conferences to discuss the patient's plan of care. After the initial period of the diet, most of the workload involves recalculation or changing of meal plans. Many of our families have access to fax machines or e-mail and prefer to communicate with our dietitian by these means, which is convenient for everyone.

2.8. Fine-Tuning the KD

A feature of our program of which we are particularly proud is our "fine-tuning" of the diet. Our dietitian or nurse maintains daily telephone contact with each patient's family during the first month, then as needed until the patient is stable and doing well on the diet. This close follow-up is essential for several reasons.

First, many questions arise despite our intensive training program. These questions are addressed as they occur, before they can cause problems and reduce the ketosis. Common topics include fussy eating habits, constipation, and nausea.

Second, it is not trivial to locate all the items in a meal plan. Recently the US Food and Drug Administration ruled that carbohydrates (CHOs) need to be listed on food packaging only if they comprise 1 g or more per serving. This allows manufacturers to label many products that contain a small amount of CHO as "carbohydrate free." Also, many products are labeled incorrectly. Thus when a specific product is purchased that is outside our experience, it is essential that the dietitian or caregiver call the manufacturer to get the exact product specifications.

Third, during any exacerbation of seizures, usually owing to a concurrent infection or fever, a visit to the ER or primary physician is essential. If the patient is prescribed a medication with a significant amount of CHO in the delivery vehicle, the diet's balance can be altered. This is especially problematic with elixir medications, which we try to avoid if possible. Most health-care workers are unaware of the complexities of the KD and may inadvertently prescribe such medications or even give the child D5W intravenously, rapidly reversing ketosis and hurtling the child into status epilepticus.

Fourth, daily monitoring of ketosis is essential. Once the diet has been established, the dietitian sees the patient in clinic at least every 3 mo for the first year. Many centers are monitoring β-hydroxybutyrate levels to assure ketosis.

Fifth, even with snacks, some patients may have trouble complying with the strictness of the diet. Palatability is a key issue. With the advances in nutritional science, it is becoming easier to develop more creative meal plans.

The nurse and dietitian communicate often, even daily, to ensure patient safety, especially during the first month of the diet and during intermittent illnesses. The number of professional hours spent on each patient on the KD is estimated as 60–80 h/yr.

2.9. The Nurse's Role

It is the nurse's responsibility to work closely with the dietitian and the ketogenic diet physicians. It is the nurse who must schedule the routine labs and make sure that the results are seen by the physician. When a patient is having a difficulty that arises from the KD, the nurse will troubleshoot with the family to determine whether the problem is dietary or medical. Often the nurse will contact the patient's primary physician or dentist to coordinate care.

If the patient is undergoing a surgical or dental procedure, it is the nurse's responsibility to make sure that everyone on the team is aware. If the patient is having surgery, a copy of our Ketogenic Diet Surgery Protocol is given to the surgeon so that he or she is aware of the diet and the precautions to be taken (*see* Appendix 3 of this chapter). Our physician is always available for questions.

Finally, the nurse serves as the coordinator and liaison for any clinical research project in which a patient may be involved.

2.10. The Pharmacist's Role

It is important to work with a pharmacist who understands the KD and is willing to assist with its management. We have identified pharmacies in several states that are used by ketogenic diet centers and are willing to formulate medications according to prescribed criteria that are compatible with the KD. These pharmacies will often ship medications by express mail, and the patient will have the medication within 24–48 h.

2.11. Outpatient or Inpatient Initiation of the Diet

There has been much discussion lately about whether it is safe to initiate the diet outside the hospital setting. Our feeling is that in certain circumstances it is possible and safe, and we have begun several patients on the KD as outpatients. Sometimes an insurance company will not cover the KD even when deemed medically indicated. If the patient has responsible caregivers, no medical contraindication, no history of status epilepticus, and is at least 8 yr old, we consider initiation of the KD on an outpatient basis. In such a situation, the physician, nurse, and dietitian are available around the clock for the first few nights to take calls from the family. Typically, the patient is fed enterally or has been on the diet before.

The outpatient initiation of the diet is gradual, starting at a very low ratio and increasing over several weeks. The parents are provided with a glucometer, trained to obtain finger-stick blood sugars, and educated about the symptoms of hypoglycemia and how to treat it. Children who are fed by gastrostomy tube are much easier to begin as outpatients because the parents can make sure the fluid intake is sufficient, and the child cannot refuse the diet.

2.12. Hyperlipidemia

We require outpatient lab tests to ensure that there is no electrolyte imbalance or hyperlipidemia during the first few days of the diet. We had one documented case of hyperlipidemia after initiating the KD. The patient, a 3-yr-old boy, had presented with medically intractable mixed seizures, including at least four generalized tonic–clonic seizures per week. He had failed five antiepileptic drugs (AEDs). He was evaluated extensively for a metabolic disorder prior to KD initiation; all laboratory screening was normal. He was started on the diet in hospital, became ketotic, and experienced a reduction in seizures. The results of his blood studies were normal on discharge from the hospital. According to our standard protocol, daily follow-up phone calls occurred between the mother and the dietitian. On d 4, in the routine daily phone call, the mother noted that the child was a little bit more sleepy than usual. On d 5 the mother said he was still sleepy and a bit fussier with his diet. These symptoms continued the following day. As a result of the consistent and documented daily change in mental status without medical improvement and because of the high index of suspicion attaching to any significant changes in a patient's mental status, the dietitian (after conferring with our physician) instructed the mother to take her child to the emergency room for evaluation and a panel of routine blood studies. The patient's private neurologist stated that "his blood drawn in the ER looked like a strawberry daiquiri, his triglycerides are 19,000…" The ketogenic diet was terminated. The child's triglycerides returned to normal, and he suffered no ill effects. Because we follow these children so closely, the boy's hyperlipidema was detected quickly.

This case of a hyperlipidemic 3-yr-old demonstrates dramatically the problems that can occur if the KD is not monitored closely. Pancreatitis can occur with triglycerides of 2000, and ischemia could have occurred in the range attained by this patient . Further delay in the child's evaluation could have resulted in irreversible neurological damage. The high index of suspicion, daily phone calls, and close follow-up all helped to detect a serious problem early.

This example highlights the serious nature of the ketogenic diet: it is not holistic therapy or a natural homeopathic remedy, but a most powerful medical treatment for intractable epilepsy that markedly affects the body's metabolic regulation. We must monitor for potential complications closely.

Because children are especially labile when they become sick and cannot always convey that they are not feeling well, we prefer to initiate the diet in the hospital and almost always do this. Another important consideration about initiating the diet for an outpatient is the potential medical–legal liability, should any complication occur. Only rarely does an insurance company or HMO refuse to pay when provided with extensive documentation on the advantages of the diet. Our usual inpatient stay is about 3 d; because we start eliminating sweets before patients are admitted, a more gentle induction of ketosis is possible.

2.13. Surgery

Occasionally, it is necessary for a patient on the KD to undergo a surgical procedure. When this occurs, it is important for the consulting physician to be aware of what the ketogenic diet is, the normal expected laboratory values, and common problems that may arise and how to manage them. We have developed a surgery protocol to facilitate surgery in patients on the KD (*see* Appendix 3 of this chapter).

3. MAINTAINING A PROGRAM AND USEFUL RESOURCES

3.1. Ketogenic Diet Coaches

The Pediatric Epilepsy Center at Johns Hopkins Hospital originated the idea of using parents of children on the diet as nonmedical "coaches." Because so many of the same questions come up with all new families, it is beneficial to have parents who are already knowledgeable about the diet and have been trained by our own staff to serve as support persons for new families. We put families who are considering the diet in touch with a "coach." With other parents, new families tend to feel more at ease about asking questions. The coach program also averts many repetitive phone calls to our staff.

3.2. Support Groups

Support groups are always helpful for the families. They are useful especially for parents first contemplating the diet. It is also fun for children to interact with others who understand their situation. During these meetings, parents discuss new foods they have discovered that may be useful on the diet as well as new recipes they have developed. Our dietitian is always present, and we try to hold the meetings at someone's house or at a park where the children can play. Another means of support is the Internet. There are several "keto groups" available online, and many of our families communicate with each other and with other families across the country by means of e-mail.

3.3. Internet for the Professionals

Medical professionals can join the ketogenic diet list serve sponsored by Stanford University Medical Center. This electronic medium allows those delivering the diet to communicate with each other about problems and successes and is a way to gather information on concerns such as osteoporosis, growth and developmental delays, and side effects of the diet. It is also a quick way to learn about what other centers are doing.

3.4. American Epilepsy Society

Every year the American Epilepsy Society (AES) holds a ketogenic roundtable at its annual meeting. New scientific research and clinical advances are shared. Because this session is attended by full-time laboratory scientists as well as nurses, dietitians, and neurologists, a lively interchange of ideas occurs.

3.5. Scientific Research

Although the KD has been implemented effectively for over 80 yr, little is known about how and why it controls seizures. Through the efforts of the Charlie Foundation and other organizations that support epilepsy research, scientists throughout the world have become interested in finding the mechanisms of KD action. Many chapters of this volume are devoted to such questions. Likewise, it is crucial for clinical centers to pose and evaluate unknown aspects about the KD, the type of patient for whom it is best suited, and the clinical setting in which is likely to be most effective.

3.6. Cost-Effectiveness of a Ketogenic Diet Program

Most KD centers are in a university setting. Our program is unique in that we are private. Therefore, we are particularly attuned to the costs of a KD program and the reimbursement provided. Because the KD is such a labor-intensive therapy and so few patients can be followed at any one time, the costs typically far outweigh the insurance reimbursement. We rely on donations and grants to help defray costs. But because we believe that it would be an injustice not to offer this effective therapy, we continue to offer the KD regardless of financial constraints. We hope that through dedicated efforts, the mechanisms that make the diet work will be uncovered and that many more patients can be helped. Until then, we will continue our efforts to help those who want to try this intensive but effective epilepsy diet treatment.

4. CONCLUSION

The KD is an extremely useful tool in the arsenal against epilepsy, especially in young children where diet can be controlled. It is most effective when there is a designated dietitian who works only with KD patients and when done in a center that uses a team approach.

ACKNOWLEDGMENTS

We thank The Charlie Foundation for continued assistance and the Zeilstra Foundation for generous, ongoing support. We are indebted to Dr. John Freeman, Millicent Kelly, Diana Pillas, and all the staff at the Pediatric Epilepsy Center at Johns Hopkins

Hospital who have answered our many questions through the years. Most of all, we thank our staff at the Epilepsy and Brain Mapping Program and Huntington Memorial Hospital, who always strive for the highest level of patient care.

REFERENCES

1. Sutherling JN, Hayes DM, Braganza MG, Huf RL, Sutherling WW. Long term follow-up of the ketogenic diet. Epilepsia 2000;41:103.
2. Freeman JM, Freeman JB, Kelly MT. The Ketogenic Diet: A Treatment for Epilepsy, 3rd ed. Demos, New York, 2000 pp. 33–36, 70–72, 76–84.

APPENDIX 1
KETOGENIC DIET STEPS

1. Complete the enclosed patient information forms, sign and return to our office at:
2. Enclose with the forms a brief letter on why you are interested in the ketogenic diet for you or your child along with a small picture.
3. Watch the Charlie Foundation's "Introduction to the Ketogenic Diet" if you have not already done so. You may get a copy of this tape by sending $10.00 to:
   The Charlie Foundation to Help Cure Pediatric Epilepsy
   1223 Wilshire Blvd.
   Box 815
   Santa Monica, CA 90403
4. You will need to purchase a book titled "THE KETOGENIC DIET", third edition, by John M. Freeman, MD, Jennifer B. Freeman, Millicent T. Kelly, RD, LD. To do so call Demos Vermande at 1-800-532-8663. It is important that you thoroughly read through this book.
5. If after you have read the book and have seen the video you feel you are interested in the diet for you or your child, please contact one of our nurses by calling 1-626-792-7300.
6. If after talking with you we think you or your child may be a candidate for the diet, you will need to be seen by one of our pediatric neurologists or adult neurologists.
7. After the steps above have been completed, we would like you to speak with one of our ketogenic diet coaches. Please make a list of questions or concerns you might have before calling them. We will put you in contact with a parent or patient who is well informed about the diet and can help answer some of your questions.
8. You will receive in the mail a preadmission package which will include a nutrition and food preference history that is required by the dietitian. A checklist to help you prepare the home for the diet will also be included. Please complete and return to our office. You will be scheduled for an appointment once this has been done and your insurance has been approved.

APPENDIX 2
TABLE OF CONTENTS OF OUR KETOGENIC DIET HANDBOOK

I. KETOGENIC DIET
   A. Purpose
   B. Background
   C. Description
   D. Basic Nutrition

Note: The original framework of our Handbook was the first edition of the book by J. M. Freeman, M. T. Kelly, and J. B. Freeman, *The Epilepsy Diet Treatment: Introduction to the Ketogenic Diet.* Demos, New York, 1994.

APPENDIX 3
KETOGENIC DIET SURGERY PROTOCOL

Patient:
Re: Upcoming Surgery
Ketogenic Diet

_____ has been on the Ketogenic Diet for Epilepsy since _____. His weight is approximately ___ kg. The Ketogenic Diet is a mathematically calculated and rigid metabolic diet. The patient is kept in a state of ketosis by an extremely high fat, low protein and low carbohydrate diet. Fluids are restricted as well. _____'s last blood ketones done on _____ were _____.

_____'s fasting serum glucose runs _____ but some patients can have it run as low as the 40s when fasting. We will treat if the patient has symptomatic hypoglycemia, pale sweaty, lethargic and difficult to arouse, rapid pulse, dizziness, nauseated, vomiting or if the patient has asymptomatic hypoglycemia with a blood sugar of less than 46/dL. The concern with these patients is that if they are given too much glucose after having been restricted, they may then start to have seizures. **THE FIRST CONCERN IS ALWAYS THE WELL-BEING OF THE PATIENT. IN THE EVENT OF A LIFE-THREATENING EMERGENCY THE CHILD's NEED FOR IMMEDIATE STABILIZATION COMES FIRST, DIET SECOND!**
When there is concern about the patient being hypoglycemic:

- give 30 cc's of apple juice if patient is able to take PO fluids
- if the patient is unable to have PO fluids then give D5W intravenously until the blood sugar reaches 60–70 mg/dL
- glucose monitoring should be done via glucometer q 20 min or until symptoms of hypoglycemia are resolved

When the patient must remain NPO following surgery:

- Hang one half NS with KCl per doctor
- Glucose monitoring should continue q 4 h via glucometer
- Should the patient exhibit signs and symptoms of hypoglycemia, D5W should be given to keep blood sugar between 60–70 mg/dL
- If the patient can take PO fluids, give Pedialyte until patient is able to take his regular ketogenic diet meal
- The family will be bringing in food from home that has been approved by our ketogenic dietitian
- Serum CO_2 may run lower than the normal values, usually if it is below 15 and there are concerns, our ketogenic team doctor should be notified
- The patient on the diet is usually **fluid restricted.** This patient's fluids have been restricted to _____ **cc's per 24 h.** After surgery, if the patient becomes hypovolemic, hypotensive, febrile, etc., the doctor should increase the fluids as necessary to stabilize the patient.
- With children for antibiotics or pain medication **no elixirs or suspensions** should be given as they contain too much carbohydrate

  - pharmacy may make a low carbohydrate, sugar-free solution by using the tablet, crushing it and adding water, or emptying the capsule into water, then dosing according to

patient's weight (suppositories may be given if approved by the surgeon) **Do not use chewable tablets** as they also have too much carbohydrate.
- tablets or capsules are usually fine to give or at least through the surgical period
- IV pain medications may be used

Should you have any questions or concerns please contact our ketogenic diet team.

6

Efficacy of the Ketogenic Diet

James E. Rubenstein and Eileen P. G. Vining

1. INTRODUCTION

Multiple yet different therapeutic strategies designed to induce ketosis are effective in treating intractable seizures. The clinical details to support this notion are reviewed in this chapter. In the following discussion, the term "efficacy" is defined as "the extent to which a specific intervention, procedure, regimen, or service provides a beneficial result under ideal conditions" *(1)*. This medical definition of efficacy is a restrictive one, requiring not only a beneficial result, but also additional "ideal conditions." This last requirement is perhaps the critical linchpin in any discussion of the efficacy of the ketogenic diet (KD) because the methodology of different centers and providers varies so greatly regarding the "ideal conditions" under which the diet is initiated, undertaken, and maintained. The following list enumerates some of these "ideal requirements."

1. Some centers initiate the KD after a fast of varying length, whereas others believe that fasting is of no benefit and may even cause harm.
2. Variable proportions of fat in the diet are used in different patient populations.
3. Various types of fat are used to create a diet plan.
4. Different techniques are used to assess ketosis.
5. There is no agreement about the seizure types and syndromes that are likely to respond to the diet.
6. Possible predictors of treatment success before or early on in diet therapy have not been defined.
7. Long-term use of the diet and the duration of its efficacy are not documented.
8. No study to date has matched patients for basic demographic characteristics such as age, gender, and race.

Furthermore, measuring and evaluating diet efficacy have not been accomplished using consistent standards or parameters. Several essential questions remain.

1. Do seizure counts represent the gold standard, and if so, how do these vary with the specific seizure syndrome involved?
2. What roles do electroencephalographic (EEG) changes (with or without clinical improvement) play in evaluating success or failure of treatment?
3. How significant is cognitive improvement in these patients, and how is it measured?

From: *Epilepsy and the Ketogenic Diet*
Edited by: C. E. Stafstrom and J. M. Rho © Humana Press Inc., Totowa, NJ

4. Can the side effects of antiepileptic drugs (AEDs) be measured pre- and postdiet, to account for their potential major impact on a child's quality of life?
5. What other side effects must be documented and taken into account. (Changes in general health indices such as somatic growth, head circumference, and lipid profile are a few examples.)

The goals of this chapter are to review a number of reports about KD efficacy and to examine the critical questions for future clinical research. If indeed the KD is "a therapy in search of an explanation" *(2)*, then the approaches used to date to study efficacy have been inadequate to solve this essential conundrum. Certainly, the unrecognized, indiscriminate, and uncontrolled use of ketosis as a means of controlling seizures has undergone a significant change since biblical times, when most observers believe the initial evidence of using starvation as an antiepileptic therapy is first documented *(3)*.

2. EARLY STUDIES OF KETOGENIC DIET EFFICACY

Because epilepsy was supposedly caused by overindulgences of some sort by its victims, the early twentieth-century solution of fasting and prayer evolved, with the initial practitioners comprising a team of a physical fitness guru, Bernarr Macfadden, and an osteopath, Hugh Conklin *(4)*. In 1921 H. R. Geyelin, a physician, published results of his protocol for the treatment of unclassified patients with convulsive episodes who, in general, were markedly improved after fasting for 3 wk and in some cases remained so when normal dietary allowances were reinstituted *(5)*.

That same year, Dr. R. M. Wilder of the Mayo Clinic proposed manipulating the ratio of dietary fat to proteins plus carbohydrates in a variety of ratios from 2:1 to 3:1 as a method of creating ongoing ketonemia that could mimic the metabolic effects provided by lengthy starvation and dehydration *(6)*.

These observations were then refined in 1925 by M. G. Peterman, who established minimal daily requirements of protein intake in association with the ketosis provided by excessive fat intake and carbohydrate restriction, and published results suggesting that more than half of his patients were seizure-free and another third had a 50% reduction in seizures *(7)*.

During the following two decades, the KD remained a primary and effective treatment modality, and only with the discovery and utilization of diphenylhydantoin in the 1940s was it relegated to the background, since its lifestyle limitations were obviously unattractive in comparison to the "miraculous" and simple-to-use pharmaceutical product.

3. RECENT STUDIES OF KETOGENIC DIET EFFICACY

Although various other medications became available in the ensuing years, clinical researchers continued to publish KD efficacy results *(8–11)*. Livingston *(9)* reported that 54% of his patients on the "classic" KD achieved complete seizure control, and an additional 26% achieved "partial" control. The Sills study *(10)* featured a modification of the classic KD by substituting medium-chain triglycerides (MCTs) in an emulsion form for better palatability. MCTs served as the primary source of calories from fat, after the changes proposed by Huttenlocher *(8)*, and this diet was a viable alternative method of achieving ketonemia. Forty-four children of 50 who started on the Sills diet tolerated it, with the following results: 8 achieved complete, i.e., 100%, control and half were able to stop all anticonvulsants; 4 had "excellent" (>90%) control; 10 had "good" (50–90%) control; 13 had "poor" (<50 %) control; and 9 showed no improvement (10).

Later, Kinsman and colleagues (11) retrospectively reviewed the use of the KD in an era when anticonvulsants such as valproate and carbamazepine had become readily available. They showed that 29% of the patients had "near total" seizure control, and an additional 38% had at least a 50% reduction in seizures. These findings, consistent with those of Peterman six decades earlier, sparked continued interest in the use of the diet.

Initial prospective studies by Schwartz et al. (12) compared three dietary modalities: the classic 4:1 diet, the MCT diet, and a modification that combined the incorporation of MCT with the classic diet and was known as the Radcliffe Infirmary diet. After 6 wk, 40% of patients showed greater than 90% improvement in seizure frequency, another 40% showed greater than 50% improvement, and only 20% had less than 50% improvement. The classic diet was the most effective and best tolerated of the three options. Again, the overall efficacy in the Schwartz study was consistent with previously published retrospective data.

In the early 1990s, the group from Johns Hopkins led by Freeman and Vining began a collaborative effort to educate a variety of centers and practitioners about the classic KD (13) and coordinated a prospective seven-center study to evaluate its efficacy (14). Fifty-one patients between 1 and 8 yr old (mean age 4.7 yr), who had multiple seizure types, an average of 230 seizures per month in the prestudy baseline month, and had failed an average of seven AEDs, were enrolled in the study and hospitalized to start the diet using a standard protocol.

Diet impact was studied at 3, 6, and 12 mo. Using as the standard for minimal efficacy the 50% responder rate, i.e., a decrease in seizure frequency by half, the researchers found the following results: 54% improvement at 3 mo, 53% at 6 mo, and 40% at 12 mo. There was a corresponding inverse relationship in discontinuation of the diet, with 88, 73, and 47% of patients remaining on the diet in their respective groups over time, and an obvious positive correlation in diet efficacy with the willingness of the patients or their families to continue with the program.

These results led to a prospective study of 150 consecutive patients who entered a standardized, "classic" KD program at Johns Hopkins between 1994 and 1996 and were followed for a minimum of one year (15). The mean age of this study population was 5.3 yr (range 1–16 yr); the patients averaged 410 seizures per month of varying types prediet and had been exposed to an average of 6.2 AEDs prior to diet therapy. Of greatest significance, after one year, 27% of the original group had a decrease in seizures of over 90%, and 50% had a decrease of over 50%, with slightly more than half (55%) remaining on the diet. In addition, almost all the Hopkins subjects had failed multiple modern AEDs; thus the population was highly skewed toward children with relatively severe, intractable seizures.

The same investigators reported in 2001 on the 3- to 6-yr follow-up of the initial study group of 150 children (16). A total of 142 (95%) of families responded, 4 were lost to follow-up, and 4 children had died (from causes unrelated to the diet). Of the original cohort, 20 patients (13%) were seizure free, and an additional 21 (14%) had over 90% reduction. Twenty-nine (19.3%) were off all AEDs, and another 28 (18.6%) remained on only one drug. Fifteen children (10%) remained on the diet.

In addition to these studies, several other clinical series have been reported recently. A 1999 retrospective chart review of 52 cases from Ottawa (17) showed that 6 patients demonstrated complete abolition of their seizures, and "improvement" was seen in another 29 patients. The KD was successfully utilized at the Children's Hospital of Philadelphia as a treatment alternative in 3 patients with acquired epileptic aphasia who had failed both traditional and unconventional treatments such as standard AEDs, steroids, intravenous immunoglobulins, and/or surgery (18). The group at Children's Hospital of Pittsburgh reported on 48 patients. Thirty-four children (71%) had a reduction in seizures of 50% or more, and 18 of those had a over 90% reduction during a short-term (45-d) period (19). A retrospective analysis at Connecticut Children's Medical Center between 1994 and 1999 with 48 patients (ages 1–15 yr) showed that 8.5% were seizure free at 6 and 12 mo, with 35 and 23% sustaining better than 50% reduction in seizures at 6 and 12 mo. This study also reported EEG background improvement (31%) and reduction in paroxysmal features (38%) (20).

Nordli and colleagues (21) retrospectively reviewed 32 infants with refractory epilepsy. Six infants (19%) became seizure free, and an additional 11 infants (35%) achieved over 50% reduction in seizures. The investigators concluded that the diet is as useful in infants as it is in older children, with no additional problems in achieving or maintaining ketosis. Appropriate somatic growth parameters were documented in 96% of the infants. Subjective improvement in alertness, activity level, and socialization was reported by most parents.

Kossoff and coworkers (22) treated 23 infants with infantile spasms (West syndrome), ages 5–24 mo, during a 4-yr period. Nine patients (39%) had symptomatic spasms and 16 (70%) had hypsarrhythmia on EEG. Prediet AED exposure was 3.3 medications, with 2 patients enrolled as a first-line therapeutic intervention. Thirteen babies (56%) remained on the diet after 12 mo: 6 (46%) of whom were improved more than 90%, and 13 (100%) were improved more than 50%. Thirteen infants had reduced or discontinued medications at 12 mo, and 13 had subjectively improved development, which correlated with seizure control. The authors concluded that the KD was a potentially effective, first-line alternative to other, more traditional therapies for West syndrome.

Numerous additional clinical reports of KD efficacy have emerged from Japan, Thailand, Taiwan, Italy, Spain, and Argentina. These varied from isolated case reports to a prospective study from Buenos Aires, Argentina, of 18 children ages 2–11 yr (23). In this latter study, 9 patients remained on the diet for 6–24 mo (average 16 mo), with 3 showing a reduction in seizures of 50–75% and an additional 4 with a 75–100 % reduction.

Another Argentine group prospectively evaluated 13 patients ages 1–19 yr, who remained on the KD for 22 mo. There was reduction of over 50% in seizure frequency in 11 patients (84.5%) and complete control in four patients (30.8%). EEG recordings showed nonspecific "improvement" in 100% (24).

In a report from Thailand (25), 35 children (16 boys and 19 girls, ages 2 mo to 13 yr), were placed on a Thai-based version of the classic 4:1 diet for an average duration of 7.7 mo. At 1, 3, 6, and 12 mo after starting treatment, 90% seizure reduction was achieved by 62.5, 68.2, 75, and 66.7%, respectively, of those remaining on the program. There was also a reported reduction in the number of AEDs required in all remaining on the diet, a critical factor in Thailand, where AEDs are very expensive.

An Italian study of 56 patients ages 1–23 yr (mean 10.4 yr), had the classic 4:1 diet added as adjunctive therapy for 1–18 mo (mean 5 mo). Their results were markedly worse than other studies, with over 50% reduction in only 37.5, 26.8, and 8.9 at 3, 6, and 12 mo (26).

4. CRITICAL CLINICAL QUESTIONS ABOUT KETOGENIC DIET EFFICACY

Reviewing a large number of efficacy studies published through 2002 clearly indicates that no investigator has successfully controlled for the numerous variables interfering with the creation of "ideal conditions" as required by the medical definition of efficacy. Several major questions remain.

4.1. Studying Ketogenic Diet Efficacy in Specific Seizure Types and Epilepsy Syndromes

Although in its early use, the KD was used to treat any and all seizure types, contemporary practitioners tend to restrict the use of the diet to treating patients with symptomatic or cryptogenic generalized seizures, usually in the form of generalized myoclonic, atonic, or atypical absence seizures. Older reports indicated either ineffectiveness in partial seizures (9) or no predictability in efficacy based on seizure semiology (11,12,14,15).

As a result, many practitioners do not use the KD in refractory partial seizures. However, in a retrospective report from the Cleveland Clinic, Maydell and colleagues (27) found no statistically significant difference in seizure reduction between patients with focal versus generalized seizures. The patients were classified by ictal EEG results or a combination of clinical semiology and interictal EEG. The children had a mean age of 7.5 yr, and the outcomes were statistically better for the patients under age 12 after 6 mo on the diet. The investigators concluded that the KD was a reasonable option if epilepsy surgery was not possible, such as in younger patients with medically refractory focal seizures.

There are still no published studies in which patients with specific, individual seizure types or syndromes have been treated with the KD as first-line, primary treatment and compared with an age-, gender-, and race-matched group treated with drug therapy. A 1999 study by Freeman and Vining (28) proposed a protocol for developing a short-term, blinded crossover study of KD efficacy in patients with atonic and/or myoclonic seizures in which the patient-subject effectively serves as his or her own control by utilizing glucose to stop or reverse the diet's effects. It may once have seemed impossible to blind such studies; yet there is no way to compare efficacy of the KD with efficacy of AEDs until long-term studies based on this concept are developed and accomplished.

In an era in which parents are increasingly wary of pharmacologic intervention in the treatment of their children, it seems reasonable to offer a nonpharmacologic first-line, primary alternative, i.e., the KD, if it can be clearly demonstrated that the efficacy, side-effect profile, and cost are comparable (or nearly so) to those of AEDs. When there is demonstrable, albeit subjective, improvement in a child's alertness, mental function, and activity level off medications, the families should be allowed to judge what their initial antiepilepic treatment choice implies in terms of quality of life.

Indeed, Seidel et al. (29) and Pulsifer et al. (30) have shown that KD treatment is associated with an improvement in the mean developmental quotient, with concurrent improvements in social function and attention span. Surely such neuropsychological variables weigh critically in making decisions about possible long-term treatment choices in childhood epilepsy.

Only by understanding the potential uses of the KD (if implemented earlier in the treatment algorithm, even in nonrefractory epilepsy) can the existing practice that restricts the diet to use in "intractable" or "refractory" epilepsy be logically and scientifically modified. Why have we continued to keep the diet "in reserve" and only used it as a "treatment of last resort," even though we know that the efficacy of a newly introduced anticonvulsant is less than 10% after two drug failures?

4.2. Clarifying Ages at Which Patients Can Be Started on the KD

A corollary example is our reluctance to use the KD in infants under 2 yr of age, although there are no clear data supporting a contraindication, even in early infancy. The studies by Nordli and Kossoff and their colleagues (21,22) demonstrate both the safety and efficacy of the diet, especially in West syndrome and the myoclonic epilepsies.

At our center, there are no age restrictions to initiating the diet. We plan to lead a multicenter, prospective trial to evaluate its efficacy as the first-line, primary treatment in such particularly devastating infantile encephalopathic syndromes. We have also begun a trial of a modified version of the diet in adolescents and adults with varying types of refractory, nonlesional epilepsy (31). Although there are currently no plans to use the KD as primary therapy in this older population, if a blinded crossover study could demonstrate efficacy, such a strategy may be attractive to a segment of that group.

There may also be opportunities to create animal models where the ketonemia of the diet may be mimicked through regulation of the endocrine and metabolic pathways of glycolosis and gluconeogenesis, with the ultimate goal of manipulating them to create non-diet-induced ketonemia, which can be attractive to certain patient populations that cannot or will not tolerate the diet itself.

4.3. Using EEGs in Evaluating Efficacy

There is no still clear relationship between EEG improvement and KD efficacy. Older retrospective work by Janaki et al. in 1976 (32) suggests that EEG improvement correlates with clinical efficacy. These investigators studied 15 "recalcitrant" patients: 3 with "minor motor" seizures (absence and/or myoclonic) achieved "good," i.e., >70%, control with "significant" EEG improvement; 12 with "major motor" seizures (generalized tonic–clonic and/or complex partial) had only "partial" (50–70%) improvement and no significant EEG changes. It is unclear, however, whether this difference related to seizure type more than any other factor.

In 1985 Ross et al. (33) demonstrated a statistically significant decrease in the mean number of epileptiform discharges immediately after the ingestion of MCT oil and initial evidence of ketosis; but 10 wk later, the EEGs had reverted close to baseline despite satisfactory seizure control in 6 of the 9 patients in the study group.

Schwartz and colleagues (12) randomly assessed baseline EEGs and 62 follow-up tracings in children on the KD. The 14 cases of EEG improvement (9 on the MCT diet and 5 on the classic diet) were all associated with over 50% seizure decrease. The tracings demonstrating deterioration (2 on the MCT diet and 3 on the classic diet) were also all associated with over 50% seizure improvement, including two with clinical improvement exceeding 90%. There were 43 EEGs with no significant change.

In the large multicenter study (14), EEG criteria including normal or abnormal background, focal EEG changes, multifocal spikes, and/or generalized spike-wave abnormalities, were correlated with outcome (either less than or greater than 50% seizure reduction) at 3, 6, and 12 mo. The only statistically significant finding was that children with a multifocal spike pattern had a poorer 3-mo clinical response, which subsequently resolved at the later dates.

In 1999, Freeman and Vining *(28)* utilized 24-h ambulatory EEG tracings to document the rapid decrease in clinical events correlating with decreased electrical abnormalities after fasting in children with atonic seizures. The EEG tracings also revealed that the prediet seizures reported by the parents represented only a fraction of the true number of electrical events.

It is necessary to study EEGs prospectively in patients with different seizure types who will be started on the diet, matched for age, gender, and race. This will enable us to determine how to use the EEG as a tool for predicting both long- and short-term response to the KD. Different EEG techniques, e.g., routine tracings, sleep records, and video EEGs of varying lengths may turn out to be valuable assets for predicting KD efficacy. Ideally, some simpler and less expensive objective predictors will emerge for clinical use.

5. CONCLUSION

There is ample evidence that the KD can and should play a significant role in epilepsy therapeutics. But despite years of accumulating data, a number of central questions remain unresolved. It seems as though the maximum efficacy of the diet remains elusive because as clinicians and scientists we have been unable to refine techniques that can define accurately the seizure types that will likely respond to the KD, ascertain safety and standardize initiation and implementation of the KD, and understand the diet's long-term usefulness. Detailed longitudinal studies of diet effectiveness are necessary to understand better the differences between efficacy immediately after the preliminary fast and long-term maintenance therapy. We also need to design better studies that answer basic questions, such as, "What aspects of the diet program are critical to seizure control?" For example, is one specific type of fat superior to another? Or, is calorie restriction necessary (or sufficient) to achieve ideal body weight for height? These are just a few examples of the questions that need to be explored to achieve clinical progress with the KD.

REFERENCES

1. Pugh, MB (ed). Stedman's Medical Dictionary, 27th ed. Lippincott Williams & Wilkins, Baltimore, 2000.
2. Stafstrom CE, Spencer S. The ketogenic diet. Neurology 2000;54:282.
3. Matthew 17:14–21.
4. Swink TD, Vining EPG, Freeman JM. The ketogenic diet 1997. Adv Pediatr 1997;44:297–329.
5. Geyelin, HR. Fasting as a method for treating epilepsy. Med Record 1921;99:1037–1039.
6. Wilder, RM. The effect of ketonemia on the course of epilepsy. Mayo Clin Bull 1921;2:307.
7. Peterman, MG. The ketogenic diet in epilepsy. JAMA 1925;84:1979–1983.
8. Huttenlocher, PR. Ketonemia and seizures: metabolic and anti-convulsant effects of two ketogenic diets in childhood. Pediatr Res 1976;10:536–540.
9. Livingston S, Pauli LL, Pruce I. Ketogenic diet in the treatment of childhood epilepsy, Dev Med Child Neurol 1977;19:833–834.
10. Sills MA, Forsythe WI, Haidukevych D, MacDonald A, Robinson M. The medium chain triglyceride diet and intractable epilepsy. Arch Dis Child 1986;61:1168–1172.
11. Kinsman SL, Vining EPG, Quaskey SA, Mellits D, Freeman JM. Efficacy of the ketogenic diet for intractable seizure disorders: review of 58 cases. Epilepsia 1992;33:1132–1136.
12. Schwartz RH, Eaton J, Bower BD, Aynsley-Green A. Ketogenic diets in the treatment of epilepsy: short-term clinical effects. Dev Med Child Neurol 1989;31:145–151.

13. Freeman JM, Kelly MT, Freeman JB. The Epilepsy Diet Treatment: An Introduction to the Ketogenic Diet, 1st ed. Demos, New York, 1994.
14. Vining EPG, Freeman JM, Ballaban-Gil K, Camfield CS, Camfield PR, Holmes GL, Shinnar S, Shuman R, Trevathan E, Wheless JW. A multicenter study of the efficacy of the ketogenic diet. Arch Neurol 1998;55:1433–1734.
15. Freeman JM, Vining EPG, Pillas DJ, Pyzik PL, Casey JC, Kelly MT. The efficacy of the Ketogenic Diet-1998: a prospective evaluation of intervention in 150 children. Pediatrics 1998;102:1358–1363.
16. Hemingway C, Freeman JM, Pillas DJ, Pyzik PL. The ketogenic diet: a 3- to 6-year follow-up of 150 children enrolled prospectively. Pediatrics 2001;108:898–905.
17. Hassan AM, Keene DL, Whiting SF, Jacob PJ, Champagne JR, Humphreys P. Ketogenic diet in the treatment of refractory epilepsy in childhood. Pediatr Neurol 1999;21:548–552.
18. Bergqvist AG, Chee CM, Lutchka LM, Brooks-Kayal AR. Treatment of acquired epileptic aphasia with the ketogenic diet. J Child Neurol 1999;14:696–701.
19. Katyal NG, Koehler AN, McGhee B, Foley CM, Crumrine PK. The ketogenic diet in refractory epilepsy: the experience of Children's Hospital of Pittsburgh. Clin Pediatr 2000;39:153–159.
20. DiMario FJ Jr, Holland J. The ketogenic diet: a review of the experience at Connecticut Children's Medical Center. Pediatr Neurol 2002;26:288–292.
21. Nordli DR Jr, Kuroda MM, Carroll J, Koenigsberger DY, Hirsch LJ, Bruner HJ, Seidel WT, De Vivo DC. Experience with the ketogenic diet in infants. Pediatrics 2001;108:129–133.
22. Kossoff EH, Pyzik PL, McGrogan JR, Vining EPG, Freeman JM. Efficacy of the ketogenic diet for infantile spasms. Pediatrics 2002;109:780–783.
23. Caraballo R, Tripoli J, Escobal L, Cersosimo R, Tenembaum S, Palacios C, Fejerman N. Ketogenic diet: efficacy and tolerability in childhood intractable epilepsy. Rev Neurol 1998;26:61–64.
24. Panico LR, Rios VG, Demartini MG, Carniello MA. The electroencephalographic evolution of a group of patients on a ketogenic diet. Rev Neurol 2000;31:212–220.
25. Kankirawatana P, Jirapinyo P, Kankirawatana S, Wongarn R, Thamanasiri N. Ketogenic diet: an alternative treatment for refractory epilepsy in children. J Med Assoc Thailand 2001;84:1027–1032.
26. Coppola G, Veggiotti P, Cusmai R, Bertoli S, Cardinali S, Dionisi-Vici C, Elia M, Lispi ML, Sarnelli C, Tagliabue A, Toraldo C, Pascotto A. The ketogenic diet in children, adolescents, and young adults with refractory epilepsy: an Italian multicentric experience. Epilepsy Res 2002;48:221–227.
27. Maydell BV, Wyllie E, Akhtar N, Kotagal P, Powaski K, Cook K, Weinstock A, Rothner AD. Efficacy of the ketogenic diet in focal versus generalized seizures. Pediatr Neurol 2001;25:208–212.
28. Freeman JM, Vining EPG. Seizures decrease rapidly after fasting: preliminary studies of the ketogenic diet. Arch Pediatr Adolesc Med 1999;153:946–949.
29. Seidel WT, Davis K, Lin MI, Mitchell WG, Chen LS. Ketogenic diet: seizure outcome and parental reports. Epilepsia 1997;38 (Suppl 8):196–197.
30. Pulsifer MB, Gordon JM, Brandt J, Vining EPG, Freeman JM. Effects of ketogenic diet on development and behavior: preliminary report of a prospective study. Dev Med Child Neurol 2001;43:301–306.
31. Kossoff EH, Krauss GL, McGrogan JR, Kreman JM. Efficacy of the Atkins diet as therapy for intractable epilepsy. Neurology 2003;61:1789–1791.
32. Janaki S, Rashid MK, Gulati MS, Jayaram SR, Baruah JK, Saxena VK. A clinical electroencephalographic correlation of seizures on the ketogenic diet. Indian J Med Res. 1976;64:1057.
33. Ross DL, Swaiman KF, Torres F, Hansen J. Early biochemical and EEG correlates of the ketogenic diet in children with atypical absence epilepsy. Pediatr Neurol 1985;1:104–108.

7 The Ketogenic Diet in Adults

Michael R. Sperling and Maromi Nei

1. INTRODUCTION

In sporadic use since the 1920s, the ketogenic diet (KD) has enjoyed a resurgence in popularity in the past decade. Physicians have placed many hundreds of children on the diet, often with a gratifying response *(1–3)*. The diet has largely been reserved for desperately ill infants and children who had failed to respond to medical therapy. For example, in a study of 150 children who were enrolled in the diet *(2),* mean seizure frequency was 410 seizures per month of multiple types, and patients had failed an average of 6.2 antiepileptic drugs (AEDs). In another study, 143 patients averaged 23.8 seizures per day, and 111 of the patients had at least daily seizures *(3)*. Most children placed on the diet experienced the most severe types of seizure, including myoclonic, atonic, tonic, and generalized tonic–clonic seizures *(4)*. As a result of the diet, seizures stopped completely in some individuals and seizure frequency greatly diminished in others. In some cases, children no longer required antiepileptic medication. While generalized seizures appear to respond more favorably, partial seizures are reduced in frequency as well *(3)*. Consequently, the KD has gained recognition as a valuable treatment in the management of children with uncontrolled seizures *(5)*.

In contrast, few adolescents and adults have been treated with the diet. In part, this bias may relate to the perception that it is easier to control a child's diet, particularly when he or she is handicapped. Consequently, use has been customarily restricted to children under age 10 yr, and efforts to treat older individuals have been met with resistance. Schwartz et al. *(6)* reported that adults could not tolerate the dietary restrictions. Efficacy has also been questioned. While a positive response is seen in some individuals, adolescents over age 12 yr may respond less favorably than younger children *(3)*. Moreover, most patients treated with the KD had generalized epilepsy, and older individuals are more likely to experience partial seizures.

Nonetheless, for many adults and older adolescents, medications are inadequate and surgery is not an option. Patients may experience frequent uncontrolled seizures, which pose risk of injury and cause psychosocial disability. The need for an alternative therapy led us to recommend the ketogenic diet in adults with uncontrolled seizures who were willing to try a new approach. This chapter briefly reviews the rationale for diet therapy, describes the resulting experience in adults, and discusses the associated risks.

From: *Epilepsy and the Ketogenic Diet*
Edited by: C. E. Stafstrom and J. M. Rho © Humana Press Inc., Totowa, NJ

2. RATIONALE

Starvation had been observed to reduce seizure frequency early in the twentieth century *(7)*. It was then postulated that ketonemia, which occurs during fasting, could also be produced by consuming a diet containing excess amounts of fat and lacking in carbohydrate *(8)*. The mechanism of action of the KD remains unknown. The ketone bodies present in the bloodstream may not be the effective agents. Rather, they may serve as a marker of the metabolic derangements that produce the clinical effect. A full discussion of the mechanisms is beyond the scope of this review, and the reader is referred to other sources in this volume and the literature *(9–12)*.

Briefly, several mechanistic hypotheses have been advanced, based on experimental observations in animals. Alterations occur in brain energy metabolism, which may decrease brain excitability. Increased levels of acetone are seen, and there is evidence that acetone has anticonvulsant properties *(11)*. Increased levels of β-hydroxybutyrate are observed as well. One study has correlated the concentration of β-hydroxybutyrate in the serum with seizure control *(12)*. In addition, substrates in the tricarboxylic acid cycle are altered, and concentrations of γ-aminobutyric acid (GABA) may be increased in the brain as a result of enhanced conversion of glutamate to GABA. Neutral amino acids may increase in the brain as well, and aspartate levels may fall. These metabolic changes may alter the excitatory–inhibitory balance, alter the extracellular milieu, and affect synaptic transmission. The alterations in brain neurotransmitters and energy metabolism are complex, and much research must be done to better understand how the KD reduces seizure frequency.

3. KETOGENIC DIET IN ADULTS

In 1930 Barborka reported the effects of the KD in 100 adult patients *(13)*. Antiepileptic drugs were not prescribed, but the results presage modern findings: 12% of patients became seizure free, 44% improved, and 44% had no improvement after one year. Patients who improved reported increased alertness. The most common side effects were constipation and cessation of menses. Despite the findings in this report, the diet remained an oddity and was considered to be unsuitable for adults. The subsequent development of effective AEDs, beginning with phenytoin in the late 1930s, undoubtedly dampened interest in unconventional approaches that were difficult to implement.

The next systematic report regarding the KD in adults did not appear until 1999. Results were presented for 11 patients with refractory seizures treated with the KD at Thomas Jefferson University Hospital in Philadelphia *(14)*. These individuals were placed on a 4:1 ketogenic diet (4 g of fat to 1 g of combined protein and carbohydrate) at a daily caloric intake designed for each patient's ideal body weight. Fluids were restricted to the milliliter equivalent of the caloric intake; e.g., a patient on a 2000-calorie diet was allowed 2000 mL of fluids. Vitamin and mineral supplements were also prescribed.

The initial results were encouraging. Of 11 patients, 3 had a 90% reduction in seizure frequency, 3 had a 50–89% reduction, 1 had less than 50% reduction, and 4 patients discontinued the diet. Of those who discontinued, 2 patients had high levels of ketosis with no change in seizure frequency, and 2 did not maintain adequate ketosis at home, although they had done so in the hospital; in those cases, compliance with the diet was not adequate.

Table 1
Patient Data

		No. of Patients
Age	Mean: 32 yr (11–51 yr)	
Epilepsy type	Idiopathic generalized	3
	Symptomatic generalized	12
	Partial epilepsy	11
Duration of diet	Mean: 7 months (0.13–25.5 mo)	

Both partial and generalized seizures responded favorably. All patients noted constipation and bloating, and women reported menstrual irregularities. Cognitive improvement was observed, similar to what has been reported in children. Seven patients noted improved cognition and mood, whereas 2 patients reported worsened concentration. Cholesterol and triglyceride levels increased, with an increased ratio of cholesterol to high-density lipoprotein (HDL). One patient with long-standing high cholesterol discontinued the diet after 5 mo and 5 mo later experienced a myocardial infarction. Although it is doubtful that the KD was responsible for this adverse event, it must be asked whether the diet contributed to this cardiovascular morbidity.

As a consequence of the response just described, we concluded that the diet held promise in adults with either localization-related or generalized epilepsy. Patients and their families must be highly motivated to use the diet, which requires rigid compliance. How long the diet should be continued remained a question, although the plan was to replicate the pediatric experience and discontinue the diet after 1–2 yr. It was also clear that greater attention must be paid to managing serum lipids, whether by dietary manipulation or pharmacologic therapy.

Since the initial report, an additional 15 patients have been treated with the KD. Consequently, results are available for 26 patients (15 women, 11 men) with refractory epilepsy who have tried the KD at Thomas Jefferson University Hospital. Table 1 provides demographic details. Twenty-five patients were 17 yr of age or older at the time of diet initiation, and one patient was 11 yr old.

A standard set of laboratory studies was performed prior to beginning the diet. This included a complete blood count, renal and electrolyte evaluation, liver function tests, fasting lipid panel, and serum vitamin B_{12}, folic acid, carnitine, and selenium levels. All patients also had 12-lead electrocardiograms (EKGs) performed. All patients placed on the diet had normal electrolytes, blood counts, and liver function tests, although some had abnormal lipid studies (*see* below). None had evidence of ischemic heart disease by EKG or history.

Patients were initiated on a standard 4:1 ratio diet after consultation with a dietician. All diets were started in the hospital with 24–48 h of fasting. One patient could not be safely started owing to the development of metabolic acidosis. All others successfully began the diet and continued on it as outpatients. Patients received supplemental phosphorus, a multivitamin, calcium, and a stool softener.

The efficacy of the diet was similar to that reported in children. Overall, 54% of patients reported a reduction in seizure frequency. Patients with symptomatic general-

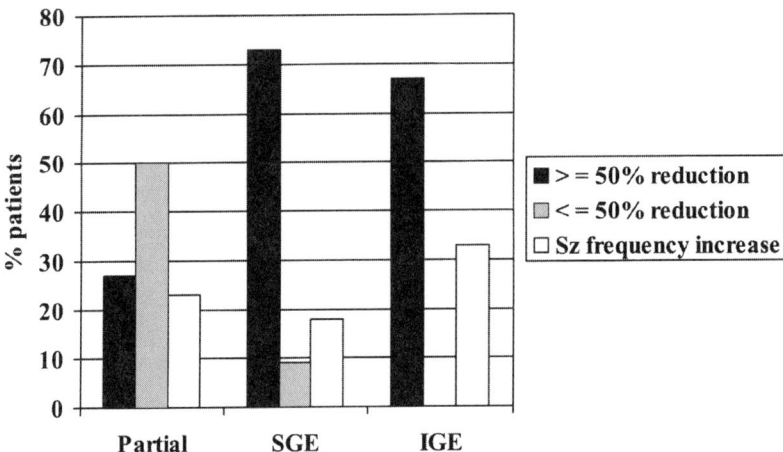

Fig. 1. Differential response of epilepsy type to ketogenic diet. The generalized epilepsies appeared to respond more favorably than the localization-related epilepsies. SZ, seizure; IGE, idiopathic generalized epilepsy; SGE, symptomatic generalized epilepsy.

ized epilepsy had the greatest response, with 73% of individuals experiencing a seizure reduction of 50% or more (Fig. 1). In contrast, only 3 of 11 patients with partial epilepsy had a seizure reduction of 50% or more. However, for some individuals with partial epilepsy, the response was dramatic. For example, a 45-yr-old man who had experienced 4–6 complex partial seizures per month before starting the KD had no seizures for 6 wk after beginning the diet and thereafter experienced a seizure reduction of 80% or more. Of the 3 patients with idiopathic generalized epilepsy, two had a significant seizure frequency reduction. One patient with a pre-diet seizure frequency of 2–3 generalized tonic–clonic seizures and 7–8 absence seizures per month was seizure free for 11 mo after diet initiation. Then a change in her domestic arrangements made it impossible to maintain dietary compliance, and she had recurrent seizures. We also observed that the response tends to be immediate. If seizures were to become less frequent, they generally diminished within the first few weeks.

The high fat content of the diet and the paucity of healthy foods such as vegetables and fruit raised concerns regarding the potential metabolic consequences of the KD. Cholesterol levels tended to rise over time in patients on the diet (mean pre-diet cholesterol 207.3 [156–304]; mean postdiet cholesterol 252.8 [123–395]; $p = 0.007$). However, the clinical significance of the elevation for a relatively short period of time, months or perhaps 2 yr, is unknown.

Clinically significant nutritional deficiencies did not occur, although asymptomatic laboratory abnormalities were found. The most common laboratory finding was a reduction in the free carnitine level, noted in 7 patients. This is a common finding in children and is of unclear clinical significance. In a few cases, there was an elevation in serum triglyceride levels that was at least partially reversed with carnitine supplementation. The serum selenium level was slightly reduced in 5 patients, but no clinically significant abnormalities occurred. Selenium supplementation was provided, which normalized levels. Slight reductions in serum magnesium, phosphorus, and potassium levels occurred transiently in one patient each. These abnormalities were also reversed with the appropriate supplementation.

Table 2
Reasons for Diet Discontinuation

Reason[a]	No. of patients
Lack of compliance	8
Ineffective	9
Weight loss	1
Fatigue	1
Metabolic acidosis	1
Lost to follow-up after 4 mo	1

[a] Three patients, all of whom had symptomatic generalized epilepsy, completed the 2-yr period established for the diet.

Although most patients had fewer seizures, few followed the ketogenic diet for 2 yr. The mean length of time that patients stayed on the diet at the time of data analysis was 7 mo (including 2 patients currently on the diet and 1 person lost to follow-up at 4 mo). Only 3 patients stayed on the diet for 2 yr; all had symptomatic generalized epilepsy and had a substantial reduction in seizure frequency once they started the diet. When the 2-yr ketogenic diet period was finished, 2 patients continued on a modified version of the Atkins diet, allowing higher protein levels and carbohydrate intake. The most common reason for discontinuing the diet was lack of efficacy, as observed in 35% of patients. Thirty-one percent of patients were unable to tolerate or continue compliance with the diet over an extended period of time. Other reasons for discontinuation included weight loss and fatigue (Table 2). Weight loss occurred in the majority of patients on the diet (mean: –6.7 kg; range –28.6 to +6.8 kg). Those with greater weight loss had desired weight reduction, and caloric intake was calculated to result in weight loss. However, some individuals did experience undesired weight loss owing to reduced appetite.

These data reveal that some adults with refractory epilepsy improve on the KD. In this series, patients with symptomatic generalized epilepsy had the best response and were able to continue the diet for a longer time than others. We are in the process of evaluating the lipid profiles in greater detail and cannot yet comment on how changing the diet corrected serum lipid abnormalities. Briefly, some patients had the fat content of the diet altered, e.g., substituting canola oil for margarine, with a resultant improvement in cholesterol/HDL ratios. Careful monitoring for nutritional deficiencies is needed to prevent the development of clinically significant abnormalities.

4. CAUTIONS AND POTENTIAL COMPLICATIONS

Several potential problems must be addressed. The risks of atherosclerosis, nephrolithiasis, metabolic acidosis, and cardiac complications are discussed in this section.

A recent study in children (15) found that the KD was associated with increases in serum lipids. This included elevations in serum low-density lipoprotein cholesterol, very-low-density lipoprotein cholesterol, triglycerides, apolipoprotein B, and apolipoprotein A-1 levels. HDL cholesterol was modestly reduced, so the mean cholesterol/HDL ratio changed from 3.36 at baseline to 5.20, a significant increase. These alterations in serum lipids persisted for 24 mo, the duration of therapy. These findings raise concern for accelerated atherogenesis, which may be particularly worrisome in middle-aged or older adults. Consequently, serum lipid levels must be carefully monitored. Another cardiac risk factor that could be worsened by the dyslipidemia, C-reactive protein, might also be measured. If necessary, changes can be made in fat content of the diet or lipid-lowering agents prescribed to reduce the risk of cardiac complications. We now advise treatment of hyperlipidemia for patients starting the KD. Dietary fat content can be changed and medications can be used to minimize undesirable lipid elevations.

Other types of cardiac abnormality may occur while patients are on the KD. Prolonged QT interval (QT_c) has been reported in children and adolescents. In a recent study, 3 of 20 patients had a prolonged QT_c. Furthermore, the degree of prolongation of the interval correlated directly with serum β-hydroxybutyrate level and inversely with serum bicarbonate level *(16)*. Prolonged QT_c poses increased risk for ventricular dysrhythmia and sudden death, and thus potentially life-threatening cardiac conduction abnormalities may be produced by the KD. It is therefore advisable to routinely monitor the EKG during treatment with the KD, and alter therapy if this complication develops.

Finally nephrolithiasis and metabolic acidosis can occur while on a KD. The consequent acidification of the urine may lead to development of stones, which can occur in 2–8% of patients *(3,17)*. In theory, concomitant use of a carbonic anhydrase inhibitor such as acetozolamide, topiramate, or zonisamide may worsen metabolic acidosis or increase the likelihood of kidney stones. Yet in practice, these outcomes have not been observed. Patients taking these medications should be carefully monitored. We have used these agents in adults without problem thus far, and one report suggests that the drugs can be safely used in children as well *(18)*. Clinically significant acidosis can be treated with bicarbonate supplements if needed.

5. CONCLUSION

The KD merits more widespread use in adults with refractory epilepsy. Based on the limited literature available, it seems reasonably safe and offers benefit for both partial and generalized seizures. The diet, which requires highly motivated patients and families, probably should be reserved for individuals who have failed at least several medications and are not candidates for a potentially curative neurosurgical procedure.

Broader application of the KD has potential societal benefits as well. There is evidence that the diet reduces medical costs in children. One study demonstrated a 46% reduction in medical costs after initiation of therapy *(19)*. The cost reduction is possibly due to improved seizure control. If this finding can be replicated, this benefit is potentially significant.

In future studies, attention must be paid to assessing the potential of the KD. In particular, dyslipidemia must be controlled. To increase popularity and improve patient compliance in adults, more palatable versions of the diet should be developed. Most important, physicians and other health-care providers must be educated in use of the diet, so that it can be more readily employed as an additional therapeutic modality.

REFERENCES

1. Vining EP, Freeman JM, Ballaban-Gil K. A multicenter study of the efficacy of the ketogenic diet. Arch Neurol 1998;55:1433–1437.

2. Hemingway C, Freeman JM, Pillas DJ, et al. The ketogenic diet: a 3- to 6-year follow-up of 150 children enrolled prospectively. Pediatrics 2001;108:898–905.

3. Maydell BV, Wyllie E, Akhtar N, et al. Efficacy of the ketogenic diet in focal versus generalized seizures. Pediatr Neurol 2001;25:208–212.

4. Vining EP. Clinical efficacy of the ketogenic diet. Epilepsy Res 1999;37:181–190.

5. Nordli D. The ketogenic diet: uses and abuses. Neurology 2002;58 (Suppl 7):S21–S24.

6. Schwartz RH, Eaton J, Bower BD, Aynsley-Green A. Ketogenic diets in the treatment of epilepsy: short-term clinical effects. Dev Med Child Neurol 1989;31:145–151.

7. Geyelin HR. Fasting as a method for treating epilepsy. Med Rec 1921;99:1037–1039.

8. Wilder RM. The effects of ketonemia on the course of epilepsy. Mayo Clin Proc 1921;2:307–308.

9. Yudkoff M, Daikhin Y, Nissim I, et al. Ketogenic diet, amino acid metabolism, and seizure control. J Neurosci Res 2001;66:931–940.

10. Schwartzkroin P. Mechanisms underlying the anti-epileptic efficacy of the ketogenic diet. Epilepsy Res 1999;37:171–180.

11. Likhodii SS, Burnham WM. Ketogenic diet: does it stop seizures? Med Sci Monit 2002;8:HY19–HY24.

12. Gilbert DL, Pyzik PL, Freeman JM. The ketogenic diet: seizure control correlates better with serum beta-hydroxybutyrate than with urine ketones. J Child Neurol 2000;15:787–790.

13. Barborka CJ. Epilepsy in adults: results of treatment by ketogenic diet in one hundred cases. Arch Neurol Psychiatr 1930;6:904–914.

14. Sirven J, Whedon B, Caplan D, Liporace J, Glosser D, O'Dwyer J, Sperling MR. The ketogenic diet for intractable epilepsy in adults: preliminary results. Epilepsia 1999;40:1721–1726.

15. Kwiterovitch PO Jr, Vining EP, Pyzik P, et al. Effect of a high-fat ketogenic diet on plasma levels of lipids, lipoproteins, and apolipoproteins in children. JAMA 2003;290:912–920.

16. Best TH, Franz DN, Gilbert DI, et al. Cardiac complications in pediatric patients on the ketogenic diet. Neurology 2000;54:2328–2330.

17. Herzberg GZ, Fivush BA, Kinsman SL, Gearhart JP. Urolithiasis associated with the ketogenic diet. J Pediatr 1990;117:743–745.

18. Takeoka M, Riviello JJ Jr, Pfeifer H, Thiele EA. Concomitant treatment with topiramate and ketogenic diet in pediatric epilepsy. Epilepsia 2002;43:1072–1075.

19. Mandel A, Ballew M, Pina-Garza JE, et al. Medical costs are reduced when children with intractable epilepsy are successfully treated with the ketogenic diet. J Am Diet Assoc 2002;102:396–398.

20. Katyal NG, Koehler AN, McGhee B, et al. The ketogenic diet in refractory epilepsy: the experience of Children's Hospital of Pittsburgh. Clin Pediatr (Phila) 2000;39:153–159.

Indications and Contraindications of the Ketogenic Diet

Anna Gunhild Christina Bergqvist

1. INDICATIONS

1.1. Intractable Epilepsy

The ketogenic diet (KD) has historically been used in the treatment of medically refractory epilepsy. It is currently not recommended for new-onset seizures because antiepileptic drugs (AEDs) are easier to use and are effective in approx 70–80% of patients. The KD requires a significant commitment of time and effort by the patient, his or her family, the KD health-care team, and the institution that supports the KD program. Determining precisely when intractability occurs in a child with epilepsy continues to be a subject of discussion among epidemiologists *(1–5)*. Generally, epilepsy centers will not offer the KD treatment until a patient has failed two or three standard AEDs. Most patients who start the KD have failed at least three times as many AEDs. The KD is not recommended to some patients until all other options have failed *(6)*. Current treatments available to patients with intractable epilepsies include a plethora of conventional AEDs, the vagus nerve stimulator, epilepsy surgery, and the KD. The optimal hierarchy of these treatments in the course of intractable epilepsy should be continually reevaluated based on efficacy, side effects, and safety. For example, epilepsy surgery (the "gold standard" for lesional temporal lobe epilepsy) is often ineffective in nonlesional, nontemporal causes of epilepsy and may result in significant morbidity. The use of the KD prior to epilepsy surgery treatment in these patients has been suggested *(7,8)*.

1.2. Seizures Types

There has been no prospective blinded clinical trial comparing the KD with other treatments, nor any trial specifically designed to compare seizure types or etiologies. Epilepsy is a heterogeneous disorder with multiple etiologies capable of causing the same type of seizure. To answer these questions definitively, large groups of patients need to be studied.

Initially, because there were few other treatments available, the KD was used for seizures of all types. Gradually KD use was shifted to generalized seizure types, such as absence, atonic, and myoclonic seizures *(9,10)*. In more recent studies, subjects with partial seizures were less common, and children with purely partial seizures were some-

From: *Epilepsy and the Ketogenic Diet*
Edited by: C. E. Stafstrom and J. M. Rho © Humana Press Inc., Totowa, NJ

times excluded *(11–13)*. However, some recent data demonstrated the effectiveness of the KD for partial seizure types. At a large epilepsy center, 134 children (100 generalized seizures and 34 partial seizures) were studied, and the KD was found to be equally efficacious between the two groups *(14)*. A recent meta-analysis, combining 11 KD studies, did not find a difference in effectiveness based on seizure types *(6)*.

1.3. Symptomatic and Asymptomatic Epilepsy

Applying the terms "symptomatic" and "asymptomatic" to seizures denotes our ability to identify specific central nervous system (CNS) pathology as the cause of the epilepsy. Most of these patients have comorbid disabilities such as mental retardation and cerebral palsy. Symptomatic epilepsy is, by definition, more difficult to treat. Whether the KD is more or less effective in the treatment of symptomatic or asymptomatic epilepsy has not been proven. The KD was initially thought to be less effective in symptomatic epilepsy; however, early follow-up data from both Keith *(10)* and Livingston *(9)* indicated success in children with symptomatic epilepsy. Later studies have uniformly supported the efficacy of the KD in this group of patients *(12,13,15–19)*. Recent studies indicate that the KD may have equal efficacy even in patients with cerebral dysgenesis *(16)*.

1.4. Age

Whether the age of the patient is an important prognostic factor in the decision to prescribe the KD is unclear. As the use of the KD increased in the 1990s, the efficacy in infants and adults was questioned. It was argued that ketosis was more difficult to sustain in infants and that compliance with the diet in adult patients was more difficult.

Successful use of the KD in infants with intractable epilepsy or inborn errors of metabolism has been demonstrated. In one study of 32 infants, 19% became seizure free and an additional 36% had more than 50% reduction in seizure frequency *(20)*. Infants utilize ketone bodies well but have higher cerebral and overall metabolic rates *(21)*. Therefore, a gradual introduction, more frequent medical and laboratory evaluations, and adjustment in the diet are often necessary to use the KD safely in this age group *(20)*. The KD has not been used in large numbers of adults, but the adult epilepsy centers offering the KD have reported efficacy equal to that seen in children (*see* Chapter 7, this volume, and refs. *22* and *23*).

1.5. Epilepsy Syndromes

Good efficacy with the KD for treatment of several epilepsy syndromes has been reported. Patients with Lennox–Gastaut syndrome with multiple seizure types (tonic, atonic, myoclonic, atypical absence, etc.), slow spike wave, and a worsening epileptic encephalopathy are known to respond well to the KD *(24–27)*. More recent studies confirmed success in this population with the KD, particularly in patients with myoclonic and atonic drop seizures *(28)*. Infantile spasms, which are associated with clusters of spasms, hypsarrythmia, and psychomotor retardation (the triad defining West syndrome), invariably result in poor outcomes if treatments fail. Success with the KD in a few cases of infantile spasms was noted in some of the general studies of efficacy *(12,13,20)*. Specific success with the KD and infantile spasms was recently shown in a study of 23 infants and children *(29)*. The majority of these children had failed traditional treatments for infantile spasms and, on average, had failed 3.3 AEDs prior to the

KD. After 12 mo of treatment with the KD, 56% remained on the diet, 26% had a greater than 90% reduction in seizures; 13% were seizure free *(29)*.

The KD has been used successfully in other less common epileptic and genetic disorders, including acquired epileptic aphasia, acquired epileptiform opercular syndrome, and Rett syndrome *(30–32)*.

1.6. Side Effects of AEDs

Most AEDs are tolerated well in monotherapy. The risk of side effects increases with polytherapy and high therapeutic dosing, which are the clinical situations frequently encountered in patients with intractable epilepsy. Both a history of poor tolerance and the appearance of significant side effects from AEDs are strong considerations in deciding whether to use the KD. In contrast to AEDs, the KD appears to improve both cognition and behavior in children. This KD-associated improvement has not been thoroughly studied but is often reported by parents and caregivers prior to discontinuation of the AEDs *(20,33)*.

Ketogenic diet efficacy studies have shown that almost all patient-responders (defined at 3 mo, > 50% reduction in seizures) are able to discontinue some AEDs while on the KD. From 20 to 60% of the responders may be successfully treated with the KD only *(12,13,20)*.

The KD is our oldest and one of our most effective treatments for patients with intractable epilepsy. The KD appears be equally effective regardless of patient age, type of seizure, or cause (symptomatic or asymptomatic) of the epilepsy. In addition, significant scientific data indicate that the KD may have antiepileptogenic properties *(see* Chapter 22, this volume). The KD should be considered earlier in the course of treatment for a child with intractable epilepsy, rather than after all other options have failed *(34,35)*.

1.7. Inborn Errors of Metabolism

The major use of the KD is as a treatment for intractable epilepsy. In a few inborn errors of metabolism, however, the metabolic defects in carbohydrate metabolism are "bypassed" by using ketone bodies as the primary energy source. We discuss these disorders because the KD, with the steady production of ketone bodies, is the treatment of choice, and early diagnosis and treatment may prolong life and reduce morbidity in these patients.

1.7.1. FACILITATED GLUCOSE TRANSPORTER PROTEIN DEFICIENCY

Glucose transporter protein deficiency is a group of recently recognized disorders resulting in impaired glucose transport across blood–tissue barriers *(36,37)*. Facilitated glucose transporter protein type 1 *(GLUT1)* deficiency syndrome results from impaired glucose transport across the blood–brain barrier *(38)*. Although a rare disorder, it is now increasingly recognized and over 70 cases have been reported in the literature *(39)*.

The brain has limited abilities to use alternative nonglucose energy sources; ketone bodies can be metabolized, but not fatty acids *(40)*. D-Glucose is therefore an essential fuel for the brain. The adult brain utilizes 20% of whole-body glucose, whereas the neonatal brain has a much higher requirement, and up to 80% of whole-body glucose is utilized *(41)*. An impaired glucose supply to the developing brain, without sufficient alternative fuels, will therefore affect both brain function and development *(42)*.

The clinical presentation of GLUT1 deficiency syndrome is nonspecific and heterogeneous. The pregnancy, delivery, and neonatal period are usually normal. In infancy or early childhood, seizures develop that are difficult to control with anticonvulsant medications. There is variation in seizure type, frequency, and character. During infancy, cyanotic, atonic, and partial seizures predominate. Myoclonic and generalized seizures develop later in childhood (43). Peculiar eye movements, developmental delay, acquired microcephaly, hypotonia with ataxia, dysmetria, dystonia, and spasticity are also common clinical features. The degree of intellectual impairment varies from profound mental retardation to normal cognitive abilities and may diminish with time (44). Clinical symptoms worsen with fasting, are often seen in the preprandial setting, and improve with food intake (45,46).

There are no specific anatomical brain abnormalities associated with GLUT1 deficiency syndrome, and brain imaging is usually normal or may show nonspecific findings. Electroencephalographic (EEG) changes include both focal and generalized epileptiform discharges and slowing, which may be reversible with food intake (47). Hypoglycorrhachia (low cerebral spinal fluid [CSF] glucose concentration) in the presence of a normal blood glucose (or a CSF/blood glucose ratio < 0.4) is the hallmark of the disease. The lumbar puncture should be performed during the metabolic steady state, such as 4–6 h after the last meal. In children, blood glucose should be determined before the lumbar puncture to avoid stress-related serum hyperglycemia. The CSF should be examined for cells, glucose, protein, and lactate and pyruvate concentrations. In GLUT1 deficiency syndrome, CSF concentrations of lactate are usually low to normal. For other causes of hypoglycorrhachia (meningitis, subarachnoid hemorrhage, sarcoidosis, trichinosis, lupus erythematosus), CSF lactate is usually elevated.

The human erythocyte glucose transporter is immunochemically identical to brain GLUT1. Therefore, the defect is in the GLUT1 gene and can be diagnosed by means of erythocyte glucose uptake studies (48). The glucose transport may be impaired from either a functional or a quantitative GLUT1 defect. GLUT1-specific immunoreactivity in the erythocyte membrane will help in distinguishing the two. A normal GLUT1 immunoreactivity suggests a functional impairment, whereas reduced immunoreactivity indicates a reduced number of transporters at the cell membrane.

The gene for GLUT1 has been identified on chromosome 1 (p35–31.3), and 21 different mutations have been detected. Prenatal diagnosis is currently not available unless a mutation has been identified in an affected child in the family. Two families with an autosomal dominant transmission of the GLUT1 disease have been described; but in other children, all mutations have been de novo, with family members unaffected. As this is a rare and novel disorder, long term outcomes are not known.

The only established treatment for GLUT1 deficiency syndrome is the KD, in which the ketone bodies β-hydroxybutyrate and acetoacetate are generated from fatty acid oxidation and provide an adequate supply of alternative fuel for brain metabolism. Patients placed on the KD usually have a quick cessation of seizure activity and concurrent improvement in the EEG. Ominously, however, one child with GLUT1 deficiency syndrome developed fatal pancreatitis while on the KD (49).

The duration of treatment with the KD in the GLUT1 deficiency syndrome is debated. Positron emission tomography studies suggest that cerebral glucose demand in children exceeds that is adults. The transition to greater glucose demand occurs during adolescence *(50)*. It is therefore currently recommended that the KD be maintained into adolescence, to ensure adequate brain development in children with *GLUT1* deficiency.

1.7.2. PYRUVATE DEHYDROGENASE DEFICIENCY

Defects in the pyruvate dehydrogenase (PDH) complex are an important cause of lactic acidemia and represent relatively common inborn errors of metabolism in children (>200 cases described). PDH complex is a mitochondrial enzyme that catalyzes the irreversible oxidation of pyruvate to acetyl-Co A. PDH is the rate-limiting enzyme connecting glycolysis with the tricarboxylic acid cycle and oxidative phosphorylation. It therefore plays an important role in energy metabolism *(51,52)*.

The PDH complex comprises three catalytic component enzymes, E1, E2, and E3, and a protein-X, necessary for the interactions of the E2 and E3 enzymes. The E1 component is a heterotetramer composed of two α and two β-subunits; there is also a cofactor (TPP) binding site. The activation of the PDH complex is tightly regulated through phosphorylation of the E1α subunit by a specific deactivating kinase and an activating phosphatase. The PDH complex is present in all tissues. The vast majority of patients with PHD complex deficiency have a defect in the PDH-E1α subunit. Defects in the other complex components have also been reported *(53,54)*.

The PDH-E1α subunit has been localized to the X chromosome (Xp22.1) *(55)*. In males, all cells are affected, and the severe form of PDH deficiency is not compatible with life. In females, the X-chromosome inactivation pattern determines the tissue-specific PDH complex cellular activity *(56)*. Most abnormalities are *de novo* point mutations, and asymptomatic carriers have been identified.

The clinical manifestations of the PDH-E1α deficiency are unusually heterogeneous. In general, the degree of clinical impairment correlates with the overall PDH complex activity. The severe neonatal form presents with overwhelming lactic acidemia, coma, and early death. These infants have a low birth weight and are hypotonic, with a weak suck, apnea, lethargy, and failure to thrive, usually they experience partial-onset seizures. Dysmorphic features, present in 25% of the children, include a broad nasal bridge, upturned nose, micrognathia, low-set and posteriorly rotated ears, short fingers and arms, simian creases, hypospadias, and anterior-placed anus. The less severe/moderate form presents at 3–6 mo of age with hypotonia, psychomotor retardation, intermittent ataxia and apnea, pyramidal signs, cranial nerve palsies, optic atrophy, deceleration of somatic and head growth, seizures (partial seizures and infantile spasms), and similar dysmorphic features. The milder form presents in childhood with intermittent ataxia, postexercise fatigue, and transient paraparesis, with normal neurological status in between episodes. Asymptomatic carriers have also been identified *(57–60)*.

Neuropathological abnormalities include a small brain with gross dilatation of the ventricles, absent corpus callosum and medullary pyramids, olivary heterotopias, hypomyelination and cavitating cystic lesions in the brainstem, basal ganglia, and cortex *(61)*.

The diagnosis of PDH deficiency is made by documenting an elevation of lactate and pyruvate (with a normal ratio) in blood and CSF, or in CSF only. Blood lactate levels may be elevated intermittently in children with less severe forms of PDH. Magnetic resonance spectroscopy may be helpful as an adjunctive test and will show lactic acid accumulation in the brain. Testing PDH complex residual activity in cultured fibroblasts is diagnostic in boys but is less reliable in girls owing to the tissue-specific variability.

Currently used treatments for PDH include high doses of the thiamine cofactor, attempts to activate the PDH complex with dichloroacetate (an inhibitor of PDH kinase), and use of a carbohydrate-restricted, high-fat KD *(62–64)*. There are no large outcome studies comparing these interventions. However, individual case reports and a small case series suggest that early intervention with the KD is related to increased longevity and improved mental development *(65,66)*.

2. CONTRAINDICATIONS

2.1. Is There a True Dietary Reference Intake for Carbohydrates?

The amount of dietary carbohydrate needed for optimal health in humans is unknown. In the few older studies of populations that consume low-carbohydrate and high-fat and high-protein diets for their lifetime (the Masai, Greenland natives, Inuits, and indigenous people of the South American Pampas), there were no apparent effects on health or longevity *(67,68)*. The new dietary reference intake (DRI) for carbohydrates is set at 130 g/d for adults and children *(69)*. This amount was based on the average minimum amount of glucose utilized by the brain. The average American eats two to three times this amount of carbohydrate daily.

The typical KD consists of 80–90% calories from fat, protein prescribed at recommended daily allowance (RDA, if possible), and the remaining calories as carbohydrates. The total carbohydrate content per day in the KD is often under 10 g (much more restrictive than the popular Atkins diet, which tries to keep the carbohydrate content under 40 g) *(70)*. The KD treatment period is typically limited to 3 yr (2-yr treatment, 1-yr wean), but some patients have been treated for significantly longer periods (up to 10–20 yr). The long-term effects of the KD on children's overall health have not been studied well and will need further investigation (*see* Chapter 9, this volume).

2.2. Inborn Errors of Metabolism in Which the KD Is Contraindicated

There are definitive contraindications to the use of the KD. These include defects in fat metabolism and disorders that require high carbohydrate contents. Failure to diagnose these disorders before starting the KD could result in significant morbidity and may be fatal. These contraindications should therefore be considered in every child before the KD treatment is started.

2.2.1. β-OXIDATION DEFECTS

β-Oxidation defects were first described in 1973, and since then at least 22 additional inborn errors of metabolism have been identified. The defects may involve fatty acid transport and activation, the carnitine cycle, enzymes of β-oxidation, and finally, ketone body production *(71–73)*. The mechanism of fatty acid oxidation is complicated. Free fatty acids (FFA) are released into the blood from dietary sources or as a result of catabolism of fat stores during fasting and stress. FFAs are then metabolized in two intracellular compartments. FFAs with a carbon length of 20 or less are metabolized by β-oxidation in the mitochondria, whereas longer-chain fats are metabolized via the peroxisomal pathway. Mitochondrial β-oxidation involves transport of activated acyl-CoA, with the help of carnitine, into the mitochondria, sequential removal of two carbon acyl-CoA units that becomes fuel for the tricarboxylic acid cycle or the production of ketone bodies *(74)*.

There is tremendous clinical heterogeneity in fatty acid oxidation defects. Patients may be asymptomatic between attacks or severely affected from a young age. Attacks are brought on by illness, stress, and prolonged fasting. The spectrum of clinical symptoms may include hypotonia, myopathy, cardiomyopathy, recurrent rhabdomyolysis with myoglobinuria, Reye-like syndrome with liver failure, intermittent altered levels of consciousness, neuropathy, and seizures. Concurrent with the symptoms are often a nonketotic hypoglycemia, unexplained metabolic acidosis, hyperammonemia, dicarboxylic aciduria, elevated creatinine kinase, and carnitine deficiency.

Metabolic testing utilized to diagnose fatty acid oxidation defects includes urine organic acids, plasma acylcarnitine profile, free fatty acid profile, plasma lactate/pyruvate, fibroblast oxidation and flux studies, specific enzyme analysis, and, finally, a challenge testing that may or may not include a period of fasting *(75,76)*.

Treatment consists of avoidance of fasting, limiting the fat content in meals (often to DRI or <25%), and using a high percentage of complex carbohydrates in the diet *(74,77)*. Continuous nasogastric or gastrostomy tube feedings are often used during the night. Other supplementation of the diet in these patients depends on the exact diagnosis and enzymatic defect, for example, carnitine (carnitine cycle defect), riboflavin (multiple acyl co-A dehydrogenase deficiencies), and medium-chain triglycerides (long-chain fatty acid defects).

2.2.2. PORPHYRIAS

Porphyrias are a related group of diseases caused by inherited blocks in heme biosynthesis. Acute intermittent porphyria results from deficiency of porphobilinogen (PBG) deaminase. It is an autosomal dominant disorder, and the gene is located on chromosome 11 *(78)*. There is great variability in the phenotypic expression, and 90% of affected individuals never have clinical symptoms. Attacks are triggered by hormonal changes and exposure to certain drugs, particularly barbiturates *(79)*. Clinical symptoms are often gastrointestinal (severe abdominal pain, vomiting, constipation, or diarrhea), but neurological symptoms (pain, muscle weakness, hyporeflexia secondary to neuropathy, altered mental status and seizures) are also common *(80,81)*. Diagnosis is made by increased amounts of aminolevulinic acid and PBG during attacks or measurement of PBG deaminase activity in erythrocytes. Carbohydrates reduce porphyrin synthesis and are therefore used at high doses (300–500 g/d) intravenously during an attack *(82,83)*. The KD could potentially worsen the condition and should not be used to treat seizures in a patient with acute intermittent porphyria *(84)*.

2.3. Medications and the KD

There are no absolute contraindications to using a medication while a child is treated with the KD (see Appendix A). Children on the KD will have the normal myriad childhood diseases (otitis media, strep throat, etc.), which will require treatment with antibiotics and other medicines. However, the need for absolute control over the daily carbohydrate intake to maintain maximal ketosis makes these "outside drugs" the KD team's nightmare. The US Food and Drug Administration does not require the pharmaceutical industry to reveal the content of carbohydrates used as "fillers" in their medications. In addition, the composition of these fillers is frequently changed. The success of any KD program, therefore, depends on support from pharmacists and their ability to obtain reliable information about carbohydrate contents from pharmaceutical manufacturers. In general, suspensions are avoided because they are mixed with large amounts (grams/per milliliter) of carbohydrates, but even capsules and chewable tablets may contain sufficient amounts of carbohydrate to alter the degree of ketosis. Then it becomes necessary to decide whether to incorporate that amount of carbohydrate (in the medications) into the daily diet plan or to cover with extra fat while the child is ill.

Steroids are antiketogenic and will result in lower ketosis; therefore, steroids are not recommended while a child is treated with the KD. It is our center's experience that even inhaled steroids will alter the degree of ketosis significantly.

There has been little written about the concomitant use of AEDs and the KD. Is there a KD/AED rational polytherapy combination? Which AEDs work better, or worse, with the KD? There is no information about absorption, malabsorption, and adjustment in medication dosing to help guide treatment with this very-high-fat diet.

Diuretics, which may worsen dehydration and acidosis, should be used with caution in patients on the KD. Similarly, concerns have been raised about using AEDs, e.g., topiramate and zonisamide, that, as a secondary effect, cause acidosis. Bicitra can be successfully used to correct the acidosis in patients who need to remain on these AEDs while on the KD (85,86).

3. CONCLUSION

The primary indication for using the KD is medically refractory epilepsy. Seizure type, epilepsy syndrome, underlying etiology, and age do not appear to alter the effectiveness of the KD. The need for poly-therapy with recurrent AED side effects is also an indication for trying the KD. The KD is medically indicated for inborn errors of carbohydrate metabolism including pyruvate dehydrogenase deficiency and facilitated glucose transporter protein deficiency. Absolute contraindications for using the KD includes inborn errors of fat metabolism (β-oxidation defects, etc.) and any disorder that requires a high carboydrate intake. Relative contraindications include steroids, diuretics, and medications with a secondary effect of increasing acid load. They should all be used with caution.

REFERENCES

1. Engel J Jr. Intractable epilepsy: definition and neurobiology. Epilepsia, 2001;42(Suppl 6):3.
2. Dlugos DJ, et al. Response to first drug trial predicts outcome in childhood temporal lobe epilepsy. Neurology, 2001;57:2259–2264.
3. Keranen T, Riekkinen P. Severe epilepsy: diagnostic and epidemiological aspects. Acta Neurol Scand Suppl 1988;117:7–14.
4. Berg AT, et al. Predictors of intractable epilepsy in childhood: a case-control study. Epilepsia 1996;37:24–30.
5. Camfield PR, Camfield CS. Antiepileptic drug therapy: when is epilepsy truly intractable? Epilepsia 1996;37(Suppl 1):S60–S65.
6. Lefevre F, Aronson N. Ketogenic diet for the treatment of refractory epilepsy in children: a systematic review of efficacy. Pediatrics 2000;105:E46.
7. Benbadis SR, Tatum WO. Advances in the treatment of epilepsy. Am Fam Phys 2001;64:91–98.
8. Wheless JW, Baumgartner J, Ghanbari C. Vagus nerve stimulation and the ketogenic diet. Neurol Clin 2001;19:371–407.
9. Livingston S. The Diagnosis and Treatment of Convulsive Disorders in Children. Charles C. Thomas, Springfield, IL, 1954.
10. Keith HM. Convulsive Disorders in Children with Reference to Treatment with the Ketogenic Diet. Little, Brown, Boston, 1963.

11. Vining EPG, et al. A multicenter study of the efficacy of the ketogenic diet. Arch Neurol 1998;55:1433–1437.
12. Kinsman SL, et al. Efficacy of the ketogenic diet for intractable seizure disorders: review of 58 cases. Epilepsia 1992;33:1132–1136.
13. Freeman JM, et al. The efficacy of the ketogenic diet–1998: a prospective evaluation of intervention in 150 children. Pediatrics 1998;102:1358–1363.
14. Maydell BV, et al. Efficacy of the ketogenic diet in focal versus generalized seizures. Pediatr Neurol 2001;25:208–212.
15. Hemingway C, et al. The ketogenic diet: a 3- to 6-year follow-up of 150 children enrolled prospectively. Pediatrics 2001;108:898–905.
16. Coppola G, et al. The ketogenic diet in children, adolescents and young adults with refractory epilepsy: an Italian multicentric experience. Epilepsy Res 2002;48:221–227.
17. DiMario FJ Jr, Holland J. The ketogenic diet: a review of the experience at Connecticut Children's Medical Center. Pediatr Neurol 2002;26:288–292.
18. Hassan AM, et al. Ketogenic diet in the treatment of refractory epilepsy in childhood. Pediatr Neurol 1999;21:548–552.
19. Katyal NG, et al. The ketogenic diet in refractory epilepsy: the experience of Children's Hospital of Pittsburgh. Clin Pediatr 2000;39:153–159.
20. Nordli DR, Jr, et al. Experience with the ketogenic diet in infants. Pediatrics 2001;108:129–133.
21. Persson B, Settergren G, Dahlquist G. Cerebral arterio-venous differences of acetoacetate and D-betahydroxybutyrate in children. Acta Paediatr Scand 1972;61:273–278.
22. Barborka CJ. Epilepsy in adults: results of treatment by ketogenic diet in one hundred cases. Arch Neurol Psychiatr 1930;23:904.
23. Sirven J, et al. The ketogenic diet for intractable epilepsy in adults: preliminary results. Epilepsia 1999;40:1721–1726.
24. Gordon N. Medium-chain triglycerides in a ketogenic diet. Dev Med Child Neurol 1977;19:535–538.
25. Huttenlocher PR. Ketonemia and seizures: metabolic and anticonvulsant effects of two ketogenic diets in childhood epilepsy. Pediatr Res 1976;10:536–540.
26. Livingston S, Pauli LL. Ketogenic diet and epilepsy. Dev Med Child Neurol 1975;17:818–819.
27. Berman W. The ketogenic diet, West and Lennox syndromes. Dev Med Child Neurol 1975;17:255.
28. Freeman JM, Vining EPG. Seizures decrease rapidly after fasting: preliminary studies of the ketogenic diet. Arch Pediatr Adolesc Med 1999;153:946–949.
29. Kossoff EH, et al. Efficacy of the ketogenic diet for infantile spasms. Pediatrics 2002;109:780–783.
30. Bergqvist AG, et al. Treatment of acquired epileptic aphasia with the ketogenic diet. J Child Neurol 1999;14:696–701.
31. Shafrir Y, Prensky AL. Acquired epileptiform opercular syndrome: a second case report, review of the literature, and comparison to the Landau–Kleffner syndrome. Epilepsia 1995;36:1050–1057.
32. Haas RH, et al. Therapeutic effects of a ketogenic diet in Rett syndrome. Am J Med Genet 1986;24(Suppl 1):225–246.
33. Pulsifer MB, et al. Effects of ketogenic diet on development and behavior: preliminary report of a prospective study. Dev Med Child Neurol 2001;43:301–306.
34. Freeman JM, Vining EPG. Ketogenic diet: a time-tested, effective, and safe method for treatment of intractable childhood epilepsy. Epilepsia 1998;39:450–451.
35. Nordli DR Jr, DeVivo DC. The ketogenic diet revisited: back to the future. Epilepsia 1997;38:743–749.
36. Kayano T, et al. Evidence for a family of human glucose transporter–like proteins. Sequence and gene localization of a protein expressed in fetal skeletal muscle and other tissues. J Biol Chem 1988;263:15245–15248.
37. Maher F, Vannucci SJ, Simpson IA. Glucose transporter proteins in brain. FASEB J 1994;8:1003–1011.
38. DeVivo DC, et al. Defective glucose transport across the blood–brain barrier as a cause of persistent hypoglycorrhachia, seizures, and developmental delay. N Engl J Med 1991;325:703–709.
39. Klepper J, Voit T. Facilitated glucose transporter protein type 1 (GLUT1) deficiency syndrome: impaired glucose transport into brain—a review. Eur J Pediatr 2002;161:295–304.
40. Clark DD, Sokoloff L. Basic Neurochemistry: Molecular, Cellular and Medical Aspects. Raven, New York, 1994.

41. Vannucci RC, Vannucci SJ. Glucose metabolism in the developing brain. Semin Perinatol 2000;24:107–115.
42. Cremer JE. Substrate utilization and brain development. J Cereb Blood Flow Metab 1982;2:394–407.
43. Klepper J, et al. Glucose transporter protein syndrome. Neuropediatrics 1998;29:A9.
44. Klepper J, et al. GTPS: Defining a new syndrome. Neurology 1998;50:A6.
45. Brockmann K, et al. Autosomal dominant glut-1 deficiency syndrome and familial epilepsy. Ann Neurol 2001;50:476–485.
46. Klepper J, et al. Defective glucose transport across brain tissue barriers:a newly recognized neurological syndrome. Neurochem Res 1999;24:587–594.
47. Brockmann K, Korenke CG, von Moers A. Epilepsy with seizures after fasting and retardation:the first familial cases of glucose transporter protein (GLUT 1) deficiency. Eur J Paediatr Neurol 1999;3:A90–A91.
48. Klepper J, et al. Erythocyte 3-O-methyl-D glucose uptake assay for diagnosis of glucose transporter protein syndrome. J Clin Lab Anal 1999;13:116–121.
49. Stewart WA, Gordon K, Camfield P. Acute pancreatitis causing death in a child on the ketogenic diet. J Child Neurol 2001;16:682.
50. Chugani HT. Development of regional brain glucose metabolism in relation to behavior and plasticity. In: Dawson G, Fisher KW (eds.). Human Behavior and the Developing Brain. Guilford, New York 1994, pp. 153–175.
51. Robinson B. Lactic acidemia. Biochim Biophys Acta 1993;1182:231–244.
52. Brown GK, et al. Pyruvate dehydrogenase deficiency. J Med Genet 1994;31:875–879.
53. Robinson B, MacKay N, Petrova-Benedict R. Defects in the E2 lipoyltransacetylase and the X-lipoyl-containing components of the pyruvate dehydrogenase complex in patients with lactic acidemia. J Clin Invest 1990;85:1821–1824.
54. Brown RM, Head RA, Brown GK. Pyruvate dehydrogenase E3 binding protein deficiency. Hum Genet 2002;110:187–191.
55. Brown RM, Dahl HH, Brown GK. X-chromosome localization of the functional gene for the E1 alpha subunit of the human pyruvate dehydrogenase complex. Genomics 1989;4:174–181.
56. Dahl HH. Pyruvate dehydrogenase E1 alpha deficiency: males and females differ yet again. Am J Hum Genet 1995;56:553–557.
57. Stansbie D, Wallace SJ, Marsac C. Disorders of the pyruvate dehydrogenase complex. J Inher Metab Dis 1986;9:105–119.
58. DeVivo DC. The expanding clinical spectrum of mitochondrial diseases. Brain Dev 1993;15:1–22.
59. DeVivo DC. Leigh syndrome:historical perspective and clinical variations. Biofactors 1998;7:269–271.
60. Canafoglia L. et al. Epileptic phenotypes associated with mitochondrial disorders. Neurology 2001;56:1340–1346.
61. Chow CW, Thorburn DR. Morphological correlates of mitochondrial dysfunction in children. Hum Reprod 2000;15(Suppl 2):68–78.
62. Di Rocco M, et al. Outcome of thiamine treatment in a child with Leigh disease due to thiamine-responsive pyruvate dehydrogenase deficiency. Eur J Paediatr Neurol 2000;4:115–117.
63. Morten KJ, et al. Dichloroacetate stabilizes the mutant E1 alpha subunit in pyruvate dehydrogenase deficiency. Neurology 1999;53:612–616.
64. Naito E, et al. Thiamine-responsive pyruvate dehydrogenase deficiency in two patients caused by a point mutation (F205L and L216F) within the thiamine pyrophosphate binding region. Biochim Biophys Acta 2002;1588:79–84.
65. Falk RE, et al. Ketonic diet in the management of pyruvate dehydrogenase deficiency. Pediatrics 1976;58:713–721.
66. Wexler ID, et al. Outcome of pyruvate dehydrogenase deficiency treated with ketogenic diets. Studies in patients with identical mutations. Neurology 1997;49:1655–1661.
67. Du Bois EF. The control of protein in the diet. J Am Diet Assoc 1928;4:53–76.
68. Heinbecker P. Studies on the metabolism of Eskimos. J Biol Chem 1928;80:461–475.
69. Trumbo P, et al. Dietary reference intakes for energy, carbohydrate, fiber, fat, fatty acids, cholesterol, protein and amino acids. J Am Diet Assoc 2002;102:1621–1630.
70. Atkins RC. Dr Atkins' New Diet Revolution, rev. ed. Avon, New York, 1998.

71. Vockley J, Singh RH, Whiteman DA. Diagnosis and management of defects of mitochondrial beta-oxidation. Curr Opin Clin Nutr Metab Care 2002;5:601–609.

72. Vockley J, Whiteman DA. Defects of mitochondrial beta-oxidation: a growing group of disorders. Neuromuscular Dis 2002;12:235–246.

73. Vianey-Liaud C, et al. The inborn errors of mitochondrial fatty acid oxidation. J Inher Metab Dis 1987;10 (Suppl 1):159–200.

74. Rinaldo P, Matern D, Bennett MJ. Fatty acid oxidation disorders. Annu Rev Physiol 2002;64:477–502.

75. Rabier D, et al. Do criteria exist from urinary organic acids to distinguish beta-oxidation defects? J Inher Metab Dis 1995;18:257–260.

76. Coates PM. New developments in the diagnosis and investigation of mitochondrial fatty acid oxidation disorders. Eur J Pediatr 1994;153 (7 Suppl 1):S49–S56.

77. Bennett MJ, Rinaldo P, Strauss AW. Inborn errors of mitochondrial fatty acid oxidation. Crit Rev Clin Lab Sci 2000;37:1–44.

78. Schuurmans MM, et al. Influence of age and gender on the clinical expression of acute intermittent porphyria based on molecular study of porphobilinogen deaminase gene among Swiss patients. Mol Med 2001;7:535–542.

79. Andersson C, Innala E, Backstrom T. Acute intermittent porphyria in women: clinical expression, use and experience of exogenous sex hormones. A population-based study in northern Sweden. J Intern Med 2003;254:176–183.

80. Wikberg A, Andersson C, Lithner F. Signs of neuropathy in the lower legs and feet of patients with acute intermittent porphyria. J Intern Med 2000;248:27–32.

81. Sykes RM. Acute intermittent porphyria, seizures, and antiepileptic drugs: a report on a 3-year-old Nigerian boy. Seizure 2001;10:64–66.

82. Regan L, Gonsalves L, Tesar G. Acute intermittent porphyria. Psychosomatics 1999;40:521–523.

83. Yano Y, Kondo M. Acute intermittent porphyria (AIP). Ryoikibetsu Shokogun Shirizu 1998;19(Pt 2):136–138.

84. Zadra M, et al. Treatment of seizures in acute intermittent porphyria: safety and efficacy of gabapentin. Seizure 1998;7:415–416.

85. Takeoka M, et al. Concomitant treatment with topiramate and ketogenic diet in pediatric epilepsy. Epilepsia 2002;43:1072–1075.

86. Kossoff EH, et al. Kidney stones, carbonic anhydrase inhibitors, and the ketogenic diet. Epilepsia 2002;43:1168–1171.

9 Complications of the Ketogenic Diet

Karen R. Ballaban-Gil

1. INTRODUCTION

The ketogenic diet (KD) is a high-fat, low-carbohydrate, low-protein diet used in the treatment of pediatric epilepsy since the 1920s *(1)*. Currently, it is being used primarily for refractory childhood epilepsy. There have been numerous uncontrolled clinical trials, mostly retrospective, which have demonstrated the diet's efficacy in reducing seizure frequency in children with refractory epilepsy *(2)*. However, adverse events have not been consistently reported in these studies, and few serious complications caused by the classic or modified KD have been reported. This chapter reviews the literature regarding adverse events that have been associated with the KD.

2. ADVERSE EFFECTS DURING INITIATION OF THE KETOGENIC DIET

Short-term complications during the initiation of the KD include dehydration, hypoglycemia, acidosis, vomiting, diarrhea, and refusal to eat *(3)*. These complications may be secondary to either the fast or the diet itself. Fluid restriction, which remains a controversial aspect of the KD, contributes to the dehydration and metabolic acidosis, which in turn can cause vomiting and lethargy. Children should therefore be monitored carefully during the initiation of the KD, so that these complications can be avoided and treated if necessary.

In children with undiagnosed underlying metabolic abnormalities, including porphyria, pyruvate carboxylase deficiency, carnitine deficiency, fatty oxidation defects, and mitochondrial disorders, the fasting phase can cause a life-threatening decompensation *(4)*. In their series of 32 infants treated with the KD, Nordli et al. *(5)* reported one infant who became hypoglycemic and comatose 8 d after diet initiation. DeVivo and colleagues *(6)* also reported one case of mental status changes and coma.

3. ADVERSE EFFECTS DURING MAINTENANCE OF THE KETOGENIC DIET

Minor side effects of the KD that have been reported include metabolic derangements (hyperuricemia [2%], hypocalcemia [2%], decreased amino acid levels, acidosis

From: *Epilepsy and the Ketogenic Diet*
Edited by: C. E. Stafstrom and J. M. Rho © Humana Press Inc., Totowa, NJ

[2–4%]), gastrointestinal symptoms (vomiting, constipation, diarrhea, abdominal pain) *(12–50%)* irritability, lethargy (4–9%), and refusal to eat *(2,7–12)*. Carnitine deficiency has also been demonstrated in some children on the KD *(13–15)*. Hypercholesterolemia has been reported in 29–59% of children on the KD *(10–12)*. Theda et al. *(16)* found an elevation of very-long-chain fatty acids in 13 of 22 plasma samples from KD patients.

3.1. Renal Calculi

Kidney stones have been reported in 3–7% of children on the KD *(7,17–22)*. This is significantly greater than the overall rate of urolithiasis in children. The average time on the diet prior to development of stones is approx 18 mo *(19,20)*, but stones have been reported within the first month on the diet. The few studies that have looked more carefully at the composition of the stones *(20,21)* have reported uric acid stones, (approx 50% of the stones analyzed), calcium oxalate, calcium phosphate, and mixed calcium/uric acid stones.

The high rate of uric acid stones in KD patients is notable because uric acid stones account for only 1.3–7.6% of stones in children *(19)*. It seems that the KD particularly predisposes to the formation of these stones. Kielb *(20)* and Herzberg *(19)* and their colleagues hypothesized that the KD results in low urinary pH, which facilitates the formation of uric acid crystals because the solubility of uric acid decreases greatly as pH falls. In addition, the KD has been associated with uric acidemia and/or increased urinary uric acid *(20,21)*, which further predisposes to the development of uric acid stones. Fluid restriction compounds this, by producing more acidic urine and by decreasing urine flow, resulting in the precipitation of urate crystals.

Calcium crystal formation may be related to hypercalciuria, which also frequently results from the KD *(21,23)*. Additionally, the KD causes hypocitruria *(20,21)*, as a result of the chronic metabolic acidosis. Because urinary citrate is an important inhibitor of calcium crystal formation, the low urinary levels increase the risk of calcium stone formation. Fluid restriction similarly compounds the risk of calcium stone formation.

The majority of children with renal calculi present with gross or microscopic hematuria *(19,20)*. Therefore, patients on the KD should be regularly screened with urinalysis. Some researchers have suggested periodic evaluation of urinary calcium/creatinine ratios *(19)* and renal ultasonography *(20)*. Treatment and prevention of future renal calculi includes fluid liberalization and/or urinary alkalization with bicitrate.

3.2. Growth on the KD

There are anecdotal reports suggesting that linear growth is retarded in children on the KD *(17)*. Couch et al. *(24)* retrospectively evaluated the nutritional status and growth of 21 children treated for 6 mo with the KD. They found a significant increase in both height and weight after 6 mo on the diet. Six children had a decrease in mean percentile standard weight for height, but no child fell below his or her original height for age percentile after 6 mo on the diet. The investigators concluded that linear growth was maintained at 6 mo in patients on the KD but suggested that longer follow-up was needed to assess whether linear growth was maintained beyond 6 mo *(24)*.

Williams et al. *(25)* reported a retrospective review of linear growth velocity in 21 children treated with the KD for 9.6 mo to 2 yr (median 1.2 yr). Eighteen of the children (86%) experienced a fall from their original height percentiles while on the diet. The authors concluded that growth may be retarded while on the KD, and this effect was independent of mean age, length of time on the diet, or protein and energy intake per body weight *(25)*. The authors also surmised that decreased linear growth may be secondary to poor nutritional status. Although children received the recommended nutrient intake for protein, energy (calories) was generally restricted to 75% of recommended daily intake. These investigators postulated that dietary protein was therefore being used for energy and gluconeogenesis, resulting in insufficient protein to support growth *(25)*.

Vining and colleagues *(26)*, who reported prospectively on the growth of 237 children treated with the KD, found that the oldest children "appear to grow taller almost normally"; but there was a suggestion that younger children fell more than 2 SD below the mean in height or stature change—that is, they grew poorly.

3.3. Increased Infections

Increased infections have been reported in 2–4% of children on the KD *(8,27,28)*. Woody et al. *(28)*, who evaluated neutrophil function in 9 children on the KD, demonstrated that while ketotic, patients had significantly less bacterial phagocytosis and killing. These effects reversed upon discontinuation of the diet. Similar impairments in neutrophil responses have been reported in patients with ketosis from other etiologies, including diabetes mellitus, alcoholism, glycogen storage disease, protein-calorie malnutrition, intralipid infusions, and carbohydrate-restricted weight reduction diets in adults *(28)*. The mechanism of the neutrophil dysfunction is not fully understood but is thought to be related to serum metabolites that affect early events in phagocytosis *(28)*. Only one of Woody's 9 patients experienced serious bacterial infections.

3.4. Bleeding Abnormalities

Bruising and easy bleeding have been anecdotally reported in patients on the KD *(29)*. Berry-Kravis and colleagues *(29)* prospectively and retrospectively evaluated the incidence of bruising and abnormal bleeding in 51 KD patients. Sixteen (31.4%) reported increased bruising, and 3 (5.9%) reported bleeding problems. There was no relationship between the occurrence of these side effects and the use of other antiepileptic drugs (AEDs), and some patients with these complaints were on no other AEDs. Six of the 15 patients with increased bruising/bleeding were studied in detail, including testing for platelet count, prothrombin time (PT), partial thromboplastin time (PTT), bleeding time, platelet function, and Von Willebrand disease. Five of the six had prolonged bleeding times, and all had abnormalities of platelet aggregation. One of the six patients was reevaluated off the diet, with normalization of bleeding time and platelet aggregation tests. The authors postulated that this dysfunction may be related to direct effects of ketosis on platelet effector systems or to changes in platelet membrane lipid composition, with resulting changes in the function of membrane-embedded proteins *(29)*. None of their patients experienced serious clinical complications as a result of the bleeding tendency.

3.5. Cardiac Complications

Cardiac abnormalities in children on the KD have been reported, including cardiomyopathy and prolonged QT interval (QT_c) *(30–32)*. Ballaban-Gil *(31)* reported 2 children who developed severe, life-threatening dilated cardiomyopathy while on the KD. In both cases, the cardiomyopathy resolved following discontinuation of the KD. Bergqvist et al. *(30)* reported one child with cardiomyopathy in association with selenium deficiency and others who had KD-induced lowering of selenium levels. Best and colleagues *(32)* screened 20 patients on the KD and found that 3 patients (15%) had prolongation of the QT_c interval. Pre-KD electrocardiograms (ECGs) were available on 2 of the 3 patients, and these confirmed that the QT_c abnormalities developed while the children were on the KD. Two of these patients had left atrial and left ventricular enlargement, and one had severe ventricular dilatation and dysfunction with associated clinical symptoms of heart failure. All the patients in Best's series had normal selenium levels. Best postulated that a greater degree of acidosis and higher β-hydroxybutyrate levels may be associated with the development of cardiac complications. The authors suggested that children on the KD should have ECGs and echocardiograms performed before initiation of the diet and while maintained on the KD regimen.

3.6. Optic Neuropathy

A symmetrical, bilateral optic neuropathy has been reported in two children on the KD *(33)*. Both patients were found to have thiamine deficiency, and both had recovery of normal visual acuity following thiamine administration. Supplementation with vitamin B can prevent this adverse event.

3.7. Pancreatitis

Stewart et al. *(34)* reported a case of a 9-yr-old girl who died from acute hemorrhagic pancreatitis while on the KD. There was no definitive proof that the pancreatitis was secondary to the diet, but the authors presented a potential pathophysiologic mechanism. Hyperlipidemia and hypertriglyceridemia are risk factors for the development of pancreatitis, and the ketogenic diet can be associated with hyperlipidemia. Unfortunately, these levels were not measured in this patient prior to her death.

3.8. Hypoproteinemia

Ballaban-Gil et al. *(35)* reported two children on the KD who developed severe hypoproteinemia, one of whom also developed lipemia and hemolytic anemia. Both patients were receiving adequate dietary protein and had no evidence of protein loss. Although a possible underlying inborn error of metabolism could result in breakdown of body proteins for energy metabolism, no such inborn errors of metabolism were identified.

3.9. Potentiation of Valproate Toxicity

Ballaban-Gil and colleagues *(35)* reported three patients who apparently developed valproate (VPA) toxicity after initiation of the KD. All had been on stable doses of VPA prior to initiation of the KD. One of the patients developed a Fanconi renal tubular acidosis within 1 mo of diet initiation. Renal function normalized after discontinuation of VPA while the patient remained on the KD. Two additional patients developed marked elevation of liver function tests on the combination of VPA and the KD. One patient developed these abnormalities during diet initiation, while the other developed these 7 mo after starting the KD, in association with a viral illness. Both patients remained on the KD and recovered when VPA was discontinued. The mechanism of potentiation of VPA toxicity was not known. The authors postulated that the hepatotoxicity may have involved impairment of fatty acid oxidation by VPA and/or the additive effects of VPA and the KD in the development of carnitine deficiency.

4. VERY-LONG-TERM (>2 YR) COMPLICATIONS

There have been no reports of the adverse events associated with the continuation of the KD for more than 2 yr, but there is only one report in the literature looking at this small subgroup of children *(18)*. In particular, long-term effects of this high-fat diet on the cardiovascular system remain to be determined.

5. CONCLUSION

The KD is an effective treatment for refractory childhood epilepsy. However, as with all other medical therapies, there are potential adverse effects. Physicians need to be aware of these potential risks so that they can properly counsel parents and monitor children for development of these complications. It is also critical that clinicians continue to report serious adverse events associated with the diet, even if the diet's causative role is uncertain.

REFERENCES

1. Wilder RM. The effect of ketonemia on the course of epilepsy. Mayo Clin Proc 1921;2:307–308.
2. Lefevre F, Aronson N. Ketogenic diet for the treatment of refractory epilepsy in children: a systematic review of efficacy. Pediatrics 2000;105:E46.
3. Peterman MG, The ketogenic diet in epilepsy. JAMA 1925;84:1979–1983.
4. Wheless JW. The ketogenic diet: an effective medical therapy with side effects. J Child Neurol 2001;16:633–635.
5. Nordli DR Jr, Kuroda MM, Carroll J, et al. Pediatrics 2001;108:129–133.
6. DeVivo DC, Pagliara AS, Prensky AL. Ketotic hypoglycemia and the ketogenic diet. Neurology 1973;23:640–649.
7. Kinsman SL, Vining EPG, Quaskey SA, et al. Efficacy of the ketogenic diet for intractable seizure disorders: review of 58 cases. Epilepsia 1992;33:1132–1136.
8. Summ JM, Woch MA, McNeil T, et al. Success and complications of the ketogenic diet for intractable childhood epilepsy. Epilepsia 1996;37 (Suppl 5):109.
9. Schwartz RH, Boyes S, Aynsley-Green A. Metabolic effects of three ketogenic diets in the treatment of severe epilepsy. Dev Med Child Neurol 1989;31:152–160.
10. Vining EPG, Kwiterovich P, Hsieh S et al. The effect of the ketogenic diet on plasma cholesterol. Epilepsia 1996;37 (Suppl 5):109.
11. Chesney D, Brouhard BH, Wyllie E, Powaski K. Biochemical abnormalities of the ketogenic diet in children. Clin Pediatr 1999;38:107–109.
12. Delgado MR, Mills J, Sparagana S. Hypercholesterolemia associated with the ketogenic diet. Epilepsia 1996;37 (Suppl 5):108.
13. Demeritte EL, Ventimiglia J, Coyne M, Nigro MA. Organic acid disorders and the ketogenic diet. Ann Neurol 1996;40:305.
14. Rutledge SL, Kinsman SL, Geraghry MT, Vining EPG, Thomas G. Hypocarnitinemia and the ketogenic diet. Ann Neurol 1989;26:472.
15. Berry-Kravis E, Booth G, Sanchez AC, Woodbury-Kolb J. Carnitine levels and the ketogenic diet. Epilepsia 2001;42:1445–1451.
16. Theda C, Woody RC, Naidu S, et al. Increased very long chain fatty acids in patients on a ketogenic diet: a cause of diagnostic confusion. J Pediatr 1993;122:724–726.
17. Hopkins IJ, Lynch BC. Use of ketogenic diet in epilepsy in childhood. Aust Paediatr J 1970;6:25–29.
18. Hemingway C, Freeman JM, Pillas DJ, Pyzik PL. The ketogenic diet: a 3 to 6 year follow-up of 150 children enrolled prospectively. Pediatrics 2001;108:898–905.
19. Herzberg GZ, Fivush BA, Kinsman SL, Gearhart JP. Urolithiasis associated with the ketogenic diet. J Pediatr;117:743–745.
20. Kielb S, Koo HP, Bloom DA, Faerber GJ. Nephrolithiasis associated with the ketogenic diet. J Urol 2000;164:464–466.

21. Furth SL, Casey JC, Pyzik PL et al. Risk factors for urolithiasis in children on the ketogenic diet. Pediatr Nephrol 2000;15:125–128.
22. Kossoff EH, Pyzik PL, Furth SL. Kidney stones, carbonic anhydrase inhibitors, and the ketogenic diet. Epilepsia 2002;43:1168–1171.
23. Dodson WE, Prensky AL, DeVivo DC, et al. Management of seizure disorders: selected aspects. Part 2. J Pediatr 1976;89:695–703.
24. Couch SC, Schwarzman F, Carroll J, et al. Growth and nutritional outcomes of children treated with the ketogenic diet. J Am Diet Assoc 1999;99:1573–1575.
25. Williams S, Basualdo-Hammond C, Curtis R, Schuller R. Growth retardation in children with epilepsy on the ketogenic diet: a retrospective chart review. J Am Diet Assoc 2002;102:405–407.
26. Vining EP, Pyzik P, McGrogan J, et al. Growth of children on the ketogenic diet. Dev Med Child Neurol 2002;44:796–802.
27. Vining EPG, Freeman JM, Ballaban-Gil K, et al. A multicenter study of the efficacy of the ketogenic diet. Arch Neurol 1998;55:1433–1437.
28. Woody RC, Steele RW, Knapple WL, Pilkington NS Jr. Impaired neutrophil function in children with seizures treated with the ketogenic diet. J Pediatr 1989;115:427–430.
29. Berry-Kravis E, Booth G, Taylor A, Valentino LA. Bruising and the ketogenic diet: evidence for diet-induced changes in platelet function. Ann Neurol 2001;49:98–103.
30. Bergqvist AGC, Chee CM, Lutchka L, Rychik J, Stallings VA. Selenium deficiency associated with cardiomyopathy: a complication of the ketogenic diet. Epilepsia 2003;44:618–620.
31. Ballaban-Gil KR. Cardiomyopathy associated with the ketogenic diet. Epilepsia 1999;40 (Suppl 7):129.
32. Best TH, Franz DN, Gilbert DL, et al. Cardiac complications in pediatric patients on the ketogenic diet. Neurology 2000;54:2328–2330.
33. Hoyt CS, Billson FA. Optic neuropathy in ketogenic diet. Br J Ophthalmol 1979;63:191–194.
34. Stewart WA, Gordon K, Camfield P. Acute pancreatitis causing death in a child on the ketogenic diet. J Child Neurol 2001;16:682.
35. Ballaban-Gil K, Callahan C, O'Dell C, et al. Complications of the ketogenic diet. Epilepsia 1998;39:744–748.

10

Measuring and Interpreting Ketosis and Fatty Acid Profiles in Patients on a High-Fat Ketogenic Diet

Kathy Musa-Veloso and Stephen C. Cunnane

1. INTRODUCTION

Despite over 80 yr of clinical experience with high-fat ketogenic diets (KDs) in the treatment of refractory seizures, we do not understand their anticonvulsant mechanism. In addition, it is difficult to monitor the efficacy of the diet and predict seizure outcome. Patients usually follow the diet for up to 3 mo before deciding whether to continue with it *(1)*. Like many aspects of the KD, this 3-mo "trial period" has been set arbitrarily. There are no clear scientific predictors of which patients will and will not eventually respond to the diet. Unfortunately, without reliable markers of seizure outcome, we cannot adequately predict seizure response or which patient will benefit from the diet.

At present, ketone bodies (ketones) are widely used as markers of seizure control. However, the association between ketosis and seizure control is controversial; thus, a comprehensive review of the assessment and interpretation of ketone measures is presented here. A review of the measurement and interpretation of fatty acid profiles in KD patients is also presented, because certain fatty acids may be important in reducing seizure susceptibility and predicting seizure outcome.

2. MEASURING KETOSIS IN PATIENTS ON THE KETOGENIC DIET

One of the immediate consequences of consuming a high-fat KD is an increase in the hepatic production of ketones, namely acetoacetate (AcAc), β-hydroxybutyrate (β-HBA), and acetone (ACET). Since ketosis is a hallmark of the KD, attempts to quantify ketone levels in KD patients have been made since the 1920s, when the KD's anticonvulsant properties were first being demonstrated. Though the relationship between ketosis and seizure control remains undefined, quantification of ketones is necessary for several reasons. Before the initiation of the KD, the hospitalized patient is usually fasted for 24–48 h *(1);* the objectives of this preliminary fast are to deplete liver and muscle glycogen stores and to "jump-start" ketogenesis as the body begins to utilize

From: *Epilepsy and the Ketogenic Diet*
Edited by: C. E. Stafstrom and J. M. Rho © Humana Press Inc., Totowa, NJ

fatty acids for energy production. During this fasting period, the assessment of ketosis is crucial for determining whether the patient is becoming too ketotic and when he or she is ready to begin KD feeding. Furthermore, during the at-home maintenance of the KD, measures of ketosis are necessary for monitoring patient dietary compliance. Several methods of monitoring ketones exist; the following discussion summarizes the advantages and disadvantages of each type of measure and introduces novel approaches for measuring ketosis.

2.1. Urinary Dipstick Ketone Test

The ketone test that is most widely commercially available is the urinary dipstick test. This test utilizes reagent strips that contain the compound nitroprusside. If AcAc is present in the urine, it will react with the nitroprusside, resulting in the development of colors ranging from buff-pink to maroon. The color that develops is matched (as well as possible) to a color chart, and the corresponding AcAc concentration is then chosen from an exponential scale.

There are several drawbacks to using the urinary dipstick ketone test. Although we found a significant positive relationship between urinary AcAc measured enzymatically and with the dipsticks in mildly ketotic adults, the dipsticks significantly overestimated the level of AcAc in the urine (2). Consequently, we suggested that a correction factor be applied to dipstick values (2). Others found that the dipstick test did not accurately reflect actual blood ketone concentrations (3–6). This is most likely because factors such as state of hydration and acid–base balance have complex effects on renal hemodynamics, urine volume, and excretion of ketones (7). Also, because a urine sample is required for this test, frequent ketone testing is not possible; this is particularly problematic in fluid-restricted KD patients. Finally, because the urinary dipstick test is specific for AcAc, the levels of the other, potentially important, ketones, β-HBA and ACET, remain unknown. Despite the inadequacies of the urinary dipstick ketone test, it is used widely in hospital clinics and serves as the sole ketone measure in home settings.

2.2. Plasma Ketone Analyses

Plasma ketone analyses provide more accurate quantifications of ketones than the urinary dipstick ketone test but also have their shortcomings. Because these analyses require a blood sample, they are invasive, and frequent blood sampling from pediatric patients presents both logistical and ethical challenges. Also, because plasma ketones are analyzed in a laboratory, there is often a delay between collecting the sample and generating the result. Finally, the analytical requirements for the quantification of each plasma ketone are different. Consequently, data for all plasma ketones are rarely reported in a single study. The quantification of plasma β-HBA is a relatively straightforward procedure; there are enzymatic kits available for this, and even an experimental device (Stat-Site Meter, GDS Diagnostics, Elkhart, IN) that can assess β-HBA from the blood of a finger-prick. The quantification of plasma AcAc and plasma ACET, however, is not simple. Because AcAc is a very unstable molecule, either plasma samples must be analyzed for AcAc immediately after collection or the AcAc must be stabilized by derivatization for later analysis. There is no enzymatic assay available for plasma ACET. Rather, the analysis of this volatile ketone requires that the sample and standards be prepared and analyzed either by gas chromatography (8,9), or by high-performance liquid chromatography (HPLC) (10).

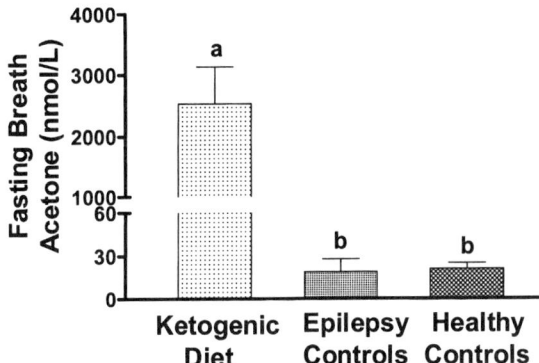

Fig. 1. Fasting breath acetone in ketogenic diet children, epilepsy controls, and healthy controls. Mean ± SEM; $n = 10$–13/group. Bars with different letters are significantly different ($p < 0.05$). At the time of the study, ketogenic diet children were consuming the classic ketogenic diet for a minimum of 1 mo. Epilepsy controls had epilepsy and were not being treated by a ketogenic diet but by anticonvulsant drugs. Healthy controls had no history of seizures and were not consuming any medications. (Reproduced with permission from ref. *16*.)

2.3. Breath Acetone as a Measure of Systemic Ketosis

Whereas AcAc, β-HBA, and ACET can all be measured in urine and plasma, ACET is distinct in that it is volatile and can be measured in the breath. Dietary manipulations such as fasting and KD consumption cause an increase in breath ACET *(2,11–16)*. Because blood ACET equilibrates readily with alveolar air *(7)*, we have been exploring breath ACET as a noninvasive measure of systemic ketosis in children with refractory seizures on a KD. In a recent study, we showed that children on a "classic" KD (based on dairy fat) had about 115 times more ACET in their breath than healthy or epilepsy controls (Fig. 1). In that study, we also documented that breath ACET levels in KD children ranged from 555 to 6671 nmol/L, although more recent studies we have conducted in KD children have revealed that the range is actually much larger (approx 100–20,000 nmol/L; unpublished). We have also found that in chronically ketotic rats and mildly ketotic adults, breath ACET is a significant predictor of plasma ketones *(2,15)*. Thus, it is possible to estimate the level of a plasma ketone from breath ACET by using an equation describing the specific relationship *(2,15)*.

Initially, we collected breath samples from children on a KD at home and transported them to the lab for ACET analysis by gas chromatography (*see* refs. *2* and *16* for analytical details). Once the potential to use breath ACET as a noninvasive marker of ketosis had become clear *(2,16)*, a collaboration was formed with Alcohol Countermeasure Systems Company (Mississauga, Ont, Canada) to develop a handheld breath acetone analyzer (HHBAA). The HHBAA is a battery-operated, rechargeable unit with a light-emitting display. It is activated by an on/off switch and has a warm-up time of approx 30 s. When the unit is warmed up, a beeping sound is heard, and the message, "blo" is displayed, indicating that the instrument is ready for a breath sample. The child provides a breath sample by blowing into a disposable mouthpiece that is inserted directly into the instrument. An ACET reading is then displayed, in nanomoles per liter. We have calibrated breath ACET measurements by the HHBAA against those analyzed by gas chromatography and have shown that the unit can accurately and reliably measure breath ACET levels exceeding 500 nmol/L *(17)*. The HHBAA was later used in a small multicenter clinical study including Bloorview MacMillan Children's Hospital (Toronto, Ont, Canada), The Hospital for Sick Children (Toronto), and Hôpital Ste-Justine (Montreal, Quebec, Canada) to assess the relationship between ketosis and seizure control, the results of which are pending.

Breath ACET has several advantages as an indicator of ketosis. Breath samples can be collected noninvasively, and the results are generated instantly. Also, breath samples can be collected and analyzed frequently with minimum discomfort and inconvenience to the patient—a property necessary for determining the relationship between ketosis and seizure control. At present, there are four important drawbacks of the current HHBAA prototype:

1. It is insensitive to breath ACET levels under 500 nmol/L.
2. Patients who are severely cognitively/developmentally delayed cannot use it.
3. It needs to be calibrated at least once a month to ensure optimal functioning.
4. It cannot discriminate between ACET and other volatile compounds, e.g., isopropanol, a metabolite of acetone, that may be emitted in large quantities.

Work is under way to deal with these shortcomings. Once a prototype more specific to ACET is developed, a large clinical study, perhaps including several KD clinics in North America, can be conducted to evaluate the importance of ketosis to seizure control.

3. ASSESSING KETONE LEVELS: CLINICAL CHALLENGES

The difficulty in reliably measuring the three different ketones has resulted in difficulties in interpreting the significance of elevation of individual ketones to seizure control. AcAc, β-HBA, and ACET are distinct, and an evaluation of the importance of ketosis to seizure control necessitates the quantification and comparison of all three ketones, not just one. For instance, the ratio of β-HBA to AcAc can be a useful marker of the patient's mitochondrial redox state, and this ratio may be more informative than the quantification of any one ketone *(18,19)*. Furthermore, all the methods of ketone analysis share a significant drawback: they assume that the ketone being measured is indicative of its concentration in the brain. Although ACET may readily cross the blood–brain barrier by diffusion, there is selective uptake of AcAc and β-HBA via a monocarboxylate transporter. Thus, the assumption that blood ketone concentrations are reflective of brain ketone concentrations may be incorrect.

To our knowledge, only Huttenlocher *(20)* has examined the relationship between plasma ketones and cerebrospinal fluid (CSF) ketones in humans on a KD. This analysis was done in only two KD patients, 4 d after the start of a KD based on medium-chain triglyceride (MCTs) oil. The results suggested that the CSF/plasma ratio of AcAc may be higher than that of β-HBA, an interesting observation inasmuch as plasma β-HBA exceeded plasma AcAc *(20)*. Further studies are needed to understand ketone uptake by the brain and the relationship between plasma and CSF ketone levels. Because the extraction of CSF from pediatric patients on a KD is quite invasive and ethically questionable, noninvasive proton magnetic resonance spectroscopy (^{1}H-MRS) can be employed to assess brain ketone concentrations in these patients *(21)*. Only then can systemic measures of ketosis be compared with brain ketone levels.

4. INTERPRETING KETONE LEVELS

Despite the lack of a commercially available, accurate, and reliable ketone test, the monitoring of ketosis is an established and integral aspect of the KD regimen. Unfortunately, the precise interpretation of ketone measures is perplexing and, at times, frustrating. Ketone measurements are useful in assessing patient dietary compliance, but their usefulness in predicting seizure outcome is unclear. Our current understanding of the importance of ketosis to seizure control is inadequate. As early as 1931, with only 10 yr of clinical experience with the KD, the importance of ketosis to seizure control was challenged when Bridge and Iob *(22)* observed that "Frequently no improvement results in spite of severe ketosis, and at times good results are obtained without the formation of ketone bodies … it has been impossible to establish any constant correlation." A comprehensive review of published clinical studies *(20,23–27)* indicates that ketosis is not always sufficient for seizure control, and that the precise role of ketones in conferring seizure resistance remains a conundrum (*see* Table 1). Interestingly, two of the six studies listed in Table 1 document a correlation between seizure reduction and an elevation in plasma lipids *(23,25)*. A closer look at these observations reveals that the KD can, in fact, lead to alterations in plasma lipid profiles, some of which may contribute to the efficacy of the KD.

5. EFFECTS OF LONG-CHAIN POLYUNSATURATED FATTY ACIDS (LC-PUFAS) ON SEIZURE SUSCEPTIBILITY

LC-PUFAs are essential for normal neurological and visual function in mammals *(28)*. Clinical, animal, and in vitro studies conducted within the last 10 yr cumulatively suggest that several LC-PUFAs (linoleic acid [LA] 18:2ω6; α-linolenic acid [ALA], 18:3ω3; eicosapentaenoic acid [EPA], 20:5ω3; docosahexaenoic acid [DHA], 22:6ω3; arachidonic acid [AA] 20:4ω6) may be beneficial in reducing seizure susceptibility *(29–34)* (*see* Table 2).

5.1. Clinical Studies

Schlanger et al. *(29)* evaluated the effects of ω3 PUFA in patients who had epilepsy secondary to another primary central nervous system disease (West syndrome, cerebral palsy, or Angelman syndrome). Five patients, all of whom were being treated with anticonvulsant drugs, were given 5 g of the supplement daily for 6 mo. The supplement was in the form of a semisolid bread spread of different flavors, and contained 65% ω3 PUFA (46% DHA, 18% EPA, 1% ALA) and 100 IU of vitamin E. All patients exhibited a reduction in the frequency of generalized tonic–clonic (grand mal) seizures and absence (petit mal) seizures, with no adverse effects noted in any. This was the first clinical study to attribute anticonvulsant effects to the consumption of ω3 PUFA.

5.2. Animal Studies

Yehuda et al. *(30)* evaluated the membrane-stabilizing and anticonvulsant potential of a mixture of nonesterified ALA and LA in four rat models of epileptic seizures. Treatment with 40 mg/kg of LA and ALA in a 4:1 ratio for 3 wk prior to each seizure challenge resulted in significant anticonvulsant effects in each of the four seizure models. Beneficial changes in membrane lipid composition and membrane fluidity of brain neurons were attributed to the consumption of PUFA.

Table 1
Relationship Between Ketosis and Seizure Control: Review of Clinical Studies

Study	Sample size	Type of ketogenic diet	Ketone measure	Main findings
No Association Between Ketosis and Seizure Control				
Dekaban, 1966 (23)	11 Children	Classic 3:1, classic 4:1	Pooled plasma ketones (β-HBA + AcAc)	Ketosis, *per se*, was not responsible for the beneficial effects obtained. Seizure reduction was attributed to a rise in plasma lipids.
Schwartz et al., 1989 (24)	55 Children 4 Adults	Classic 4:1, MCT, modified MCT	Pooled blood ketones (β-HBA + AcAc)	Seizure control was not directly related to ketone levels; the classic KD induced significantly greater ketosis than the other diets, but not significantly greater seizure control.
Fraser et al., 2003 (25)	9 Children	Classic 4:1	Plasma β-HBA	No correlation was found between seizure reduction and plasma β-HBA. Seizure reduction and serum total arachidonate were positively correlated.
Positive Association Between Ketosis and Seizure Control				
Huttenlocher, 1976 (20)	22 Children	Classic 3:1, MCT	Plasma β-HBA and plasma AcAc	A plasma β-HBA >2.0 mmol/L and a plasma AcAc >0.6 mmol/L were required for optimal reduction in seizure frequency.
Whedon et al., 1999 (26)	15 Adults	Classic 4:1	Serum β-HBA	A serum β-HBA >2.4 mmol/L was required for optimal reduction in seizure frequency.
Gilbert et al., 2000 (27)	54 Children	Classic 4:1	Blood β-HBA	Seizure control correlated with blood β-HBA and was more likely with blood β-HBA values > 4 mmol/L.

AcAc, acetoacetate; β-HBA, β-hydroxybutyrate; MCT, medium-chain triglyceride.

Table 2
Review of In Vitro, Animal, and Clinical Studies Finding Beneficial Effects of PUFA on Neuronal Excitability

Studies	Ref.	Dosage and type of PUFA	Model	Main findings
Clinical	Schlanger et al., 2002 (29)	ω3 PUFA (2.3 g of DHA + 0.9 g of EPA + 0.05 g of ALA) daily for 6 mo	Five patients with epilepsy secondary to a central nervous system disease	Reduction in the frequency of generalized tonic–clonic and absence seizures in all subjects with no adverse effects noted in any of the patients.
Animal	Yehuda et al., 1994 (30)	40 mg/kg of a mixture of LA and ALA (4:1) daily for 3 wk	Adult male Sabra or Sprague-Dawley albino rats	Anticonvulsant effects in four rat models of epileptic seizures.
In vitro	Voskuyl et al., 1998 (31)	40 µmol/L of DHA, infused	Adult male Wistar rats	Demonstrated a 15–20% increase in the seizure threshold using the cortical stimulation model.
	Fraser et al., 1993 (32)	1–30 µmol/L of AA	Cultured central neurons	Hyperpolarization of resting membrane potential, reduction in action potentials, and reduction in neurotransmitter release.
	Xiao et al., 1999 (33)	20 µmol/L of DHA or EPA	CA1 neurons of hippocampal slices	DHA and EPA caused hyperpolarization of the resting membrane potential, reduction in the frequency of action potentials, and increase in the stimulatory threshold of action potentials. EPA reduced pentylenetetrazole- or glutamate-induced neuronal excitability to control levels.
	Young et al., 2000 (34)	50 µmol/L of DHA	CA1 neurons of rat hippocampal slices	Frequency-dependent inhibition of neuronal excitability (induced by bicuculline or a Mg^{2+}-free medium).

AA, arachidonic acid; ALA, α-linolenic acid; DHA, docosahexaenoic acid; EPA, eicosapentaenoic acid; LA, linoleic acid; PUFA, polyunsaturated fatty acid.

135

Subsequently, using the cortical stimulation model, Voskuyl et al. *(31)* demonstrated that the infusion of 40 μmol/L of free (nonesterified) DHA resulted in a 15–20% increase in the seizure threshold. Infusion of DHA esterified to phospholipid was noted to be ineffective in controlling seizures in this model, suggesting that brain uptake of the free form of this LC-PUFA is selective.

5.3. In Vitro Studies

Fraser et al. *(32)* demonstrated a significant inhibition of voltage-gated sodium channels with the application of 1–30 μmol/L of AA to cultured striatal neurons. The results included hyperpolarization of the resting membrane potential, reduction in action potentials, and subsequent reduction in neurotransmitter release. The antiepileptic drugs carbamazepine, phenytoin, and valproate have similar effects on sodium channels, indicating that LC-PUFAs, like AA, may be endogenous ligands mimicked by some anticonvulsants *(31)*.

Subsequently, Xiao et al. *(33)* demonstrated a significant reduction in the frequency of electrically evoked action potentials in CA1 neurons of hippocampal slices with the exogenous application of 20 μmol/L of DHA or EPA. DHA and EPA were also associated with a significant hyperpolarization of the resting membrane potential and a significant increase in the stimulatory threshold of action potentials. EPA was also able to reduce pentylenetetrazole (PTZ) or glutamate induced neuronal excitability to control levels.

Xiao et al. *(33)* reported that DHA has stabilizing effects on neuronal membrane stability, but it has also been found to increase *N*-methyl-D-aspartate (NMDA) responses *(35)* and to block K^+ channels *(36,37)*, therefore predisposing neurons to epileptiform bursting and an aggravation in seizure activity. To rule out the possibility that DHA may indiscriminately increase neuronal excitability, Young et al. *(34)* examined the effect of DHA on the epileptiform activity of CA1 neurons of rat hippocampal slices induced by bicuculline or a Mg^{2+}-free medium. Instead of provoking epileptiform activity, DHA inhibited neuronal excitability in a frequency-dependent fashion. DHA was suggested to elicit its seizure inhibitory effects by blocking sodium channels, thereby stabilizing presynaptic membranes and decreasing the release of glutamate. These results indicate that despite some neuronal excitatory effects, DHA may be beneficial for patients with epilepsy.

6. LONG-CHAIN POLYUNSATURATED FATTY ACIDS: THEIR ROLE IN A KETOGENIC DIET

Dekaban *(23)* was the first to suggest that seizure reduction was directly related to the elevation of plasma total lipids, cholesterol, and, to a lesser extent, total fatty acids. He observed that in children, ketones increase rapidly during the consumption of a KD, whereas plasma lipids reach their highest plateaus only after 2–3 wk. Dekaban *(23)* argued that optimal improvements in seizure frequency do not occur immediately, i.e., parallel to elevations in ketones, but between 10 d and 3 wk after the initiation of the KD, i.e., parallel to elevations in plasma lipids. Though suggesting that raised total free fatty acids may be useful in predicting seizure outcome, Dekaban *(23)* did not define which plasma fatty acids were significantly elevated and which were significantly associated with seizure control.

Although several types of KD are being used in the treatment of childhood refractory seizures (classic, MCT, modified MCT) *(38)*, none contains a particularly high proportion of dietary LC-PUFA. Thus, at first glance, the possibility that KDs exert their anticonvulsant effects via an LC-PUFA-based mechanism seems unlikely. Interestingly, however, an elevation in LC-PUFAs has been reported in subjects fed a KD. Anderson et al. *(39)* reported significantly elevated serum levels of ALA, docosapentaenoic acid (DPA, 22:5ω6), docosapentaenoic acid (DPA, 22:5ω3), and docosatetraenoic acid (DTA, 22:4ω6) in rats fed a KD. More recently, Fraser et al. *(25)* documented a significant increase in LA, AA, and DHA in serum free fatty acids, triglycerides, and phospholipids in nine pediatric patients on a KD for treatment of refractory seizures. Seizure reduction in these patients was positively and significantly correlated with serum total AA ($r^2 = 0.53$, $p < 0.05$), and a similar relationship between seizure reduction and serum total DHA approached significance ($r^2 = 0.41$, $p = 0.09$). Taken together, these two studies indicate that the high-fat KD elevates serum LC-PUFA and that these LC-PUFAs may be important in predicting seizure outcome and understanding the anticonvulsant mechanism of the KD.

Studies documenting a beneficial effect of LC-PUFA on seizure susceptibility are descriptive; that is, they may suggest a correlation, but they do not indicate a mechanism by which LC-PUFAs confer seizure resistance. The in vitro studies conducted thus far are mechanistic but have involved exposure of cultured neurons (usually hippocampal brain slices) to individual LC-PUFAs. Although both types of study are valuable, neither allows us to conclude with certainty that LC-PUFAs cross the blood–brain barrier and gain entry into the brain during KD/LC-PUFA consumption.

Some models suggest that long-chain fatty acids have ready access to the brain via proteins that exist at the blood–brain barrier and are able to bind fatty acids *(40)*. Nevertheless, Dell and colleagues *(41)* have shown that despite raised plasma free fatty acids in rats fed KDs of differing fatty acid content and composition, brain DHA and AA do not change significantly. These results suggest that the mature rat brain is resistant to changes in plasma and dietary fatty acids *(28)*. The infant brain, however, may more readily acquire fatty acids from the circulation *(28)*. The same may be true of the epileptic brain.

If the brain is resistant to changing its fatty acid composition, then an increase in plasma LC-PUFAs may reduce seizure susceptibility via an alternate mechanism. Fatty acid mobilization from adipose tissue and subsequent β-oxidation do not occur at the same rate for all fatty acids *(42,43)*. In general, ALA and LA are more easily mobilized and β-oxidized than AA or saturated fatty acids; also, EPA and DHA are relatively easily mobilized and β-oxidized *(42,44)*. Except for AA, the most easily mobilized and β-oxidized dietary long-chain fatty acids are the same as those (DHA, EPA, ALA) that are most effective in inhibiting seizures *(28)*. Because fatty acids that are more easily β-oxidized are generally more ketogenic *(28)*, it is possible that LC-PUFAs exert their anticonvulsant effects, in part, by being β-oxidized to ketones, which can then cross the blood–brain barrier and exert antiseizure effects. The KD is believed to work best in pediatric epilepsy patients, and it is well known that during starvation and consumption of high-fat KDs, infants and children have a greater capacity than adults to produce, extract, and use ketones as primary energy substrates in the brain *(45)*.

7. DIETARY LONG-CHAIN POLYUNSATURATED FATTY ACIDS IN A KETOGENIC DIET: CLINICAL CHALLENGES

The data outlined thus far regarding LC-PUFAs can be summarized as follows:

1. Supplementation/exposure to LC-PUFAs may reduce seizure susceptibility.
2. Increased serum levels of LC-PUFAs have been observed in subjects consuming a KD.

Although incorporating LC-PUFAs into a KD may enhance the diet's efficacy, there are several clinical challenges that must first be addressed.

The optimal dosage and composition of the LC-PUFA supplement must be determined. Preliminary evidence suggests that only nonesterified forms of these fatty acids are effective (31), and this needs to be considered. Only one clinical study has assessed the antiseizure effects of a PUFA supplement in epilepsy patients (29). In this study, patients were given 3.25 g of an ω3 PUFA supplement (2.3 g of DHA, 0.9 g of EPA, and 0.05 g of ALA) daily. Although this dosage resulted in a reduction in seizure frequency and was not associated with any adverse effects, the epilepsy patients studied were not being treated with a KD. Because bruising is one of the common side effects of the KD, being experienced by 31% of KD patients (46), it is possible that ω3 PUFA supplementation may exacerbate this condition. Thus, the acute and long-term effects of various doses of ω3 LC-PUFA on factors such as platelet count, platelet aggregation, and bleeding time in KD subjects must be defined. Berry-Kravis et al. (46) have speculated that the KD causes changes in platelet membrane lipid composition and resultant changes in the function of membrane-embedded proteins, thus leading to alterations in platelet function. It would therefore be interesting to assess the composition of ω3 LC-PUFA in platelet membranes of children on a KD.

Another area that needs to be addressed is the potential for ω3 LC-PUFA to improve other health risks associated with the KD. An increase in plasma lipids in children on a classical KD is well documented (23,25,47–49) but not always observed (50). These increases are not of great concern in the pediatric population; but in the adult population, KD-induced hyperlipidemia may predispose patients to an increased risk of cardiovascular disease (51). In a recent animal study, rats fed a KD based on flaxseed oil, which contains a large proportion of ALA and LA, had significantly lower plasma and liver triglycerides than rats fed KDs containing butter and experienced reductions in seizure susceptibility similar to those posted by the butter-based KD group (41). Although the beneficial effects of PUFAs and MCTs on plasma lipid profiles in KD subjects have been documented (20,23,50), the effects of LC-PUFAs (DHA, EPA, AA) have not yet been explored.

8. CONCLUSION

The characterization and selection of appropriate candidates for the KD necessitates the development of reliable markers/indicators of seizure response. The controversy regarding the usefulness of ketone measures in assessing seizure outcome persists because no conclusion can be drawn from the current literature on this area. More research is needed to understand the relationship between plasma and brain ketone levels. There should be a strong initiative in the future to quantify all plasma ketone concentrations and examine relatively the levels of, e.g., β-HBA/AcAc.

The development of an accurate and noninvasive measure of ketosis is necessary to properly address the importance of ketosis to seizure control. Preliminary work suggests that breath ACET may have an important role in this area. However, because LC-PUFAs exert antiseizure effects and are elevated in KD patients, attempts should be made to routinely examine fatty acid profiles in KD patients to determine whether KD responders have elevated LC-PUFAs compared with nonresponders. Such studies may enhance both the way KD patients are monitored and our understanding of the diet's mechanism.

ACKNOWLEDGMENTS

Dairy Farmers of Canada, the Natural Sciences and Engineering Research Council of Canada, Bloorview Children's Hospital Foundation, Stanley Thomas Johnson Foundation, and the University of Toronto (Awards Division) are thanked for financial support. Alcohol Countermeasure Systems Company (Mississauga, Ont, Canada) and Mary Ann Ryan are thanked for their technical support.

REFERENCES

1. Freeman JM, Freeman JB, Kelly MT. The Ketogenic Diet: A Treatment for Epilepsy, 3rd ed. Demos, New York, 2000.
2. Musa-Veloso K, Likhodii SS, Cunnane SC. Breath acetone is a reliable indicator of ketosis in adult volunteers consuming ketogenic meals. Am J Clin Nutr 2002;76:65–70.
3. Freund G. The calorie deficiency hypothesis of ketogenesis tested in man. Metabolism 1965;14:985–990.
4. Livingston S. Dietary treatment of epilepsy. In: Comprehensive Management of Epilepsy in Infancy, Childhood and Adolescence. Charles C Thomas, Springfield, IL, 1992, pp. 378–405.
5. Schwartz RM, Eaton J, Bower BD, Aynsley-Green A. Ketogenic diets in the treatment of epilepsy: short-term clinical effects. Dev Med Child Neurol 1989;31:145–151.
6. Laffel L. Ketone bodies: a review of physiology, pathophysiology and application of monitoring to diabetes. Diabetes Metab Res Rev 1999;15:412–426.
7. Freund G. The calorie deficiency hypothesis of ketogenesis tested in man. Metabolism 1965;14:985–990.
8. McDonald LA, Hackett LP, Dusci LJ. The identification of acetone and the detection of isoproanol in biological fluids by gas chromatography. Clin Chim Acta 1975;63:235–237.
9. Cheung ST, Lin WN. Simultaneous determination of methanol, ethanol, acetone, isopropanol and ethylene glycol in plasma by gas chromatography. J Chromatogr 1987;414:248–250.
10. Brega A, Villa P, Quadrini G, Quadri A, Lucarelli C. High-performance liquid chromatographic determination of acetone in blood and urine in the clinical diagnostic laboratory. J Chromatogr 1991;553:249–254.
11. Freund G, Weinsier RL. Standardized ketosis in man following medium chain triglyceride ingestion. Metabolism 1966;15:980–991.
12. Rooth G, Ostenson S. Acetone in alveolar air and the control of diabetes. Lancet 1966;1102–1105.
13. Tassopoulos CN, Barnett D, Fraser TR. Breath acetone and blood sugar measurements in diabetes. Lancet 1969;1282–1286.
14. Jones AW. Breath acetone concentrations in fasting male volunteers: further studies and effect of alcohol administration. J Anal Toxicol 1988;12:75–79.
15. Likhodii SS, Musa K, Cunnane SC. Breath acetone as a measure of systemic ketosis assessed in a rat model of the ketogenic diet. Clin Chem 2002;48:115–120.
16. Musa-Veloso K, Rarama E, Comeau F, Curtis R, Cunnane S. Epilepsy and the ketogenic diet: assessment of ketosis in children using breath acetone. Pediatr Res 2002;52:443–448.
17. Musa-Veloso K, Likhodii SS, Ramana E, Comeau F, Cunnane SC. The assessment of breath acetone using a hand-held acetone analyzer (abstr). Proc Can Fed Biol Sci 2002; F040.
18. Mitchell GA, Kassovska-Bratinova S, Boukaftane Y, et al. Medical aspects of ketone body metabolism. Clin Invest Med 1995;18:193–216.
19. Veech RL, Chance B, Kashiwaya Y, Lardy HA, Cahill GF Jr. Ketone bodies, potential therapeutic uses. Life 2001;51:241–247.
20. Huttenlocher, PR. Ketonemia and seizures: metabolic and anticonvulsant effects of two ketogenic diets in childhood epilepsy. Pediatr Res 1976;10:536–540.
21. Seymour KJ, Bluml S, Sutherling J, Sutherling W, Ross BD. Identification of cerebral acetone by ^{1}H-MRS in patients with epilepsy controlled by ketogenic diet. MAGMA 1999;8:33–42.
22. Bridge EM, Iob LV. The mechanism of the ketogenic diet in epilepsy. Johns Hopkins Med J 1931;48:373–389.

23. Dekaban AS. Plasma lipids in epileptic children treated with the high fat diet. Arch Neurol 1966;15:177–184.
24. Schwartz RM, Boyes S, Aynsley-Green A. Metabolic effects of three ketogenic diets in the treatment of severe epilepsy. Dev Med Child Neurol 1989;31:152–160.
25. Fraser DD, Whiting S, Andrew RD, Macdonald EA, Musa-Veloso K, Cunnane SC. Elevated polyunsaturated fatty acids in blood serum obtained from children on the ketogenic diet. Neurology 2003;60:1026–1029.
26. Whedon B, Sirven JI, O'Dwyer J, Sperling MR. Therapeutic serum β-OH butyrate levels in adult ketogenic diet patients. Epilepsia 1999;40 (Suppl. 7):221.
27. Gilbert DL, Pyzik PL, Freeman JM. The ketogenic diet: seizure control correlates better with serum β-hydroxybutyrate than with urine ketones. J Child Neurol 2000;15:787–790.
28. Cunnane S, Musa K, Ryan M, Whiting S, Fraser D. Potential role of polyunsaturates in seizure protection achieved with the ketogenic diet. Prostaglandins Leukotrienes Essent Fatty Acids 2002;67:131–135.
29. Schlanger S, Shinitzky M, Yam D. Diet enriched with omega-3 fatty acids alleviates convulsion symptoms in epilepsy patients. Epilepsia 2002;43:103–104.
30. Yehuda S, Carasso RL, Mostofsky DI. Essential fatty acid preparation (SR-3) raises the seizure threshold in rats. Eur J Pharmacol 1994;254:193–198.
31. Voskuyl A, Vreugdenhil M, Kang JX, Leaf A. Anitconvulsant effects of polyunsaturated fatty acids in rats using the cortical stimulation model. Eur J Pharmacol 1998;341:145–152.
32. Fraser DD, Hoehn K, Weiss S, MacVicar BA. Arachidonic acid inhibits sodium currents and synaptic transmission in cultured striatal neurons. Neuron 1993;11:633–644.
33. Xiao YF, Li X. Polyunsaturated fatty acids modify mouse hippocampal neuronal excitability during excitotoxic or convulsant stimulation. Brain Res 1999;846:112–121.
34. Young C, Gean PW, Chiou LC, Shen YZ. Docosahexaenoic acid inhibits synaptic transmission and epileptiform activity in the rat hippocampus. Synapse 2000;37:90–94.
35. Nishikawa M, Kimura S, Akaike N. Facilitatory effect of docosahexaenoic acid on N-methyl-D-aspartate response in pyramidal neurons of rat cerebral cortex. J Physiol (Lond) 1994;475:83–90.
36. Poling JS, Karanian JW, Salem N Jr, Vicini S, Time- and voltage-dependent block of delayed rectifier potassium channels by docosahexaenoic acid. Mol Pharmacol 1995;47:381–390.
37. Poling JS, Vicini S, Rogawski MA, Salem N Jr. Docosahexaenoic acid block of neuronal voltage-gated K^+ channels: subunit selective antagonism by zinc. Neuropharmacology 1996;35:969–982.
38. Schwartz RM, Eaton J, Bower BD, Aynsley-Green A. Ketogenic diets in the treatment of epilepsy: short-term clinical effects. Dev Med Child Neurol 1989;31:145–151.
39. Anderson GD, Rho JM, Bough KJ, Storey TW, Szot P, Schwartzkroin PA. Rats fed a ketogenic diet exhibit significantly elevated levels of long-chain, polyunsaturated fatty acids. Epilepsia 2001;42 (Suppl 7):262–263.
40. Rapoport SI. In vivo fatty acid incorporation into brain phospholipids in relation to plasma availability, signal transduction, and membrane remodeling. J Mol Neurosci 2001;16:243–262.
41. Dell CA, Likhodii SS, Musa K, Ryan MA, Burnham WM, Cunnane S.C. Lipid and fatty acid profiles in rats consuming different high-fat ketogenic diets. Lipids 2001;36:373–378.
42. Raclot T, Groscolas R. Selective mobilization of adipose tissue fatty acids during energy depletion in the rat. J Lipid Res 1995;36:2164–2173.
43. Cunnane SC. New developments in alpha-linolenate metabolism with emphasis on the importance of β-oxidation and carbon-recycling. World Rev Nutr Diet 2001;88:178–183.
44. Sheaff-Greiner RC, Zhang Q, Goodman KJ, Guissini DA, Nathanielsz PW, Brefnna JT. Linoleate, α-linolenate and docosahexaenoate recycling into saturated and monounsaturated fatty acids is a major pathway in pregnant or lactating adults and fetal or infant rhesus monkeys. J Lipid Res 1996;37:2675–2686.
45. Swink TD, Vining EPG, Freeman JM. The ketogenic diet: 1997. Adv Pediatr 1997;44:297–329.
46. Berry-Kravis E, Booth G, Taylor A, Valentino LA. Bruising and the ketogenic diet: evidence for diet-induced changes in platelet function. Ann Neurol 2001;49:98–103.
47. Vining EPG, Kwiterovich P, Hsieh S, Casey J, Freeman J. The effect of the ketogenic diet on plasma cholesterol. Epilepsia 1996;37 (Suppl 5):107.
48. Delgado MR, Mills J, Sparagana S. Hypercholesterolemia associated with the ketogenic diet. Epilepsia 1996;37 (Suppl 5):108.

49. Chesney D, Brouhard BH, Wyllie E, Powaski K. Biochemical abnormalities of the ketogenic diet in children. Clin Pediatr 1999;38:107–109.

50. Couch SC, Schwarzman F, Koenigsberger D, Nordli DR, Deckelbaum RJ, DeFelice AR. Growth and nutritional outcomes of children treated with the ketogenic diet. J Am Diet Assoc 1999;99 (Suppl):1573–1575.

51. Sirven J, Whedon B, Caplan D, Liporace J, Glosser D, O'Dwyer J, Sperling MR. The ketogenic diet for intractable epilepsy in adults: preliminary results. Epilepsia 1999;40:1721–1726.

11

Insights From Neuroimaging Studies Into Ketosis and the Ketogenic Diet

Jullie W. Pan

1. INTRODUCTION

Over the past 15 yr, noninvasive imaging has become an increasingly key tool in the evaluation of the human brain, both clinically and scientifically. A large body of work in the methodology of imaging has broadened its base significantly beyond solely structural information to include regional metabolic and biochemical information. Thus, with the resurgence of interest in identifying the mechanisms underlying the clinical efficacy of the ketogenic diet (KD), sophisticated neuroimaging is likely to yield valuable insights into the functional and metabolic changes induced by this treatment. This chapter focuses on the application of this technology toward a mechanistic understanding of the KD.

Positron emission tomography (PET) and magnetic resonance (MR) have been used to provide critical structural, metabolic, biophysical, and biochemical evaluations of the brain. With its variety of radioligands and tracers, PET has provided a wealth of data on receptor binding, blood flow, and glucose consumption in adult brain across a wide range of diseases and normal states. Given its extensive history of applications and available reviews *(1,2)*, this chapter does not provide further background discussion on PET. Rather, the focus is on the information that PET has provided on the physiology of ketosis. However, with the more recent developments in MR, we briefly describe the more novel imaging approaches in MR and MR spectroscopy that have significantly expanded the ability to study the ketogenic diet and epilepsy. Furthermore, because of the integrative nature of imaging work, the chapter continues with a description of both PET- and MR-based studies that have examined the normal brain in ketosis. Finally, and most important, data are presented on imaging-based patient studies performed by separate research groups that have begun to provide some potentially important insights into ketosis and the ketogenic diet. Such clinical studies may be especially important given that some critical aspects of the diet and ketosis may be revealed only under conditions of actual utilization, i.e., with epilepsy patients on the diet.

From: *Epilepsy and the Ketogenic Diet*
Edited by: C. E. Stafstrom and J. M. Rho © Humana Press Inc., Totowa, NJ

2. MR IMAGING AND SPECTROSCOPY

The ability of magnetic resonance to noninvasively and nonradioactively evaluate structures, metabolites, and processes places it among the most important technologies for the evaluation of brain function. Given the very high concentration of water in the brain, and its varying environments within different brain compartments, MR imaging of water is the workhorse in the structural evaluation of the brain. However, MR imaging can readily be applied to compounds other than water, and therefore MR spectroscopy and spectroscopic imaging are being increasingly used to image compounds such as N-acetyl aspartate (NAA), lactate, adenosine triphosphate (ATP), all of which are important in neuronal function as well as in pathological processes such as neuronal damage, ischemia, and hypoglycemia.

In ^{1}H-MR spectroscopy, the compounds NAA, creatine, choline, lactate, glutamate, glutamine, acetone, γ-aminobutyric acid (GABA), myoinositol (mI), glucose, and β-hydroxybutyrate (BHB) are all relatively well detected. Compounds present in lower concentrations, approx 1mM, e.g., lactate, GABA, BHB, represent a greater challenge for measurement than those present in more abundant concentrations of approx 5–12mM, e.g., NAA, creatine (Cr), and thus have required more specialized detection approaches. ^{31}P-MR spectroscopy can evaluate high-energy phosphates (ATP, phosphocreatine), as specific assessments of the bioenergetic state. ^{13}C-MR spectroscopy, although of considerably less sensitivity than ^{1}H or ^{31}P imaging, can allow a dynamic assessment of neurotransmission and amino acid turnover in the human brain.

2.1. ^{1}H and ^{31}P Spectroscopy

NAA, as a compound synthesized predominantly in neuronal mitochondria, has been extensively regarded as an indicator of neuronal function. Because NAA levels decline with functional deterioration and rise with therapy, the original interpretation of NAA has been revised to reflect neuronal function rather than solely neuron number. Other metabolites, such as Cr and mI, are present in varying content depending on cell type, but typically they are at higher concentrations in astrocytes. Thus, the combined parameter of NAA/Cr has been highly useful in the detection of seizure foci and prognostication of outcome in mesial temporal lobe epilepsy (mTLE), finding accuracy of 85–95$^+$% for lateralization (3,4). Additionally, quantitative application of the NAA/Cr ratio (rather than use of asymmetry indices) has demonstrated a relatively high incidence of bilateral hippocampal involvement (25–50%) in surgical TLE patients (3–5). Such findings, together with other PET anomalies showing multiple subcortical abnormalities, have contributed critically toward the pathophysiologic concept that temporal lobe epilepsy is characterized by dysfunction of a metabolic network, rather than aberration of a single focus. Finally, with the high concordance between electroencephalography (EEG) and MR spectroscopy, it is evident that MR spectroscopic imaging of NAA/Cr in the hippocampus is a highly sensitive and useful measure of neuronal damage and dysfunction. Two examples of the ability of ^{1}H-MR spectroscopy to lateralize the damage seen in both temporal lobe and neocortical epilepsy are shown in Fig. 1, where the severity of abnormality of NAA/Cr is indicated by the outline (6,7).

The high-energy phosphates of ATP, phosphocreatine (PCr) and inorganic phosphate (P$_i$) are also readily measurable with ^{31}P-MR spectroscopy. However, the lower sensi-

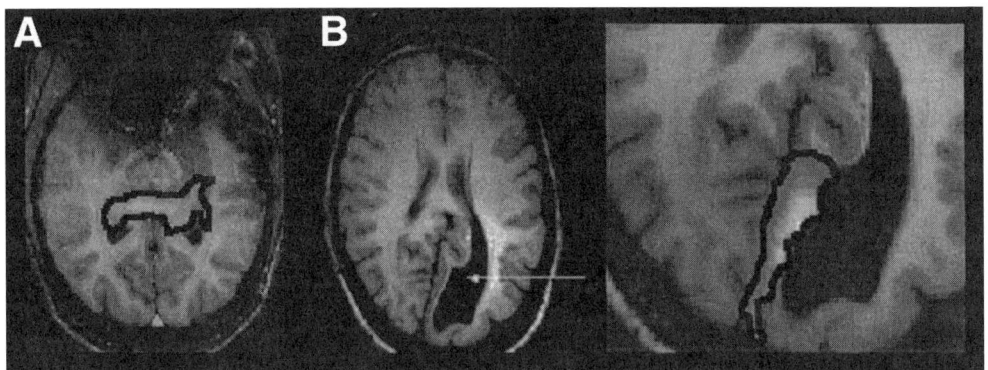

Fig. 1. Magnetic resonance images, structural and metabolic (NAA/Cr), from two epilepsy patients. **(A)** Image from a patient with bilateral hippocampal epilepsy shows highlighted abnormalities in both hippocampi, with the patient's left hippocampus more extensively involved than the right. Notably, the NAA/Cr thresholds used to define the regional abnormalities are set for cerebral gray and white matter tissue types; thus the cerebellar tissue is being detected as abnormal. **(B)** Images from a patient with a large occipital–parasagittal malformation (arrow). The NAA/Cr image (far right) is able to localize the region of neuronal dysfunction primarily to the parasagittal gray matter. Data from refs. *5* and *6*, permission provided by HP Hetherington.

tivity of the ^{31}P nucleus results in relatively poorer spatial resolution than is available by means of ^{1}H-MR spectroscopy. At present, most clinical systems are devoted to detecting only ^{1}H signals; thus, it is primarily research-level systems that have the hardware for detecting ^{31}P or ^{13}C. Nonetheless, the combined assessment of ATP, PCr, and inorganic phosphate remains a very important tissue parameter for questions of bioenergetic status. With improvements in data acquisition and analysis, the utilization of ^{31}P spectroscopy has increased and has been implemented recently to evaluate the network hypothesis of temporal lobe epilepsy. The present spatial resolution of research grade systems is 12 cm^3 *(6)*, and this is likely to improve further in the future.

2.2. ^{13}C Spectroscopy

^{13}C spectroscopy is the most informative, yet also the least sensitive, MR measure used to study human brain. In comparison to ^{1}H and ^{31}P, which are effectively 100% abundant, ^{13}C has a very low natural abundance (1.1%). Brain studies, therefore, typically require supplementation of the ^{13}C signal, through provision of [^{13}C]glucose (either through intravenous infusions or oral intake), or other metabolite such as [^{13}C]ketones. With commercial availability of such compounds with specific ^{13}C labeling, spectroscopy based on this isotope has been used to track the fate of the ^{13}C nucleus into the amino acid pools of glutamate, glutamine, and GABA *(8)*, reflecting their rapid transport, metabolic processing through glycolysis, the tricarboxylic acid (TCA) cycle, and neurotransmitter cycling. The resonances readily visualized include the label itself, e.g., [^{13}C]glucose or [^{13}C]ketone, ^{13}C-4, ^{13}C-3, ^{13}C-2 resonance positions of glutamate and glutamine, and GABA. The specific position of the label depends on the extent of metabolic processing and can be readily predicted and interpreted from the well-known glycolytic and oxidative biochemical pathways.

Although ^{13}C spectroscopy provides a wealth of peaks to evaluate, its relative insensitivity (in terms of both intrinsic sensitivity and natural abundance) compared with the

[1]H and ^{31}P forms makes it significantly more challenging to interpret accurately. For example, typically reported in vivo volume sizes in human ^{1}H spectroscopy range from 0.5 to 15 mL, but typical ^{13}C sizes are 45–125 mL *(9,10)*. Interpretation of such large volumes is complex, given the summation of gray and white matter, as well as astrocytic and neuronal compartments. An alternative approach to the large voxel sizes of ^{13}C spectroscopy is to use [1]H-[13]C (the ^{13}C nonradioactively tags the compounds; ^{1}H serves for detection) spectroscopy, which allows detection of turnover of glutamate with a spatial resolution of several cubic centimeters *(11,12)*. However, such an approach focuses on a smaller number of resonances, and thus, it may be a combination of ^{13}C and [1]H-^{13}C spectroscopy that gives the most accurate view of the brain's metabolic physiology. In both approaches, adequate models of the tissue are needed with the pool sizes of component metabolites to assess how metabolic fluxes may be coupled. For example, such data, as applied in whole rat brain, have been used to argue for a close relationship between neurotransmission cycling and TCA cycle flux *(13)*.

3. KETOSIS AND THE NORMAL BRAIN

It has long been known that the brain uses ketones in states of decreased glucose availability. However, the specifics of such a shift—e.g., the interrelationships of glucose and ketones, the requisite extent of shift for seizure control, and why such connections should result in altered neuronal excitability and improved seizure control in patients with epilepsy—remain unclear. Many questions about the mechanism of the ketogenic diet result from a lack of extensive knowledge of how ketosis affects normal brain. This section reviews the available metabolic, PET, and MR studies that have evaluated normal human brain under conditions of ketosis, with the anticipation that we may be able to conceptualize how the ketogenic diet affects the epileptic brain.

3.1. Ketone Body Consumption With Glucose and Transport in Human Brain

How does the brain make use of glucose relative to available ketones? Using fluorodeoxyglucose (FDG)-PET imaging, Redies et al. *(14)* demonstrated in obese subjects undergoing an extended fast (3 wk) that cerebral glucose use decreased to 54% of the unfasted baseline, seen over the entire brain. Haymond et al. *(15)* used deuterated glucose infusions in fasted normal children and adults, and in epileptic children on the ketogenic diet, to find an inverse relationship between estimated brain glucose consumption and plasma ketone body concentration. By correcting for brain mass differences between children and adults, the investigators were able to eliminate much of the data's variability, allowing detection of the inverse relationship. Nonetheless, the stoichiometry of the relationship between glucose and ketone utilization remains difficult to estimate. Using an acute hyperketonemic protocol, Hasselbalch et al. *(16)* reported that at 2mM plasma levels of ketones, whole-brain glucose use (arterio-venous difference and FDG-PET data) decreased approx 30%, whereas ketone consumption increased such that the total fuel use remained approximately constant. Thus, in total, it appears that ketones and glucose do trade off to support the brain's fuel needs, although the exact intercept and slope of this relationship remain unclear.

What transport features characterize ketone consumption, and does this affect overall ketone use? Blomqvist et al. *(17)* synthesized [11]C[BHB] as a PET tracer for study in human brain, finding a minimal pool of free BHB in the brain. This is consistent with the recent data from MR spectroscopic studies of BHB in acute hyperketonemia *(18)*. This report studied control adult volunteers infused with ^{d}-BHB to raise plasma levels up to 2.24mM. The MR data acquired from a 12-cm^3 brain volume located in the occipital lobe revealed minimal accumulation of brain BHB at 0.16mM. Modeling of these data implied that under nonfasted conditions with plasma BHB concentrations of up to approx 2mM, BHB entry must be rate limiting for BHB utilization.

Conditions of fasting, however, may be different. In control adult volunteers over a 3-d fasting period, plasma levels of up to 4mM were seen, and brain BHB levels rose with fasting, reaching 1mM *(19)*. Corrected for plasma and cerebrospinal fluid (CSF) contributions, this would give a minimum parenchymal BHB concentration of 0.9mM. Combined with the acute hyperketonemia data, this finding implies that BHB transport is most likely induced with fasting, consistent with extensive animal model data showing induction of transport with fasting *(20)*.

3.2. Ketone Body Metabolism in Human Brain

The availability of ^{13}C-labeled metabolites for infusion allows ^{13}C-MR spectroscopy to directly track the fate of ketones in human brain. As stated previously, [^{13}C]glucose studies in human brain have established that there is rapid entry of ^{13}C molecules into the amino acid pools such as glutamate and glutamine, the amount of which reflects the fractional enrichment of infusate and plasma, the pool size of the amino acid, and the intervening metabolic fluxes. The tissue volume sampled in the ^{13}C studies was typically between 50 and 125 cm^3. However, because the white matter concentrations of amino acids such as glutamate and glutamine are approximately half the concentration of gray matter, and because the sampled tissue regions can be biased toward a greater gray matter fraction, with adequate modeling, such large tissue voxels can still be insightful. This is particularly true for steady state studies, in which the total labeling can be attributed to known pool sizes, and concerns for differing but simultaneous fluxes are minimized given the steady state.

[^{13}C-2,4] BHB has been used to examine the fate of ketones in human brain (Fig. 2A) *(21)*. In overnight-fasted adult controls, a plasma BHB level of 2.5mM produced a small contribution to total oxidative flux of 7%. Although this may seem to contradict the earlier data from Hasselbalch et al. *(16)*, these values are within the standard deviations reported in this earlier AV-difference study. Analysis of the steady state data from these infusion studies in terms of a model that allows neurotransmitter cycling interaction between neurons and astrocytes has provided evidence that BHB is preferentially used by neurons by a factor of 1.8 ± 0.9. Finally, in a comparison of the BHB labeling pattern with equivalent studies using glucose and acetate (spectra processed to match the earlier data) *(10,22)*, the BHB labeling appearance is generally similar to that of glucose (Fig. 2B), reflect the consumption of BHB in the larger neuronal compartment. The neuronal preference for BHB, which may allow a separate energy source, independent of astrocytes, that would otherwise be modulating neuronal metabolism, may be relevant for the ketogenic diet.

4. KETOSIS AND THE KETOGENIC DIET IN EPILEPSY

The approaches described thus far to study ketosis can be informative in studying the ketogenic diet. Although there are not many MR spectroscopic studies of patients on the ketogenic diet, those few reports have presented provocative data.

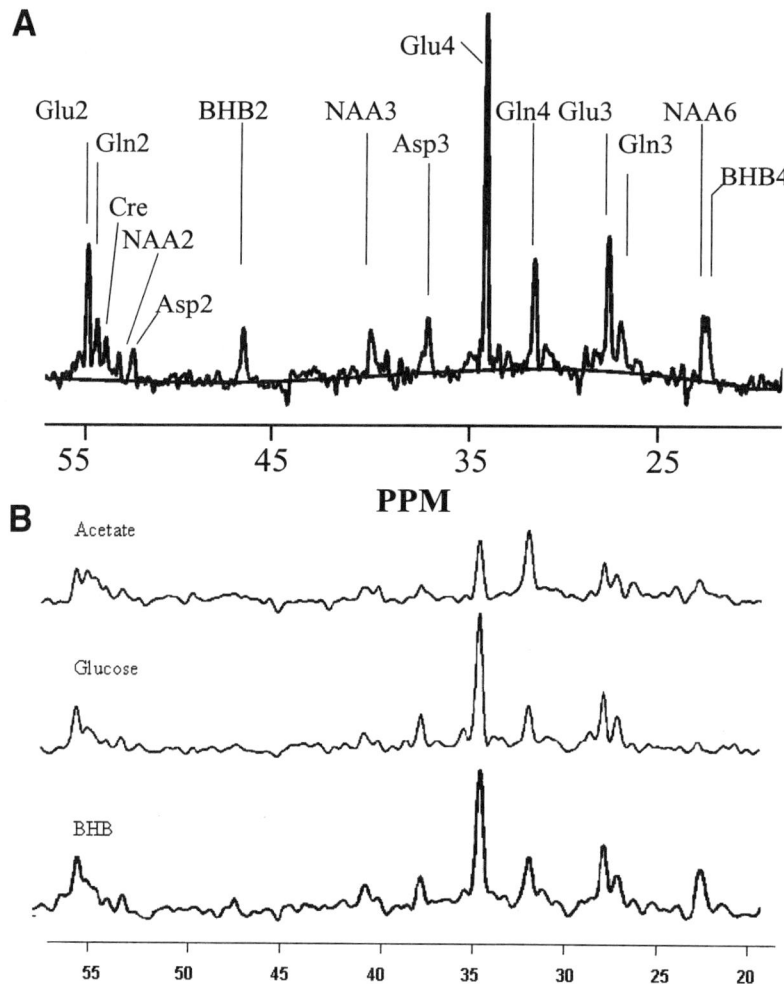

Fig. 2. **(A)** Spectrum of [^{13}C]-labeled metabolites obtained using [^{13}C]-2,4-β-hydroxybutyrate infusions from in vivo human brain. The spectrum is acquired starting 60 min into a bolus–plateau infusion protocol and acquired during the 60- to 120-min time period. **(B)** Comparison of spectra obtained using three different ^{13}C-labeled metabolites to demonstrate the pattern of labeling. [^{13}C]BHB labels broadly similar to that seen with glucose, consistent with its use by the large neuronal pool; detailed modeling of the glutamate and glutamine pools suggest that it is favored by the neuronal pool, whereas acetate is favored by the glial pool.

Given the earlier animal model data suggesting enhanced bioenergetic reserve with the ketogenic diet *(23),* the initial ketogenic diet study from Pan et al. *(24)* focused on an evaluation of the brain bioenergetic status with initiation of the diet. This study used high-field (4-tesla) ^{31}P-MR spectroscopic imaging to evaluate bioenergetic changes in a small group of patients (all younger than 13 yr), studied before initiation of the diet and after one month on the diet. Spectral data from this study are shown in Fig. 3, acquired from two children (both diagnosed with Lennox–Gastaut syndrome) who were treated with the diet. As seen in Fig. 3, there is an increase in the PCr/ATP and PCr/P$_i$ ratios that is particularly notable in the patient who did well on the diet. Data from the entire group of patients demonstrated a significant increase in the PCr/ATP and PCr/P$_i$ ratios

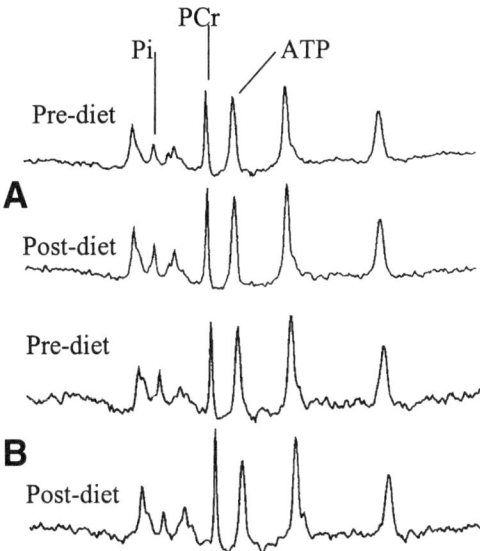

Fig. 3. ^{31}P spectra taken from two patients (A and B), both with Lennox–Gastaut syndrome, before and after initiation of the ketogenic diet. Both patients were 2 yr old at the time of study. **(A)** Patient A (top two spectra) did poorly on the diet. **(B)** Patient B (bottom two spectra) did well on the diet. The resonances of PCr, ATP, and inorganic phosphate (Pi) are marked. The ratio of PCr to ATP does not change with diet treatment in patient A, but patient B shows a post diet increase in PCr/ATP.

evaluated from voxels that were predominantly gray matter, whereas no significant difference was seen in primarily white matter voxels. This finding, together with the known volume overlap between the gray and white matter voxels, implies that the increases in the gray matter bioenergetic ratios are even larger than those reported.

The increase in PCr/ATP and PCr/P$_i$ ratios may be most simply interpreted in terms of an increased, i.e., more negative, thermodynamic potential of ATP hydrolysis, which would be consistent with the previously cited animal model data *(23)*. Such an increase in available energy presumably reflects a steady state shift in all energy-consuming processes, which, for example, may result in a hyperpolarization of membrane potentials. These patients' seizures are being treated by the diet, however, and thus the increase in the PCr ratios may simply represent the improved bioenergetic state under fewer seizures. Without understanding the intrinsic effects of the ketogenic diet and ketosis in nonepileptic brain, this will be difficult to resolve. Nonetheless, these data are consistent with a bioenergetic role for seizure control. Given its dependence on fuel availability, immediate dietary state may thus be expected to be important for seizure control, consistent with the observations that obliteration of ketosis results in an immediate decrease in seizure control *(25)*.

Single-voxel ^{1}H spectroscopy has been used by Seymour et al. to identify the presence of cerebral acetone in KD-treated patients *(26)*. This study used short-echo ^{1}H spectroscopy to evaluate seven patients on the ketogenic diet, five between the ages of 8 and 17 yr and two patients older than 20 yr. The investigators found that although all patients improved substantially on the diet, all five younger patients developed a resonance at 2.2 ppm that was subsequently identified as acetone. In this study, no other ^{1}H changes were detected in the spectra; however, as stated earlier, the detection of low concentration metabolites can be challenging in vivo. Notably, the younger patients generally had larger plasma concentrations of ketones; however, there was no correlation between plasma ketones and the amount of the cerebral acetone resonance. In this small study, no clear correlation was seen between degree of seizure control and acetone levels.

Nonetheless, given that the physicochemical effects of acetone on the brain may be similar to those of general anesthetics, it is intriguing to speculate that the seizure control effects of the ketogenic diet stem from an anesthetic-like process. However, such an anesthetic process is likely to be atypical, with the majority of patients on the diet reporting a general increase in alertness, activity, and awareness, rather than any decrease in functionality.

5. CONCLUSION

All the findings from spectroscopic studies are provocative in terms of a possible relation to efficacy of seizure control. We hope that efficacy studies will be forthcoming, for these may provide important insights into the mechanism of action of the diet, as well as its practical clinical management. Given the number of hypotheses that have been advanced regarding the mechanistic underpinnings of the ketogenic diet, e.g., the GABA hypothesis *(27)*, glutamate, energetics, and acetone, it would be helpful to have some correlative data from metabolic imaging. In such studies, the complexities of human studies should be considered, such as effects of age, seizure type, and sedation. For example, several studies have demonstrated that the values of NAA and creatine are age dependent, with the ratio of NAA/Cr declining with age. Since the diet is most frequently used for children, such age effects may be significant. The potential importance of imaging studies is clear, not only to better understand the mechanisms of action of the ketogenic diet, but also to allow a therapeutic assessment of the diet's effect (and efficacy) on the brain itself.

REFERENCES

1. Schmidt KC, Lucignani G, Sokoloff L. Fluorine-18-fluorodeoxyglucose PET to determine regional cerebral glucose utilization: a re-examination. J Nucl Med 1996;37:394–339.
2. Frankle WG, Laruelle M. Neuroreceptor imaging in psychiatric disorders. Ann Nucl Med 2002 16:437–446.
3. Cendes F, Caramanos Z, Andermann F, Dubeau F, Arnold DL. Proton magnetic resonance spectroscopic imaging and magnetic resonance imaging volumetry in the lateralization of temporal lobe epilepsy: a series of 100 patients. Ann Neurol 1997;42:737–746.
4. Hetherington H, Kuzniecky R, Pan J, Mason G, Morawetz R, Harris C, Faught E, Vaughan T, Pohost G. Proton nuclear magnetic resonance spectroscopic imaging of human temporal lobe epilepsy at 4.1 T. Ann Neurol 1995;38:396–404.
5. Kuzniecky R, Hugg J, Hetherington H, Martin R, Faught E, Morawetz R, Gilliam F. Predictive value of ^{1}H MRSI for outcome in temporal lobectomy. Neurology 1998;53:694–698.
6. Hetherington HP, Pan JW, Spencer DD. ^{1}H and ^{31}P spectroscopy and bioenergetics in the lateralization of seizures in temporal lobe epilepsy. J Magn Reson Imaging 2002;16:477–483.
7. Kuzniecky R, Hetherington H, Pan J, Hugg J, Palmer C, Gilliam F, Faught E, Morawetz R. Proton spectroscopic imaging at 4.1 tesla in patients with malformations of cortical development and epilepsy. Neurology 1997;48:1018–1024.
8. Gruetter R, Novotny EJ, Boulware SD, Mason GF, Rothman DL, Shulman GI, Prichard JW, Shulman RG. Localized ^{13}C NMR spectroscopy in the human brain of amino acid labeling from D-[$^{1-13}$C]glucose. J Neurochem 1994;63:1377–1385.

9. Gruetter R, Seaquist ER, Kim S, Ugurbil K. Localized in vivo ^{13}C-NMR of glutamate metabolism in the human brain: initial results at 4 T. Dev Neurosci 1998;20:380–388.

10. Shen J, Petersen KF, Behar KL, Brown P, Nixon TW, Mason GF, Petroff OA, Shulman GI, Shulman RG, Rothman DL. Determination of the rate of the glutamate/glutamine cycle in the human brain by in vivo ^{13}C NMR. Proc Natl Acad Sci USA 1999;96:8235–8240.

11. Rothman DL, Novotny EJ, Shulman GI, Howseman AM, Petroff OA, Mason G, Nixon T, Hanstock CC, Prichard JW, Shulman RG. ^{1}H-[^{13}C] NMR measurements of [4-^{13}C]glutamate turnover in human brain. Proc Natl Acad Sci U S A 1992;89:9603–9606.

12. Mason GF, Pan JW, Chu WJ, Newcomer BR, Zhang Y, Orr R, Hetherington HP. Measurement of the tricarboxylic acid cycle rate in human gray and white matter in vivo by [1]H-^{13}C magnetic resonance spectroscopy at 4.1T. J Cereb Blood Flow Metab 1999;19:1179–1788.

13. Sibson NR, Dhankhar A, Mason GF, Rothman DL, Behar KL, Shulman RG. Stoichiometric coupling of brain glucose metabolism and glutamatergic neuronal activity. Proc Natl Acad Sci U S A 1998;95(1):316–321.

14. Redies C, Hoffer J, Beil C, Marliss EB, Evans ACV, Lariviere F, Marrett S, Meyer E, Diksic M, Gjedde A, Hakim AM. Generalized decrease in brain glucose metabolism during fasting in humans studied by PET. Am J Physiol 1989;256:E805–E810.

15. Haymond MW, Howard C, Ben-Galim E, DeVivo DC. Effects of ketosis on glucose flux in children and adults. Am J Physiol 1983;245:E373–E378.

16. Hasselbalch SG, Madsen PL, Hageman LP, Olsen KS, Justesen N, Holm S, Paulson OB. Changes in cerebral blood flow and carbohydrate metabolism during acute hyperketonemia. Am J Physiol 1996;270 (5 Pt 1):E746–E751.

17. Blomqvist G, Alvarsson M, Grill V, Von Heijne G, Ingvar M, Thorell JO, Stone-Elander S, Widen L, Ekberg K. Effect of acute hyperketonemia on the cerebral uptake of ketone bodies in nondiabetic subjects and IDDM patients. Am J Physiol Endocrinol Metab 2002;283:E20–E28.

18. Pan JW, Telang FW, Lee JH, DeGraaf RA, Rothman DL and Hetherington HP. Acute hyperketonemia raises brain β-hydroxybutyrate. J Neurochem 2001;79:539–544.

19. Pan JW, Rothman DL, Behar KL, Stein DT, Hetherington HP. Human brain β-hydroxybutyrate and lactate increase in fasting induced ketosis. J Cereb Blood Flow Metab 2000;20:1502–1507.

20. Gjedde A, Crone C. Induction processes in blood brain transfer of ketone bodies during starvation. Am J Physiol 1975;229:1165–1169.

21. Pan JW, de Graaf RA, Petersen KF, Shulman GI, Hetherington HP, Rothman DL. [2,4-[13]C2]-β-Hydroxybutyrate metabolism in human brain. J Cereb Blood Flow Metab 2002;22:890–898.

22. Lebon V, Petersen KF, Cline GW, Shen J, Mason GF, Dufour S, Behar KL, Shulman GI, Rothman DL. Astroglial contribution to brain energy metabolism in humans revealed by ^{13}C nuclear magnetic resonance spectroscopy: elucidation of the dominant pathway for neurotransmitter glutamate repletion and measurement of astrocytic oxidative metabolism. J Neurosci 2002;22:1523–1531.

23. DeVivo DC, Leckie MP, Ferrendelli JS, McDougal DB Jr. Chronic ketosis and cerebral metabolism. Ann Neurol 1978;3:331–337.

24. Pan JW, Bebin EM, Chu WJ, Hetherington HP. Ketosis and epilepsy: [31]P spectroscopic imaging at 4 T. Epilepsia 1999;40:703–707.

25. Huttenlocher PR. Ketonemia and seizures: metabolic and anticonvulsant effects of two ketogenic diets in childhood epilepsy. Pediatr Res 1976;10:536–540.

26. Seymour KJ, Bluml S, Sutherling J, Sutherling W, Ross BD. Identification of cerebral acetone by ^{1}H-MRS in patients with epilepsy controlled by the ketogenic diet. MAGMA 1999;8:33–42.

27. Yudkoff M, Daikhin Y, Nissim I, Lazarow A, Nissim I. Ketogenic diet, amino acid metabolism, and seizure control. J Neurosci Res 2001;66:931–940.

12 Potential Applications of the Ketogenic Diet in Disorders Other Than Epilepsy

Rif S. El-Mallakh

1. INTRODUCTION

Starvation is associated with many drastic or extreme changes in energy metabolism and hormonal levels. Thus, it is not surprising that mimicking this process with the ketogenic diet (KD) may yield a wide range of effects, some potentially deleterious, others having benefits. Use of the KD in intractable epilepsy has increased the comfort level and general experience with the diet and is opening doors to potential new applications. None of these applications is as well studied or as well established as the anticonvulsant potential of the KD. Currently, all the applications discussed in this chapter are highly experimental.

2. FACILITATED GLUCOSE TRANSPORTER PROTEIN TYPE I DEFICIENCY

Under normal conditions, glucose is the preferred brain fuel source. However, glucose is polar and cannot diffuse unaided across the blood–brain barrier; it must be transported across the membrane through a special transporter. In a family of glucose transporters, a single protein transports glucose across the blood–brain barrier—the facilitated glucose transporter type I protein (GLUT1) *(1)*. In 1991 a rare genetic disorder was described in which infants present with seizures, developmental delay, acquired microcephaly, hypotonia, and motor problems *(2)*. Importantly, there is low cerebrospinal fluid glucose (hypoglycorrhachia) in the setting of normal plasma glucose *(2)*. Other than a wide range of infections and lupus erythematosus, there are no other causes of isolated hypoglycorrhachia *(1)*. The cause of this disease is absence of GLUT1 *(3–6)*.

The KD has been recommended as the major treatment for GLUT1 deficiency. Patients with this disorder achieve prompt control of seizures once placed on the diet *(4,7)*. However, other symptoms of GLUT1 deficiency, such as cognitive delay, do not appear to be affected by the KD *(4,7)*. The ketogenic diet is believed to work by converting brain energy metabolism from being glucose based to being based on ketone bodies.

From: *Epilepsy and the Ketogenic Diet*
Edited by: C. E. Stafstrom and J. M. Rho © Humana Press Inc., Totowa, NJ

3. MANIC–DEPRESSIVE ILLNESS

Bipolar, or manic–depressive, illness has been likened to a "slow seizure" *(8),* and indeed all the accepted mood-stabilizing medications for this disorder either are antiepileptic drugs (valproate, carbamazepine, lamotrigine) *(9)* or have a seizure-reducing potential (lithium) *(10,11).* Similarly, electroconvulsive therapy (ECT) and vagus nerve stimulation (VNS), both of which increase the seizure threshold *(12,13),* are useful in treating bipolar illness *(14–16).* Thus, anticonvulsant activity appears to be related to mood-stabilizing activity. However, anticonvulsant activity alone is insufficient. The anticonvulsant gabapentin actually worsens manic symptoms *(17).*

Excessive intracellular sodium accumulation has been linked with both mania and depression *(18–20).* One of the commonalities of effective mood-stabilizing agents appears to be their ability to inhibit sodium entry or accumulation in an activity-dependent manner *(9).*

The KD induces a mild extracellular acidosis, at least in the periphery. The excess of extracellular hydrogen ions would be expected to reduce intracellular sodium concentration through the sodium–proton counterexchange system *(21,22).* Additionally, acidosis has been associated with a reduction of neuronal excitability and activity of excitatory neurotransmitters *(23–26).* However, despite such conjecture, there is no direct evidence that brain pH changes are induced by the KD *(27,28).*

Finally, mania and bipolar depression have been associated with both global and focal reductions in glucose utilization *(29–33).* The KD appears to increase available energy in the form of adenosine triphosphate *(34).*

These observations have been proposed to suggest a clinical utility of the KD in the management of bipolar illness *(35).* However, one case report of a treatment-resistant bipolar woman placed on the diet for a month (but never achieving ketosis) was negative *(36).*

4. RISKS FOR OBESITY, DIABETES, AND CARDIOVASCULAR DISEASE

4.1. Obesity

Obesity is a major public health problem in the United States, with an increasing prevalence in both adults *(37,38)* and children *(39).* Obesity increases the risk of morbidity and mortality from associated diseases such as diabetes, hypertension, coronary heart disease, and cancer *(40–42).* Diets have been the traditional approach to dealing with excessive weight. Robert Atkins *(43)* popularized the use of the ketogenic diet to deal with weight gain. This type of ketogenic diet is a low-carbohydrate but high-protein formulation and consequently is fundamentally different from diets used for seizure control.

The Atkins diet is based on the premise that control of insulin is essential for weight loss and associated beneficial effects in reduction of diabetes and cardiovascular risk. By reducing carbohydrate intake to a negligible level, the diet attempts to eliminate insulin fluctuations that might occur after a typical meal. It is important to note that while this diet does not limit protein intake, many amino acids can be incorporated into the glycolysis pathways and thus can influence insulin secretion. However, this is not true for fatty acids. Consequently, a low-protein ketogenic diet is more likely to achieve the hypothesized goals of the Atkins diet than the widely used Atkins-type diet itself.

Weight loss with Atkins-type diets appears to be comparable to conventional hypocaloric diets in adults (mean loss of 5 kg in 12 wk) *(44)*. Adolescents may respond better to a very-low-calorie KD than to a low-calorie nonketogenic diet (average loss of 15.4 kg over 8 wk on the KD vs 2.3 kg over 12 wk on a low-calorie nonketogenic diet) *(45)*. Weight loss may also occur when the diet is intended to be isocaloric to the baseline diet *(46,47)*. In addition to the reduction of carbohydrates, the type of fat consumed may be important.

Papamandjaris et al. *(48)* proposed that medium-chain fatty acids may hold more potential for weight loss than long-chain fatty acids, since the former are metabolized preferentially in the mitochondria and are associated with a postprandial increase in energy expenditure.

4.2. Cardiovascular Disease

In one study, over a relatively short (12-wk) duration, there were no observed differences between varying diets in total weight, fat content, or lean body mass in adults *(44)*. Physiologically, a high-protein Atkins-type KD does not appear to alter exercise capacity. After 3 d of control or KD, healthy volunteers showed no decrement in exercise tolerance *(49)*. Markers of cardiovascular disease do not appear to be adversely affected by the diet. In obese adolescents, total cholesterol decreased from 162 ± 12 to 121 ± 8 mg/dL over 2 mo *(45)*. Both high-density lipoproteins (HDL) and low-density lipoproteins (LDL) decreased, leaving the LDL/HDL ratio unchanged at 2.5 *(45)*. In normal-weight healthy men placed on a high-protein KD for 6 wk, there were several favorable changes in markers of cardiovascular disease. Fasting triacylglycerol decreased by 33–55%; total cholesterol was unchanged; HDL tended to increase (9.7–11.5%); and serum lipemia and peak posttriacylglycerol after a fat-rich meal were also reduced (29–42%) *(50)*. In subjects with small LDL particles pattern B, a pattern that is associated with an increase of cardiovascular disease risk *(51)*, there was an increase in mean particle diameter *(50,52)*. After 10 d on the KD, there is no change in apolipoprotein AI, a protein component whose decrease is associated with worsening of atherosclerosis *(53)*.

In contrast to these observations, the low-protein, low-carbohydrate KD used in the treatment of epilepsy is associated with elevations of serum cholesterol and triglycerides *(54)*, and prolongation of the QT interval (QT_c) in as many as 15% of subjects *(55)*, both findings that would appear to increase cardiovascular risk.

4.3. Diabetes

Before the availability of insulin, the treatment of choice for diabetes was starvation. Limiting caloric intake reduced diabetics' acute problems, e.g., ketoacidosis, and prolonged life expectancy. The introduction of insulin for the treatment of diabetes made such extreme interventions obsolete, but diet continues to be a cornerstone of the management of diabetes. Unfortunately, current dietary recommendations for diabetes have been driven by the cardiovascular field and have thus focused on lowering dietary fat and cholesterol *(56)*. The high-protein Atkins-type KD may be the diet of choice for control of diabetes. In a study of non-insulin-dependent diabetics given controlled formulas that contained either high complex carbohydrate or low carbohydrate and high fat, glucose control was superior in the latter group *(57)*. Glucose, insulin, and C-peptide were all higher in the diabetics who were fed high complex carbohydrates *(57)*. In general, comparative studies find that high-fat diets improve glycemic control as long as unsaturated or monosaturated fats are used *(58,59)*.

5. RHEUMATOID ARTHRITIS

Acute starvation appears to have a beneficial effect on clinical and laboratory markers of rheumatoid arthritis disease activity *(60–62)*. This effect does not appear to be related to avoidance of specific food items *(63,64)*. However, since carbohydrate restriction mediates much of the hormonal change observed in starvation *(65)*, it follows then that the KD may also be associated with clinical improvement in arthritis. In a study of 13 subjects afflicted with rheumatoid arthritis placed on a carbohydrate-restricted (<40 g/day) but not protein-restricted ketogenic diet for 1 wk, Fraser and colleagues found no beneficial effect on either clinical *(46)* or laboratory *(46,47)* parameters of rheumatoid arthritis disease activity. Longer duration of diet and use of carbohydrate- and protein-restricted KD have not been studied.

6. CONCLUSION

The KD has an established role in the treatment of refractory seizures. In one metabolic disorder, GLUT1 deficiency, use of the KD is not only beneficial but essential—in patients with that disorder, brain energy must be obtained by noncarbohydrate sources. In addition, the KD may find a role in alleviating the symptoms of other disorders, including manic–depressive illness, obesity, cardiovascular disease, diabetes, and rheumatoid arthritis. Whether the KD works through a similar mechanism in disorders of cellular hyperexcitability (epilepsy), energy depletion (GLUT1 deficiency), and the others just listed awaits further research. Similarly, it is presently unclear whether certain patient subpopulations in the other disorders will preferentially benefit from the KD.

REFERENCES

1. Klepper J, Voit T. Facilitated glucose transporter protein type I (GLUT1) deficiency syndrome: impaired glucose transport into brain—a review. Eur J Pediatr 2002;161:295–304.
2. DeVivo DC, Trifiletti RR, Jacobson RI, Ronen GM, Behmand RA, Harik SI. Defective glucose transport across the blood–brain barrier as a cause of persistent hypoglycorrhachia, seizures, and developmental delay. N Engl J Med 1991;325:703–709.
3. Brockmann K, Wang D, Korenke CG, von Moers A, Ho YY, Pascual JM, Kuang K, Yang H, Ma L, Kranz-Eble P, Fischbarg J, Hanefeld F, De Vivo DC. Autosomal dominant glut-1 deficiency syndrome and familial epilepsy. Ann Neurol 2001;50:476–485.
4. Klepper J, Wang D, Fischbarg J, Vera JC, Jarjour IT, O'Driscoll KR, DeVivo DC. Defective glucose transport across brain tissue barriers: a newly recognized neurological syndrome. Neurochem Res 1999;24:587–597.
5. Klepper J, Willemsen M, Verrips A, Guertsen E, Herrmann R, Kutzick C, Florcken A, Voit T. Autosomal dominant transmission of GLUT1-deficiency. Hum Mol Genet 2001;10:63–68.
6. Seidner G, Alvarez MG, Yeh JI, O'Driscoll KR, Klepper J, Stump TS, Wang D, Spinner NB, Birnbaum MJ, DeVivo DC. GLUT-1 deficiency syndrome caused by haploinsufficiency of the blood–brain barrier hexose carrier. Nat Genet 1998;18:188–191.
7. DeVivo DC, Garcia-Alverez M, Ronen G, Trifiletti R. Glucose transport protein deficiency: an emerging syndrome with therapeutic implications. Int Pediatr 1995;10:51–56.
8. El-Mallakh RS. The Na,K-ATPase hypothesis for manic-depression. I. General considerations. Med Hypoth 1983;12:253–266.
9. El-Mallakh RS, Huff MO. Mood stabilizers and ion regulation. Harv Rev Psychiatr 2001;9:23–32.

10. Erwin CW, Gerber DJ, Morrison SD, James JF. Lithium carbonate and convulsive disorders. Arch Gen Psychiatr 1973;28:646–648.

11. Shukla S, Mukherjee S, Decina P. Lithium in the treatment of bipolar disorders associated with epilepsy: an open study. J Clin Psychopharmacol 1988;8:201–204.

12. Post RM, Putnam F, Uhde TW, Weiss SRB. Electoroconvulsive therapy as an anticonvulsant: implications for its mechanism of action in affective illness. N Y Acad Sci 1986;462:376–388.

13. Morris GI III, Mueller WM, and the Vagus Nerve Stimulation Study Group E01-E05. Long-term treatment with vagus nerve stimulation in patients with refractory epilepsy. Neurology 1999;53:1731–1735.

14. Milstein V, Small JG, Klapper MH, Small IF, Miller MJ, Kellams JJ. Unilateral versus bilateral ECT in the treatment of mania. Convuls Ther 1987;3:1–9.

15. Small JG, Kalapper MH, Kellams JJ, Miller MJ, Milstein V, Sharpley PH, Small IF. Electroconvulsive treatment compared with lithium in the management of manic states. Arch Gen Psychiatr 1988;45:727–732.

16. George MS, Sackeim HA, Rush AJ, Marangell LB, Nahas Z, Husain MM, Lisanby S, Burt T, Goldman J, Ballenger JC. Vagus nerve stimulation: a new tool for brain research and therapy. Biol Psychiatr 2000;47:287–295.

17. Pande AC. Combination treatment in bipolar disorders. Bipolar Disord 1999;1 (Suppl 1):17.

18. Coppen A. Shaw DM, Malleson A, Costain R. Mineral metabolism in mania. Br Med J 1966;1:71–75.

19. Shaw DM. Mineral metabolism, mania and melancholia. Br Med J 1966;2:262–267.

20. Naylor GJ, McNamee HB, Moody JP. Changes in erythrocyte sodium and potassium on recovery from
   . depressive illness. Br J Psychiatr 1971:118:219–223.

21. Siebens AW, Boron WF. Depolarization-induced alkalinization in proximal tubules. I. Characteristics and dependence on Na^+. Am J Physiol 1989:25:F342–F353.

22. Pappas CA, Ransom BR. A depolarization-stimulated, bafilomycin-inhibitable H^+ pump in hippocampal astrocytes. Glia 1993:9:280–291.

23. Konnerth A, Lux HD, Morad M. Proton-induced transformation of calcium channel in dorsal root ganglion cells. J Physiol 1987:386:603–633.

24. Balestrino M, Somjen GG. Concentration of carbon dioxide, interstitial pH and synaptic transmission in hippocampal formation of the rat. J Physiol 1988;396:247–266.

25. Tang CM, Dichter MA, Morad M. Modulation of the N-methyl-d-aspartate channel by extracellular H^+. Proc Natl Acad Sci U S A 1990;87:6445–6449.

26. Traynelis SF, Cull-Candy SG. Proton inhibition of N-methyl-d-aspartate J receptors in cerebral neurons. Nature 1990;345:347–350.

27. Al-Mudallal AS, LaManna JC, Lust WD, Harik SI. Diet-induced ketosis does not cause cerebral acidosis. Epilepsia 1996;37:258–261.

28. Novotny EJ Jr, Chen J. Rothman DL. Alterations in cerebral metabolism with the ketogenic diet. Epilepsia 1997;38 (Suppl 8):147.

29. Baxter LR Jr, Phelps ME, Mazziotta JC, Schwartz JM, Gerner RH, Selin CE, Sumida RM. Cerebral metabolic rates for glucose in mood disorders: studies with positron emission tomography and fluorodeoxyglucose F-18. Arch Gen Psychiatr 1985;42:441–447.

30. Baxter LR Jr, Schwartz JM, Phelps ME, Mazziotta JC, Guze BH, Selin CE, Gerner RH, Sumida RM. Reduction of prefrontal cortex glucose metabolism common to three types of depression. Arch Gen Psychiatr 1989;46:243–250.

31. Buchsbaum MS, Wu J, DeLisi LE, Holcomb H, Kessler R. Johnson J, King AC, Hazlett E, Langston K. Post RM. Frontal cortex and basal ganglia metabolic rates assessed by positron emission tomography with [18F]2-deoxyglucose in affective illness. J Affect Disord 1986;10:137–152.

32. Bucsbaum MS, Someya T, Wu JC, Tang CY, Bunney WE. Neuroimaging bipolar illness with positron emission tomography and magnetic resonance imaging. Psychiatr Ann 1997;27:489–495.

33. Schwartz JM, Baxter LP, Mazziotta JC, Gerner RH, Phelps ME. The differential diagnosis of depression: relevance of positron emission tomography (PET) studies of cerebral glucose metabolism to the bipolar–unipolar dichotomy. JAMA 1987;258:1368–1374.

34. Pan JW, Bebin EM, Chu WJ, Hetherington HP. Ketosis and epilepsy: ^{31}P spectroscopic imaging at 4.1 T. Epilepsia 1999;40:703–707.

35. El-Mallakh RS, Paskitti ME. The ketogenic diet may have mood-stabilizing properties. Med Hypoth 2001;57:724–726.

36. Yaroslavsky Y, Stahl Z, Belmaker RH. Ketogenic diet in bipolar illness. Bipolar Disord 2002;4:75.
37. Flegal KM, Carroll MD, Ogden CL, Johnson CL. Prevalence and trends in obesity among US adults, 1999–2000. JAMA 2002;288:1723–1727.
38. Weil E, Wachterman M, McCarthy EP, Davis RB, O'Day B, Iezzoni LI, Wee CC. Obesity among adults with disabling conditions. JAMA 2002;288:1265–1268.
39. Ogden CL, Flegal KM, Carroll MD, Johnson CL. Prevalence and trends in overweight among US children and adolescents, 1999–2000. JAMA 2002;288:1728–1732.
40. Lew EA, Garfinkel L. Variations in mortality by weight among 750,000 men and women. J Chron Dis 1979;32:563–576.
41. Bray GA. Complications of obesity. Ann Intern Med 1985;103:1052–1062.
42. Must A, Jacques PF, Dallal GE, Bajema CJ, Dietz WH. Long-term morbidity and mortality of overweight adolescents. N Engl J Med 1992;327:1350–1355.
43. Atkins RC. Dr. Atkins's New Diet Revolution, rev. ed. Avon, New York, 2002.
44. Landers P, Wolfe MM, Glore S, Guild R, Phillips L. Effect of weight loss plans on body composition and diet duration. J Okla State Med Assoc 2002;95:329–331.
45. Willi SM, Oexmann MJ, Wright NM, Collop NA, Key LL Jr. The effects of a high-protein, low-fat, ketogenic diet on adolescents with morbid obesity: body composition, blood chemistries, and sleep abnormalities. Pediatrics 1998;101:61–67.
46. Fraser DA, Thoen J, Bondhus S, Haugen M, Reseland JE, Djøseland O, Førre Ø, Kjeldsen-Kragh J. Reduction in serum leptin and IGF-1 but preserved T-lymphocyte numbers and activation after a ketogenic diet in rheumatoid arthritis patients. Clin Exp Rheumatol 2000;18:209–214.
47. Fraser DA, Thoen J, Djøseland O, Førre Ø, Kjeldsen-Kragh J. Serum levels of interleukin-6 and dehydroepiandrosterone sulphate in response to either fasting or a ketogenic diet in rheumatoid arthritis patients. Clin Exp Rheumatol 2000;18:357–362.
48. Papamandjaris AA, MacDougall DE, Jones PJ. Medium chain fatty acid metabolism and energy expenditure: obesity treatment implications. Life Sci 1998;62:1203–1215.
49. Langfort J, Pilis W, Zarzeczny R, Nazar K, Kaciuba UH. Effect of low-carbohydrate-ketogenic diet on metabolic and hormonal responses to graded exercise in man. J Physiol Pharmacol 1996;47:361–371.
50. Sharman MJ, Kraemer WJ, Love DM, Avery NG, Gómez AL, Scheett TP, Volek JS. A ketogenic diet favorably affects serum biomarkers for cardiovascular disease in normal-weight men. J Nutr 2002;132:1879–1885.
51. Austin MA, Breslow JL, Hennekens CH, Buring JE, Willett WC, Krauss RM. Low-density lipoprotein subclass patterns and risk of myocardial infarction. JAMA 1988;260:1917–1921.
52. Volek JS, Gómez AL, Kraemer WJ. Fasting lipoprotein and postprandial triacylglycerol responses to a low-carbohydrate diet supplemented with n-3 fatty acid. J Am Coll Nutr 2000;19:383–391.
53. Haas MJ, Reinacher D, Pun K, Wong NC, Mooradian AD. Induction of the apolipoprotein AI gene by fasting: a relationship with ketosis but not with ketone bodies. Metab Clin Exp 2000;49:1572–1578.
54. Sirven J, Whedon B, Caplan D, Liporace J, Glosser D, O'Dwyer J, Sperling MR. The ketogenic diet for intractable epilepsy in adults: preliminary results. Epilepsia 1999;40:1721–1726.
55. Best TH, Franz DN, Gilbert DL, Nelson DP, Epstein MR. Cardiac complications in pediatric patients on the ketogenic diet. Neurology 2000;54:2328–2330.
56. Storlien LH, Tapsell LC, Calvert GD. Diabetic diets—whither goest? Nutrition 1998;14:865–867.
57. Sanz-Paris A, Calvo L, Guallard A, Salazar I, Albero R. High-fat versus high-carbohydrate enteral formulae: effect on blood glucose, C-peptide, and ketones in patients with type 2 diabetes treated with insulin or sulfonylurea. Nutrition 1998;14:840–845.
58. Garg A, Bonanome A, Grundy SM, Zhang Z-J, Unger RH. Comparison of a high-carbohydrate diet with a high-monounsaturated-fat diet in patients with non-insulin-dependent diabetes mellitus. N Engl J Med 1988;319:829–834.
59. Campbell LV, Marmot PE, Dyer JA, Borkman M, Storlien LH. The high-monounsaturated fat diet as a practical alternative for NIDDM. Diabetes Care 1994;17:177–182.
60. Sköldstam L, Larsson L, Lindström FD. Effects of fasting and lactovegetarian diet on rheumatoid arthritis. Scand J Rheumatol 1979;8:249–255.
61. Hafström I, Ringertz B, Gyllenhammer H, Palmblad J, Harms-Ringdahl M. Effects of fasting in disease activity, neutrophil function, fatty acid composition, and leukotriene biosynthesis in patients with rheumatoid arthritis. Arthritis Rheum 1988;31:585–592.

62. Fraser D, Thoen J, Reseland J, Førre Ø, Kjeldsen-Kragh J. Decreased CD4+ lymphocyte activation and increased IL-4 production in peripheral blood of rheumatoid arthritis patients after acute starvation. Clin Rheumatol 1999;18:394–401.

63. Van der Laar MAFJ, van der Korst JK. Food intolerance in rheumatoid arthritis. I: A double blind, controlled trial of the clinical effects of elimination of milk allergens and azo dyes. Ann Rheum Dis 1992;51:298–302.

64. Haugen M, Kjeldsen-Kragh J, Førre Ø. A pilot study of the effect of an elemental diet in the management of rheumatoid arthritis. Clin Exp Rheumatol 1994;12:275–279.

65. Klein S, Wolfe R. Carbohydrate restriction regulates the adaptive response to fasting. Am J Physiol 1992;262:E631–E636.

13 Dietary Treatments for Epilepsy Other Than the Ketogenic Diet

Carl E. Stafstrom and Gregory L. Holmes

There is nothing in the world that can pass the human mouth that hasn't at some time been advocated as a remedy against epilepsy. E. H. Sieveking, 1858

1. INTRODUCTION

The prospect that epilepsy might be controlled, at least partially, by dietary intake is radical but highly appealing. The ketogenic diet (KD) is the best-known and most well-studied dietary treatment for epilepsy, but it is by no means the only nutritional intervention touted to reduce seizures. As noted by Sieveking (quoted in ref. *1*, p. 1366), numerous food substances to cure epilepsy have been tried over the course of human history. However, aside from the KD, no dietary treatment has met widespread acceptance or success. Human consumption of several specific substances can be shown to later incorporate into neuronal membranes and affect their function. Therefore, at least theoretically, dietary approaches to a disorder of neuronal hyperexcitability such as epilepsy could be feasible. However, aside from the KD, the role of diet in epilepsy has received scant attention.

This chapter reviews three dietary approaches to epilepsy other than the KD. First, choline is discussed as an example of a dietary supplement (vital amine or "vitamin") that may be potentially beneficial. Second, polyunsaturated fatty acids (PUFAs) are considered as an example of a normal dietary lipid constituent that might play a role in neuronal excitability. Third, the issue of total calorie intake (energy) is addressed, inasmuch as recent studies have shown that reduction of calorie intake has numerous health benefits including a prolonged life-span, elevated seizure threshold, and reduced injury-induced neurotoxicity. We also consider dietary alterations that could worsen seizure control. We omit discussion of the numerous dietary manipulations sometimes referred to as "alternative medicine," not because they lack potential usefulness *(2)* but, rather, because there is little if any concurrence among practitioners, and solid scientific data are unavailable. Finally, we regret that space precludes discussion of various regional or "ethnic" dietary treatments of epilepsy; this topic is reviewed in detail by Sonnen *(1)*.

From: *Epilepsy and the Ketogenic Diet*
Edited by: C. E. Stafstrom and J. M. Rho © Humana Press Inc., Totowa, NJ

2. EXAMPLES OF DIETARY TREATMENTS FOR EPILEPSY

2.1. Choline-Enriched Diets

2.1.1. FUNCTIONS OF CHOLINE

Choline is an amine that has been of interest for many years because of its critical role in brain development and response to injury. Choline is an essential nutrient for all mammals, and an adequate supply is particularly important during fetal development, when the organism grows rapidly (3). Pregnancy and lactation are the periods of highest dietary demands for choline, when large amounts of this compound are transferred from the mother to the offspring via placenta and milk. Choline serves as a precursor of phospholipids, phosphatidylcholine, lysophosphatidylcholine, choline plasmalogen, and sphingomyelin, essential components of all membranes. It is also a precursor of acetylcholine and is essential for the formation of signaling phospholipids such as platelet-activating factor and sphingosylphosphorylcholine (3).

2.1.2. BENEFICIAL EFFECTS OF CHOLINE SUPPLEMENTATION

2.1.2.1. Cognitive Function Previous studies have shown that supplementation with choline during both pre- and postnatal development in rats can result in improved cognitive function when animals are tested as adults. Choline supplementation has produced long-term facilitation of memory function in a variety of tasks including the radial arm maze, water maze, and passive avoidance test (4–7). This increase in memory capacity might constitute a "cognitive reserve" to make prenatally choline-supplemented animals resistant to memory impairment.

Choline administration may interact with other factors, such as environmental stimulation, to enhance cognitive function. Pre- and postnatal supplementation of choline enhanced spatial learning and memory in the Morris water maze (8). In that study, animals reared in a complex, enriched environment performed better than those raised in a standard environment. This improved performance was further enhanced in animals that received choline.

There are also indications that choline can aid in recovery from neurotoxic insults. Rats exposed to alcohol *in utero* performed poorly on a task involving visual–spatial discrimination. When neonatal rats exposed to alcohol were administered supplemental choline from postnatal days (P) 2–21, their performance on the visual–spatial discrimination task improved significantly over that of nonsupplemented rats (9). In an operant conditioning task in senescent rats, choline supplementation resulted in improved performance over that of nontreated controls (10).

2.1.2.2. Status Epilepticus In rats, prenatal choline supplementation reduced brain damage and cognitive dysfunction following status epilepticus (11). In that study, pregnant rats received a control or choline-supplemented diet during d 11–17 of gestation. Male offspring were tested for their ability to find a platform in a water maze before and after administration of a convulsant dose of pilocarpine on P34. The behavior, electroencephalographic (EEG) findings, and spontaneous recurrent seizures following pilocarpine resembled results seen in temporal lobe epilepsy (12). Following pilocarpine-induced status epilepticus, adolescent and adult rats had significant deficits in learning and behavior compared with controls (13). There were no differences between offspring of control or choline-supplemented dams in water maze performance prior to the seizure. One week after status epilepticus (P41–44), animals that had received the control diet prenatally had drastically impaired performance in the water maze during the 4-d testing period, whereas rats that had been supplemented prenatally with choline showed no impairment. The benefits of choline were seen only in the animals that experienced status epilepticus. No differences in water maze performance were found between the choline-supplemented and controls rats when tested prior to the status epilepticus, nor were there any differences between choline-supplemented and control animals that did not receive pilocarpine and were tested a second time.

Holmes and colleagues *(14)* also compared outcome following status epilepticus in animals that had received a normal, choline-supplemented, or choline-deficient diet starting on d 11 of gestation and continuing until P7. On P42, rats were given kainic acid (KA), a glutamate analog that acts as a potent convulsant. As with pilocarpine, the behavior, EEG findings, and spontaneous recurrent seizures in this model resembled those seen in human temporal lobe epilepsy *(15)*. In rodents, KA status epilepticus is associated with subsequent cognitive impairment, histological damage, and sponta- neous seizures *(16,17)*. Two weeks after KA-induced status epilepticus, rats underwent testing of visual–spatial memory in the Morris water maze. Rats receiving supplemental choline performed substantially better on this task than animals in the choline-deficient and control groups *(14)*.

Choline administration *after* status epilepticus has also been demonstrated to be bene- ficial *(14)*. KA was administered to P35 rats that had been fed a normal diet. Following the status epilepticus, the rats were given a choline-supplemented or control diet for 4 wk and then were tested in the water maze. Rats receiving choline supplementation per- formed far better than rats receiving a regular diet. This study demonstrated that choline supplementation prior to or following KA-induced status epilepticus can protect rats from memory deficits induced by status epilepticus. Therefore, choline supplementation could be beneficial even when administered following status epilepticus, although it is presently unclear whether there is a specific time window for this therapeutic benefit.

2.1.3. Mechanisms of Action of Choline

The mechanisms by which choline supplementation improves learning and choline deficiency impairs learning are not clear. Studies of changes in cholinergic enzymes have yielded inconsistent results. Prenatal choline supplementation reduced hippocam- pal choline acetyltransferease (ChAT) and acetylcholinesterase (AChE) activities in juvenile rats (up to P27), but these effects have not been demonstrated in older animals *(11,18,19)*. Offspring from mothers given choline-deficient diets had significantly lower ChAT levels than the animals receiving either a control diet or a choline-supplemented diet *(14)*. Since ChAT is the enzyme that converts choline into acetylcholine, reduction of ChAT presumably would decrease the amount of acetylcholine available for synaptic transmission. In this regard, mice treated with choline oxidase, a hydrolytic enzyme for choline, had impaired acquisition of passive avoidance learning, presumably secondary to decreased cerebral cholinergic neurotransmission *(20)*.

In many studies, choline is given prenatally. The period of administration, embryonic days 11–17, typically includes a critical period for development of the cholinergic sys- tem in rat brains *(21)*. The observation that prenatal choline supplementation can alter the caudal–rostral distribution and size of cells in the medial septal nucleus and the nucleus of the diagonal band of Broca is consistent with reports that choline can influ- ence forebrain cytogenesis, migration, and neuronal survivability *(22)*. Moreover, choline supplementation during this period alters multiple functional indices of the septohippocampal cholinergic system, thought to be critical for the processes of attention, learning, and memory (23,24). Loy and colleagues (25) found that pre- and postnatal choline supplementation resulted in medial septal cell bodies that were larger, rounder, and more uniform than those in controls. In addition, p75 neurotrophin receptor-positive cells (presumably cholinergic neurons) in the diagonal band of rats supplemented with choline prenatally were larger than those of controls (26).

Prenatal choline therapy can enhance excitatory neurotransmission. Montoya and Swartzwelder (27) examined hippocampal N-methyl-D-aspartate (NMDA) neurotransmission in offspring of pregnant mothers receiving control, choline-supplemented, or choline-deficient diets. Evoked NMDA receptor-mediated excitatory postsynaptic potentials (EPSPs) were enhanced in slices from prenatally choline-supplemented animals relative to controls. Furthermore, the prenatal choline-deficient group had fewer viable NMDA receptor-mediated EPSPs than controls and supplemented animals. Prenatal choline administration also prevents MK801-induced cortical neuronal degeneration (28). Functionally, prenatally adminstered choline decreased the threshold for long-term potentiation (LTP) in hippocampal area CA1 (29). These results suggest that lowering of the LTP threshold among prenatally supplemented animals could be the result of an enhancement of NMDA receptor-mediated neurotransmission in the Schaffer collateral–commissural/CA1 circuit.

2.1.4. SUMMARY AND CLINICAL USE OF CHOLINE SUPPLEMENTATION

Although there have been no clinical trials of choline supplementation in patients with epilepsy, animal studies point to the potential usefulness of this compound, both before and after epileptic insults. Likewise, there are theoretical reasons to suspect that choline may affect neuronal excitability, although the exact mechanisms by which seizures may be modulated by choline are unknown. Further study in this area is certainly warranted.

2.2. Polyunsaturated Fatty Acids (PUFAs)

2.2.1. EFFECTS OF FATTY ACIDS ON BRAIN DEVELOPMENT

The critical role of fatty acids in nervous system development has been emphasized in numerous studies (for reviews, see refs. 30–33). Essential fatty acids, especially long-chain polyunsaturated fatty acids (PUFAs) of the omega-3 (ω3 or n-3) class, are necessary for development of normal retinal and neuronal membranes (34,35) and subsequent normal behavior and cognition (36–40). PUFAs are particularly important for normal retinal and brain development in preterm infants, leading to the suggestion that infant formulas should be supplemented to achieve PUFA levels comparable to those in human breast milk (41–43). It has even been suggested that the diet of lactating mothers be supplemented with PUFAs (44,45).

The need for such supplementation remains controversial. In addition to the positive effects of PUFAs, some caveats exist as well. Deficiency of the PUFA docosahexaenoic acid (DHA, 22:6ω3) leads to cognitive, behavioral, and structural abnormalities (46). However, very high maternal levels of DHA may negatively affect myelinogenesis of central auditory pathways (47). In a recent study, Fewtrell and colleagues failed to establish the effectiveness of PUFA-enriched formula on global aspects of neural development in premature infants (48). Nevertheless, the prevailing opinion is that PUFAs are essential for optimal nervous system development.

2.2.2. EFFECTS OF FATTY ACIDS ON CELLULAR EXCITABILITY

2.2.2.1. Actions on Cardiac Myocytes In addition to their role in brain development, fatty acids exert important modulatory effects on cellular excitability *(49)* and receptor-mediated signaling pathways *(50)*. Many of the effects of PUFAs on physiological excitability were originally shown in elegant studies on cardiac muscle cells *(51)*. In cardiac myocytes, long-chain PUFAs inhibit voltage-dependent sodium channels and L-type calcium channels, thereby stabilizing the membrane, resulting in an antiarrhythmic action *(52)*.

2.2.2.2. Actions on Neurons and Seizure Activity In Vitro PUFAs also exert important modulatory actions on neurons. Fatty acids can increase or decrease the firing of neurons, alter neurotransmitter release, and modulate synaptic responses *(38,53–55)*. PUFAs have been shown to reduce neuronal sodium and calcium currents *(56)* and to inhibit or activate potassium channels *(57–59)*. DHA facilitates excitatory synaptic transmission mediated by NMDA-type glutamate receptors *(60)*. However, in some neurons, e.g., substantia nigra, DHA reduces responses to the inhibitory transmitter γ-aminobutyric acid (GABA) *(61)*. Nevertheless, most current evidence favors a role for DHA reducing neuronal excitability.

In the kainic acid (KA) model of epilepsy, intraperitoneal administration of KA results in partial seizures that rapidly generalize into convulsive status epilepticus, later causing the death of hippocampal neurons and spontaneous recurrent seizures, i.e., epilepsy. When the PUFA linolenic acid (LIN, 18:2ω6) was administered prior to KA, animals were protected against status epilepticus and subsequent excitotoxic hippocampal cell death; similar neuroprotection was seen if LIN was given shortly after KA *(62)*. Neuroprotection was not observed with palmitic acid, a saturated fatty acid. Of particular interest is that PUFAs activate a class of "background" or "leak" potassium channels (called 2-pore or 2P-domain potassium channels) that are responsible for maintaining the resting potential of neurons *(63)*. When such potassium channels are opened, the neuron hyperpolarizes, reducing glutamate release and thereby limiting glutamate-induced excitotoxicity. This scheme is appealing in that the 2P-domain potassium channels could represent a novel antiepileptic target *(64,65)*.

In cultured striatal neurons, another PUFA, arachidonic acid (AA, 20:4ω6), inhibits voltage-gated sodium channels and shifts sodium inactivation to hyperpolarized potentials *(66)*. The result of these physiological alterations is to suppress neurotransmitter release and reduce the repetitive firing of neurons, similar to the actions of the well-established anticonvulsants phenytoin and carbamazepine *(67)*. Fatty acid levels can also rise during paroxysmal activity and subsequently may alter excitability by affecting ionic homeostasis *(68)*.

Brain slice preparations can be used to assess whether direct application of a PUFA can alter ongoing epileptiform activity. In preliminary experiments, we used the zero-magnesium model, which allows excessive activation of NMDA receptor-mediated seizure activity *(69)*. Extracellular recordings were made from the CA1 subfield in hippocampal slices of P14 rats. When the magnesium was removed from the bathing medium, brief spontaneous interictal discharges appeared, followed by prolonged, intense ictal bursts (electrographic seizures). Perfusion of DHA ($100\mu M$) eliminated those ictal bursts in a reversible manner, suggesting that this PUFA blocks epileptiform events and therefore may be able to exert an antiepileptic action in the brain. Others using this model have also reported a suppressant effect of PUFA on seizure activity.

DHA (50μ*M*) enhanced inhibition and reduced bicuculline- and low-magnesium-induced seizure activity in the CA1 region of hippocampal slices, leading to the conclusion that DHA blocks seizure activity by a frequency-dependent blockade of sodium channels *(70)*, a mechanism discussed in the preceding paragraph.

Similar protective effects of the PUFAs DHA and eicosapentaenoic acid (EPA, 20:5ω3) against seizure activity were also described in hippocampal slices in vitro *(71)*. Both compounds hyperpolarized hippocampal CA1 neurons, raising their threshold for action potential generation, and reduced baseline and convulsant-induced firing rates. It is likely that PUFA effects are regionally specific and may vary according to developmental stage. Fatty acids and their derivatives may also attenuate the response to excitotoxic injury during the neonatal period *(72)*.

2.2.2.3. Actions on Seizure Activity In Vivo Based on the effectiveness of PUFAs in reducing excitability in cardiac cells, as well as their widespread actions on neurons, the idea arose that perhaps PUFAs could also suppress neuronal hyperexcitability in conditions of pathophysiological epileptic firing *in vivo*. This notion has some precedent, as Yehuda and colleagues showed that a mixture of n-3 and n-6 essential fatty acids, in a specific ratio, raised seizure threshold in several experimental models, including single and multiple subconvulsive doses of the convulsant pentelylenetetrazole (PTZ) *(73)*. Because a mixture of PUFAs was used, these experiments could not determine an exact anticonvulsant role for any specific PUFA. It was subsequently shown that long-chain PUFAs produce a transient elevation of seizure threshold in a cortical stimulation model *(74)*. In this model, seizure threshold to convulsive electrical stimuli to cortex is followed in the same animal for up to 24 h, allowing dynamic changes in seizure susceptibility to be assessed and correlated with plasma concentration. PUFAs significantly raised the threshold to both focal and generalized seizures, with seizure protection varying according to the number of double bonds in the PUFA (DHA and EPA were most effective) *(75)*. Brain PUFA levels were not measured.

Another set of preliminary experiments examined whether dietary PUFA supplementation could reduce generalized seizures in weanling rats (P21). Rats were divided into two dietary groups: standard rat chow and a diet enriched in n-3 PUFA (20% menhaden oil) *(76)*. Plasma levels of DHA and EPA were assessed chromatographically before and 2 wk into dietary therapy; rats gained weight equally, and the PUFA group exhibited 7-to 15-fold increases in plasma EPA and DHA levels. After 3 wk of dietary treatment, rats were subjected to seizures induced by inhalation of the convulsant flurothyl. The latency, duration, or severity of flurothyl seizures did not differ between standard diet and PUFA diet groups. These negative preliminary results must be interpreted with caution, and further experiments are necessary. Since brain PUFA levels were not measured, we cannot assume that incorporation occurred at the neuronal level.

Given the extensive evidence for a neuromodulatory role of fatty acids on cortical hyperexcitability, it is tempting to speculate that this class of compound might be utilized in clinical situations in which hyperexcitable neurons fire in abnormal, synchronous patterns, i.e., epilepsy. It is notable that valproic acid, a commonly used broad-spectrum antiepileptic drug, is itself a short-chain fatty acid.

2.2.3. ROLE OF LIPIDS IN THE KD

Since the KD provides an abundance of lipids, a natural hypothesis would be that hyperlipidemia diminishes seizure susceptibility by altering the lipid composition of neuronal or glial membranes, by affecting membrane protein mobility or function, or by some metabolic mechanism. It is uncertain which, if any, lipid components are essential or modulatory on neuronal excitability in the ketotic condition. The classic KD consists of approx 80% dairy fat by weight (predominantly saturated fats, such as butter and cream) *(77)*. Many studies, both human and animal, have demonstrated elevation of serum lipids in KD-fed individuals *(78–81)*. However, serum lipids rise over several weeks, and a tight correlation with seizure reduction has not been established. Discontinuation of the KD quickly causes seizure recurrence, while lipids remain elevated. It may be that lipids of certain types, chain lengths, or degrees of saturation exert an important role on seizure control. In rodents, a cholesterol-rich diet protected against seizures induced by pentamethylenetetrazole and audiogenic stimuli *(82)*, but in humans there is no consistent correlation between cholesterol level and seizure control *(83)*. In rats, seizure control was correlated with a higher ketogenic ratio, with maximal protection against PTZ seizures at a 6:1 ratio of fat to carbohydrate plus protein *(84)*. In addition to the ketogenic ratio *per se,* the type of fat comprising a ketogenic diet may play a major role in seizure protection *(85)*.

As discussed in Sections 1. and 2.2.1., exogenous fatty acids, taken parenterally, can integrate into neuronal membranes and alter their fluidity and composition *(86)*. Increasing membrane fluidity, e.g., by insertion of certain lipid constituents, increases membrane excitability. Therefore, a reasonable and testable hypothesis would be that lipid type exerts a differential effect on membrane excitability *(49,87)*. Yehuda and colleagues *(73)* reported that the ratio of dietary n-3 to n-6 PUFAs was the critical variable that afforded protection in several epilepsy models. Fatty acids of the n-3 variety reduce the excitability of cardiac myocyte membranes *(51)* and may also exert a suppressive role on the excitability of neurons *(56,71,74)*.

2.2.4. PUFAs: A Feasible Epilepsy Treatment?

The preceding discussion has established the following:

1. PUFAs are an important modulator of neuronal excitability.
2. Dietary PUFAs can alter several aspects of brain function.
3. The KD is an effective therapeutic modality for some persons with epilepsy.
4. The mechanism of the KD's seizure protective effect is unknown but may involve lipid components.
5. The classic KD is composed of a high volume of saturated fats that contain a variable but usually small proportion of PUFAs.
6. Specific serum PUFAs increase in children on a KD.

From these observations, can we make a leap to the hypothesis that PUFAs may be effective as anticonvulsants? For any agent to be considered to be a clinically useful anticonvulsant, it must be nontoxic at therapeutically effective doses, cross the blood–brain barrier, and reduce neuronal excitability, thereby suppressing seizures.

Clinical dietary trials of PUFAs to reduce disorders of cardiac excitability have been promising *(88)*, but there have been few analogous attempts to use PUFAs for seizure control, either in patients or in animal models. A single study has attempted a clinical trial of PUFA-enriched diet in patients with epilepsy. Schlanger and colleagues *(89)* administered 5 g daily of n-3 PUFA supplement (as a bread spread) to five institutionalized patients with epilepsy. The supplement was ingested on the patients' bread each morning for 6 mo. The bread spread consisted of 65% n-3 PUFAs (46% DHA, 18% EPA, and 1% α-linolenic acid); no rationale was provided to describe how this concoction was devised. Seizure counts were compared before and after the dietary treatment. Seizure frequency before the trial ranged from 1 to 14 seizures per week; after the dietary PUFA trial, seizure counts ranged from 0 to 1 per month. Although intriguing, this study has numerous serious limitations. The study was not blinded or controlled; it involved only 5 patients (16 others were enrolled but refused to eat the supplement); and there was no uniformity in many variables, including seizure type, seizure etiology, seizure history, and concurrent anticonvulsant therapy. There was no attempt to vary the composition of the supplement, and there was no crossover to a regular diet. Therefore, these results raise the possibility that PUFA supplementation may improve seizure control; but before we conclude a positive effect, the foregoing concerns must be addressed in a much larger, well-controlled prospective study.

2.2.5. Summary and Clinical Use of PUFAs

PUFAs play multiple important roles in brain development and the regulation of neuronal excitability. Exploration of their possible function in epilepsy treatment is just now beginning. The possibility that a "PUFA diet," analogous to the existing "ketogenic diet," could be effective in the battle against epilepsy is indeed tantalizing.

2.3. Calorie Restriction

2.3.1. Fasting

The original idea for a KD derived from the beneficial effect of fasting on seizures (*see* Chapter 2, this volume) (but *see* also ref. *90*). This approach is obviously impractical except for very short-term use. An additional disadvantage is depletion of essential nutrients as well as energy intake. Nevertheless, the health benefits of modest calorie restriction are becoming increasingly clear. In animals, these benefits include an increase of mean life-span, reduction of cancer and cardiovascular disease, and amelioration of the degenerative effects of aging *(91–93)*. Although studies of calorie restriction in epilepsy are limited in scope, it is worth considering the potential for calorie restriction to limit seizure occurrence.

2.3.2. Calorie Restriction: EL Mice, Humans

The effect of calorie restriction on seizure threshold in a model of genetic epilepsy (the EL mouse) is described in detail by Seyfried and colleagues (*see* ref. *94* and Chapter 19, this volume). EL mice normally develop seizures by about 50 d of age, either spontaneously or in response to handling. When EL mice are fed a KD from infancy, the onset of seizures is delayed by several weeks. However, these investigators found that simply restricting calories had as robust an effect of seizure suppression as did the KD. They postulated that calorie restriction may underlie the mechanism of the KD, either from ketosis or hypoglycemia. The authors believe that the mechanism of seizure suppression is probably related to glucose dysregulation *(95)*. Most likely, a combination of the two factors is operative; e.g., the brain metabolizes ketones better under conditions of reduced glucose.

Reliable data on caloric restriction in humans with epilepsy is lacking. Systemic glucose levels usually range from 60 to 120 mg/dL, with a wide range of "normal." The relationship between seizure threshold and plasma glucose concentration is complex, and elevated glucose concentrations can be proconvulsant *(96)*. Individuals on the KD tend to run blood glucose levels on the lower end of normal, but rarely are they hypoglycemic. Therefore, a metabolic adaptation occurs in response to the diet to maintain relative euglycemia.

Two case reports reach the opposite conclusion: that calorie restriction facilitates seizures. Generalized tonic–clonic seizures developed *de novo* in a woman on a self-imposed low-calorie diet (600–800 kcal/d for several weeks) *(97)*. Three other patients developed seizures within 2 wk of beginning a "very-low-calorie" diet (400–600 kcal/d) for weight reduction *(98)*. While any number of factors could have caused the seizures in these patients, clearly their seizures were not averted by the low-calorie intake.

2.3.3. NEUROPROTECTION

As already noted, modest restriction of calorie intake is associated with delay or reduction of the typical degenerative effects of aging. These effects include dendritic regression in pyramidal neurons, atrophy of synapses, cytoskeletal abnormalities, and reactive gliosis *(92)*. These age-related neuronal changes are attributed to alterations in the genome related to both environmental and genetic factors. The end result is enhanced production of highly reactive oxygen species that damage crucial neuronal and genetic targets, mediated through neuroinflammatory changes. It is not known how dietary restriction prevents such detrimental effects, or how a combination of environmental enrichment and calorie restriction allays their occurrence. However, multiple relevant genes are affected *(92)* that enhance neuronal survival and plasticity, while reducing neuronal degeneration and cell death. As reviewed by Mattson and colleagues *(99)*, compensatory changes in genes ordinarily increased or decreased during the aging process include maintenance of brain-derived neurotrophic factor (BDNF) production, prevention of the usual increase in proinflammatory genes such as glial fibrillary acidic protein (GFAP), and maintenance of energy-related enzymes.

Rats administered KA that results in selective neurodegeneration of hippocampal hilar and pyramidal neurons have impaired performance on tasks of spatial learning and memory such as the Morris water maze. These learning deficits and histological damage were ameliorated in rats on a calorie-restricted diet (30% fewer calories for 2–4 mo) *(100)*. It was hypothesized that this neuroprotection is secondary to reduced oxidative stress. Other studies on the effect of calorie restriction on cognition and behavior have been less dramatic, or have shown a sex-specific effect. For example, in one study, male but not female calorie-restricted mice had better performance on the water maze than controls on an *ad libitum* diet *(101)*.

2.3.4. MALNUTRITION

Malnutrition is the extreme example of calorie restriction. In addition to calorie deprivation, of course, multiple other nutrients are likely to be lacking in malnourished persons. There is evidence that malnourished children have an increased susceptibility to seizures *(102)*, but many variables likely play into such a scenario. For example, malnourished children tend to have more acute illnesses and a greater likelihood of underlying brain maldevelopment *(103)*, and it would be difficult to sort out which nutrient is primarily responsible for an increased seizure susceptibility. In particular, protein malnutrition is associated with altered brain development and excitability *(104)*. The seizure susceptibility of malnourished individuals may also be influenced by age, with greater risk during critical phases of rapid brain development *(105)*.

Some of these issues can be approached by using laboratory models. Bronzino and colleagues showed that rats with prenatal protein malnutrition (induced by feeding dams a 25% reduced low-protein diet) caused increased susceptibility to kindled seizures, with hyperexcitability of dentate granule cells *(106)*. When the KA model was used, malnourished developing rats were highly susceptible to clinical seizures and displayed EEG evidence of hyperexcitability, with epileptiform discharges at lower KA doses than normally nourished rats *(107)*. In that study, malnutrition involved all nutrients, not just protein: the litter size was doubled per dam without altering milk composition. Malnutrition alters subsequent brain growth following a prolonged seizure in developing rats and increases dentate granule cell proliferation *(108)*. These findings both raise the possibility that children with malnutrition are at higher risk for seizure-induced brain damage than normally nourished children and carry implications for international nutritional efforts *(109)*.

3. DIETARY FACTORS THAT MAY WORSEN SEIZURES

Although this chapter focuses on dietary manipulations that may alleviate seizures, it must be acknowledged that some diets or dietary constituents may worsen seizure control. Glutamate, the primary excitatory brain neurotransmitter, is clearly epileptogenic *(110,111)*; seizure exacerbation has been attributed to excess intake of glutamate (in particular, monosodium glutamate, a flavor enhancer) *(112)*. Stimulants such as caffeine have been reported to exacerbate seizures, probably owing to its blockade of adenosine A1 receptors, activation of which is anticonvulsant *(113,114)*. Alcohol ingestion can lower seizure threshold, both acutely and chronically *(115)*. This list is obviously incomplete, and worldwide, specific local dietary practices can reveal particular foods that can cause seizures, e.g., betel nuts *(116)*. It is certainly simplistic to suggest a direct link between each of these food substances and epilepsy, inasmuch as more complex regulatory mechanisms are undoubtedly involved. However, the physician must be aware of the potential for certain foods to exacerbate seizures.

4. CONCLUSION

Aside from heeding common sense, i.e., "eat a well-balanced, healthy diet," can we offer our epilepsy patients any specific advice regarding nutrition? Unfortunately, our knowledge about the relationship between nutrition and epilepsy is in its infancy. Aside from the KD, nutritional suggestions of means to treat epilepsy are premature. Nevertheless, as indicated in this chapter, there are several potential treatment adjuncts on the horizon. Further basic research is necessary before clinical trials are undertaken for any of these prospective treatments. However, clinicians should be aware that DHA, choline, and a variety of other substances are available commercially in health food stores, and *patients are using them*! Many surveys have established that patients are using "alternative medicines" regardless of advice of their physicians and often unbeknownst to their health-care providers *(117)*. Patients can easily obtain information about the wide variety of accepted and nonaccepted medicinals through the Internet. Therefore, it behooves us to inquire of our patients, not only about their compliance with recommended medicinal regimens, but also *what else* they are using/doing. When queried in a nonjudgmental and supportive manner, patients are often eager to disclose such information, and we can often provide guidance regarding their use. Until nutritional treatments of epilepsy are standard, such support should be considered to be a part of optimal clinical care.

REFERENCES

1. Sonnen AEH. Alternative and folk remedies. In: Engel JJ, Pedley TA (eds.). Epilepsy: A Comprehensive Textbook. Lippincott-Raven, Philadelphia, 1997, pp. 1365–1378.
2. Murphy PA. Treating Epilepsy Naturally. Keats, Chicago, 2002.
3. Blusztajn JK. Choline, a vital amine. Science 1998;281:794–795.
4. Meck WH, Smith RA, Williams CL. Pre- and postnatal choline supplementation produces long-term facilitation of spatial memory. Dev Psychobiol 1988;21:339–353.
5. Schenk F, Brandner C. Indirect effect of peri- and postnatal choline treatment on place-learning abilities in rat. Psychobiology 1995;35:302–313.
6. Meck WH, Williams CL. Perinatal choline supplementation increases the threshold for chunking in spatial memory. NeuroReport 1997;8:3053–3059.
7. Meck WH, Williams CL. Characterization of the facilitative effects of perinatal choline supplementation on timing and temporal memory. NeuroReport 1997;8:2831–2835.
8. Tees RC. The influences of sex, rearing environment, and neonatal choline dietary supplementation on spatial and nonspatial learning and memory in adult rats. Dev Psychobiol 1999;35:328–342.
9. Thomas JD, La Fiette MH, Quinn VRE, Riley EP. Neonatal choline supplementation ameliorates the effects of prenatal alcohol exposure on a discrimination learning task in rats. Neurotoxicol Teratol 2000;22:703–711.
10. Fundaro A, Paschero A. Behavioural effects of chronic manipulations of dietary choline in senescent rats. Prog Neuropsychopharmacol Biol Psychiatr 1990;14:949–960.
11. Yang Y, Cermak JM, Tandon P, Sarkisian MR, Stafstrom CE, Neill JC, Blusztajn JK, Holmes GL. Protective effects of prenatal choline supplementation on seizure-induced memory impairment. J Neurosci 2000;20(RC109):1–6.
12. Turski WA, Cavalheiro EA, Schwarz M, Czuczwar SJ, Kleinrok Z, Turski L. Limbic seizures produced by pilocarpine in rats: behavioural, electroencephalographic and neuropathological study. Behav Brain Res 1983;9:315–335.
13. Liu Z, Gatt A, Mikati MA, Holmes GL. Long-term behavioral deficits following pilocarpine seizures in immature rats. Epilepsy Res 1995;19:191–204.
14. Holmes GL, Yang Y, Liu Z, Cermak JM, Sarkisian MR, Stafstrom CE, Neill JC, Blusztajn JK. Seizure-induced memory impairment is reduced by choline supplementation before or after status epilepticus. Epilepsy Res 2002;48:3–13.
15. Nadler JV. Kainic acid as a tool for the study of temporal lobe epilepsy. Life Sci 1981;29:2031–2042.
16. Stafstrom CE, Thompson JL, Holmes GL. Kainic acid seizures in the developing brain: status epilepticus and spontaneous recurrent seizures. Dev Brain Res 1992;65:227–236.
17. Stafstrom CE, Chronopoulos A, Thurber S, Thompson JL, Holmes GL. Age-dependent cognitive and behavioral deficits after kainic acid seizures. Epilepsia 1993;34:420–435.
18. Cermak JM, Holler T, Jackson DA, Blusztajn JK. Prenatal availability of choline modifies development of the hippocampal cholinergic system. FASEB 1998;12:349–357.
19. Cermak JM, Blusztajn JK, Meck WH, Williams CL, Fitzgerald CM, Rosene DL, Loy R. Prenatal availability of choline alters the development of acetylcholinesterase in rat hippocampus. Dev Neurosci 1999;21:84–104.
20. Ikarashi Y, Kuribara H, Shiobara T, Takahashi A, Ishimaru H, Maruyama Y. Learning and memory in mice treated with choline oxidase, a hydrolytic enzyme for choline. Pharmacol Biochem Behav 2000;65:519–522.
21. Semba K, Fibiger HC, Organization of central cholinergic systems. Prog Brain Res 1989;79:37–63.
22. Albright CD, Tsai AY, Friedrich CB, Mar MH, Zeisel SH. Choline availability alters embryonic development of the hippocampus and septum in the rat. Dev Brain Res 1999;113:13–20.

23. Fibiger HC. Cholinergic mechanisms in learning, memory, and dementia: a review of the evidence. Trends Neurosci 1991;14:220–223.

24. Jones DNC, Barnes JC, Kirkby DL, Higgins GA. Age-associated impairments in a test of attention: evidence for involvement of cholinergic systems. J Neurosci 1995;15:7282–7292.

25. Loy R, Heyer D, Williams CL, Meck WH. Choline-induced spatial memory facilitation correlates with altered distribution and morphology of septal neurons. Adv Exp Med Biol 1991;295:373–382.

26. Williams CL, Meck WH, Heyer D, Loy R. Hypertrophy of basal forebrain neurons and enhanced visuospatial memory in perinatally choline-supplemented rats. Brain Res 1998;794:225–238.

27. Montoya D, Swartzwelder HS. Prenatal choline supplementation alters hippocampal *N*-methyl-D-aspartate receptor-mediated neurotransmission in adult rats. Neurosci Lett 2000;296:85–88.

28. Guo-Ross SX, Jones KH, Shetty AK, Wilson WA, Swartzwelder HS. Prenatal dietary choline availability alters postnatal neurotoxic vulnerability in the adult rat. Neurosci Lett 2003;341:161–163.

29. Jones JP, Meck WH, Williams CL, Wilson WA, Swartzwelder HS. Choline availability to the developing rat fetus alters adult hippocampal long-term potentiation. Dev Brain Res 1999;118:159–167.

30. Kurlak L, Stephenson T. Plausible explanations for effects of long chain polyunsaturated fatty acids (LCPUFA) on neonates. Arch Dis Child (Fetal Neonat Ed) 1999;80:F148–F154.

31. Innis SM. The role of dietary n-6 and n-3 fatty acids in the developing brain. Dev Neurosci 2000;22:474–480.

32. Uauy R, Mena P. Lipids and neurodevelopment. Nutr Rev 2001;59(8 [Pt 2]):S34–S58.

33. Gibson R. Long-chain polyunsaturated fatty acids and infant development. Lancet 1999;354:1919–1920.

34. Neuringer M, Anderson G, Connor W. The essentiality of n-3 fatty acids for the development and function of the retina and brain. Annu Rev Nutr 1988;8:517–541.

35. Carlson SE, Werkman SH. A randomized trial of visual attention of preterm infants fed docosahexaenoic acid until nine months. Lipids 1996;31:91–97.

36. Enslen M, Milon H, Malnoe A. Effect of low intake of n-3 fatty acids during development on brain phospholipid fatty acid composition and exploratory behavior in rats. Lipids 1991;26:203–208.

37. Carrie I, Clement I, Clement M, De Javel D, Frances H, Bourre JM. Learning deficits in first generation OF1 mice deficient in (n-3) polyunsaturated fatty acids do not result from visual alteration. Neurosci Lett 1999;266:69–72.

38. McGahon B, Martin DSD, Horrobin DF, Lynch MA. Age-related changes in synaptic function: analysis of the effect of dietary supplementation with ω-3 fatty acids. Neurosci 1999;94:305–314.

39. Yehuda S, Rabinovitz S, Mostofsky DI. Essential fatty acids are mediators of brain biochemistry and cognitive functions. J Neurosci Res 1999;56:565–570.

40. Takeuchi T, Fukumoto Y, Harada E. Influence of a dietary n-3 fatty acid deficiency on the cerebral catecholamine contents, EEG and learning ability in rat. Behav Brain Res 2002;131:193–203.

41. Crawford M. The role of essential fatty acids in neural development: implications for perinatal nutrition. Am J Clin Nutr 1993;57 (Suppl):703S–710S.

42. Raiten D, Talbot D, Waters J. Assessment of nutrient requirements for infant formulas. Am J Clin Nutr 1998;115:2089–2110.

43. Lucas A, Stafford M, Morley R, Abbott R, Stephenson T, MacFadyen U, Elias-Jones A, Clements H. Efficacy and safety of long-chain polyunsaturated fatty acid supplementation of infant-formula milk: a randomised trial. Lancet 1999;354:1948–1954.

44. Salvati S, Attorri L, Avellino C, DiBiase A, Sanchez M. Diet, lipids and brain development. Dev Neurosci 2000;22:481–487.

45. Yavin E, Glozman S, Green P. Docosahexaenoic acid sources for the developing brain during intrauterine life. Nutr Health 2001;15:219–224.

46. Ahmad A, Moriguchi T, Salem N Jr. Decrease in neuron size in docosahexaenoic acid-deficient brain. Pediatr Neurol 2002;26:210–218.

47. Haubner LY, Stockard JE, Saste MD, Benford VJ, Phelps CP, Chen LT, Barness L, Weiner D, Carver JD. Maternal dietary docosahexanoic acid content affects the rat pup auditory system. Brain Res Bull 2002;58:1–5.

48. Fewtrell MS, R. Morley R, Abbott RA, Singhal A, Isaacs EB, Stephenson T, MacFadyen U, Lucas A. Double-blind, randomized trial of long-chain polyunsaturated fatty acid supplementation in formula fed to preterm infants. Pediatrics 2002;110 (1 Pt 1):72–83.

49. Ordway RW, Singer JJ, Walsh JV Jr. Direct regulation of ion channels by fatty acids. Trends Neurosci 1991;14:96–100.

50. Hwang D, Rhee SH. Receptor-mediated signaling pathways: potential targets of modulation by dietary fatty acids. Am J Clin Nutr 1999;70:545–556.

51. Kang JX, Xiao Y-F, Leaf A. Free, long-chain, polyunsaturated fatty acids reduce membrane electrical excitability in neonatal rat cardiac myocytes. Proc Natl Acad Sci U S A 1995;92:3997–4001.

52. Leaf A, Kang JX, Xiao Y-F, Billman GE, Voskuyl RA. The antiarrhythmic and anticonvulsant effects of dietary n-3 fatty acids. J Membr Biol 1999;172:1–11.

53. Meves H. Modulation of ion channels by arachidonic acid. Prog Neurobiol 1994;43:175–186.

54. Bazan N, Packard MG, Teather L, Allan G. Bioactive lipids in excitatory neurotransmission and neuronal plasticity. Neurochem Int 1996;2:225–231.

55. Leaf A, Kang JX, Xiao Y-F, Billman GE, Voskuyl RA. Functional and electrophysiologic effects of polyunsaturated fatty acids on excitable tissues: heart and brain. Prostaglandins Leukotrienes Essent Fatty Acids 1999;60:307–312.

56. Vreugdenhil M, Bruehl C, Voskuyl RA, Kang JX, Leaf A, Wadman WJ. Polyunsaturated fatty acids modulate sodium and calcium currents in CA1 neurons. Proc Natl Acad Sci U S A 1996;93:12559–12563.

57. Poling J, Vicini S, Rogawski MA, Salem N Jr. Docosahexaenoic acid block of neuronal voltage-gated K+ channels: subunit selective antagonism by zinc. Neuropharmacology 1996;35:969–982.

58. Keros S, McBain C. Arachadonic acid inhibits transient potassium currents and broadens action potentials during electrographic seizures in hippocampal pyramidal and inhibitory interneurons. J Neurosci 1997;17:3476–3487.

59. Horimoto N, Nabekura J, Ogawa T. Arachadonic acid activation of potassium channels in rat visual cortex neurons. Neuroscience 1997;77:661–671.

60. Nishikawa M, Kimura S, Akaike N. Facilitatory effect of docosahexaenoic acid on N-methyl-D-aspartate response in pyramidal neurons of rat cerebral cortex. J Physiol (Lond) 1994;475:83–93.

61. Hamano H, Nabekura J, Nishikawa M, Ogawa T. Docosahexanoic acid reduces GABA response in substantia nigra neuron of rat. J Neurophysiol 1996;75:1264–1270.

62. Lauritzen I, Blondeau N, Heurteaux C, Widmann C, Romey G, Lazdunski M. Polyunsaturated fatty acids are potent neuroprotectors. EMBO J 2000;19:1784–1793.

63. Voskuyl RA. Is marine fat anti-epileptogenic? Nutr Health 2002;16:51–53.

64. Lesage F. Pharmacology of neuronal background potassium channels. Neuropharmacology 2003;44:1–7.

65. Talley EM, Sirois JE, Lei Q, Bayliss DA. Two-pore domain (KCNK) potassium channels: dynamic roles in neuronal function. Neuroscientist 2003;9:46–56.

66. Fraser DD, Hoehn K, Weiss S, MacVicar BA. Arachidonic acid inhibits sodium currents and synaptic transmission in cultured striatal neurons. Neuron 1993;11:633–644.

67. Rho JM, Sankar R. The pharmacologic basis of antiepileptic drug action. Epilepsia 1999;40:1471–1483.

68. Woods BT, Chiu T-M. Fatty acid elevation and brain seizure activity [letter]. Trends Neurosci 1991;14:405.

69. Stafstrom CE. Effects of fatty acids and ketones on neuronal excitability: implications for epilepsy and its treatment. In: Mostofsky DI, Yehuda S, Salem N Jr. (eds.). Fatty Acids—Physiological and Behavioral Functions. Humana, Totowa, NJ, 2001, pp. 273–290.

70. Young C, Gean P-W, Chiou L-C, Shen Y-Z. Docosahexaenoic acid inhibits synaptic transmission and epileptiform activity in the rat hippocampus. Synapse 2000;37:90–94.

71. Xiao Y-F, Li X. Polyunsaturated fatty acids modify mouse hippocampal neuronal excitability during excitotoxic or convulsant stimulation. Brain Res 1999;846:112–121.

72. Valencia P, Carver JD, Wyble LE, Benford VJ, Gilbert-Barness E, Weiner DA, Phelps C. The fatty acid composition of maternal diet affects the response to excitotoxic neural injury in neonatal rat pups. Brain Res Bull 1998;45:637–640.

73. Yehuda S, Carasso RL, Mostofsky DI. Essential fatty acid preparation (SR-3) raises the seizure threshold in rats. Eur J Pharmacol 1994;254:193–198.

74. Voskuyl RA, Vreugdenhil M, Kang JX, Leaf A. Anticonvulsant effect of polyunsaturated fatty acids in rats, using the cortical stimulation model. Eur J Pharmacol 1998;341:145–152.

75. Voskuyl RA, Vreugdenhil M. Effects of essential fatty acids on voltage-regulated ionic channels and seizure thresholds in animals. In: Mostofsky DI, Yehuda S, Salem N Jr (eds.). Fatty Acids—Physiological and Behavioral Functions. Humana, Totowa, NJ, 2001, pp. 63–78.

76. Stafstrom CE, Sarkisian M. A diet enriched in polyunsaturated fatty acids does not protect against flurothyl seizures in the immature brain. Epilepsia 1997;38 (Suppl 8):34.

77. Cunnane SC, Musa K, Ryan MA, Whiting S, Fraser DD. Potential role of polyunsaturates in seizure protection achieved with the ketogenic diet. Prostaglandins Leukotrienes Essent Fatty Acids 2002;67:131–135.

78. Appleton DB, DeVivo DC. An animal model for the ketogenic diet. Epilepsia 1974;15:211–217.

79. Huttenlocher PR, Wilbourn AJ, Signore JM. Medium-chain triglycerides as a therapy for intractable childhood epilepsy. Neurology 1971;21:1097–1103.

80. Dekaban AS. Plasma lipids in epileptic children treated with the high fat diet. Arch Neurol 1966;15:177–184.

81. Schwartz RM, Eaton J, Bower BD, Aynsley-Green A. Ketogenic diets in the treatment of epilepsy: short term clinical effects. Dev Med Child Neurol 1989;31:145–151.

82. Alexander GJ, Kopeloff LM. Induced hypercholesterolemia and decreased susceptibility to seizures in experimental animals. Exp Neurol 1971;32:134–140.

83. Huttenlocher PR. Ketonemia and seizures: metabolic and anticonvulsant effects of two ketogenic diets in childhood epilepsy. Pediatr Res 1976;10:536–540.

84. Bough KJ, Eagles DA. A ketogenic diet increases the resistance to pentylenetetrazole-induced seizures in the rat. Epilepsia 1999;40:138–143.

85. Dell CA, Likhodii SS, Musa K, Ryan MA, Burnham WM, Cunnane SC. Lipid and fatty acid profiles in rats consuming different high-fat ketogenic diets. Lipids 2001;36:373–378.

86. Bourre JM, Bonneil M, Clement M, Dumont O, Durand G, Lafont H, Nalbone G, Piciotti M. Function of dietary polyunsaturated fatty acids in the nervous system. Prostaglandins Leukotrienes Essent Fatty Acids 1993;48:5–15.

87. Jumpsen J, Lien EL, Goh YK, Clandinin MT. Small changes of dietary (n-6) and (n-3)/fatty acid content ratio alter phosphatidylethanolamine and phosphatidylcholine fatty acid composition during development of neuronal and glial cell in rats. J Nutr 1997;127:724–731.

88. Leaf A. Health claims: Omega-3 fatty acids and cardiovascular disease. Nutr Rev 1992;50:150–154.

89. Schlanger S, Shinitzky M, Yam D. Diet enriched with omega-3 fatty acids alleviates convulsion symptoms in epilepsy patients. Epilepsia 2002;43:103–104.

90. DeToledo JC, Lowe MR. Epilepsy, demonic possessions, and fasting: another look at translations of Mark 9:16. Epilepsy Behav 2003;4:338–339.

91. Ramsey JJ, Harper M-E, Weindruch R. Restriction of energy intake, energy expenditure, and aging. Free Radical Biol Med 2000;29:946–968.

92. Prolla TA, Mattson MP. Molecular mechanisms of brain aging and neurodegenerative disorders: lessons from dietary restriction. Trends Neurosci 2001;24(11) Suppl.:S21–S31.

93. Koubova J, Guarante L. How does calorie restriction work? Genes Dev 2003;17:313–321.

94. Greene AE, Todorova MT, McGowan R, Seyfried TN. Caloric restriction inhibits seizure susceptibility in epileptic EL mice by reducing blood glucose. Epilepsia 2001;42:1371–1378.

95. Greene AE, Todorova MT, Seyfried TN. Perspectives on the metabolic management of epilepsy through dietary reduction of glucose and elevation of ketone bodies. J Neurochem 2003;86:529–537.

96. Schwechter EM, Veliskova J, Velisek L. Correlation between extracellular glucose and seizure susceptibility in adult rats. Ann Neurol 2003;53:91–101.

97. Marinella MA. Generalized seizures associated with low-calorie dieting. Ann Emerg Med 2000;35:405.

98. Kaufman MA, Bhargava A. Dietary weight reduction and seizures. Neurology 1990;40:1905–1906.

99. Mattson MP, Duan W, Lee J, Guo Z. Suppression of brain aging and neurodegenerative disorders by dietary restriction and environmental enrichment: molecular mechanisms. Mech Ageing Dev 2001;122:757–778.

100. Bruce-Keller A., Umberger G, McFall R, Mattson MP. Food restriction reduces brain damage and improves behavioral outcome following excitotoxic and metabolic insults. Neurology 1999;45:8–15.

101. Wu A, Sun X, Liu Y. Effects of caloric restriction on cognition and behavior in developing mice. Neurosci Lett 2003;339:166–168.

102. Nunes ML, Teixeira GC, Fabris I, Gonçalves RA. Evaluation of the nutritional status in institutionalized children and its relationship to the development of epilepsy. Nutr Neurosci 1999;2:139–145.

103. DeBassio WA, Kemper TL, Tonkiss J, Galler JR. Effect of prenatal protein deprivation on postnatal granule cell generation in the hippocampal dentate gyrus. Brain Res Bull 1996;41:379–383.

104. Fukuda MTH, Francolin-Silva AL, Sebastiao SS. Early postnatal protein malnutrition affects learning and memory in the distal but not the proximal cue version of the Morris water maze. Behav Brain Res 2002;133:271–277.

105. Morgane PJ, Mokler DJ, Galler JR. Effects of prenatal protein malnutrition on the hippocampal formation. Neurosci Biobehav Rev 2002;26:471–483.

106. Bronzino JD, Austin-LaFrance RJ, Morgane PJ, Galler JR. Effects of prenatal protein malnutrition on kindling-induced alterations in dentate granule cell excitability: I. Synaptic transmission measures. Exp Neurol 1991;112:206–215.

107. Sharma SK, Selvamurthy W, Maheshwari MC, Singh TP. Kainic acid induced epileptogenesis in developing normal and undernourished rats—a computerized EEG analysis. Indian J Med Res (B) 1990;92:456–466.

108. Nunes ML, Liptakova S, Veliskova J, Sperber E, Moshe S. Malnutrition increases dentate granule cell proliferation in immature rats following status epilepticus. Epilepsia 2000;41 (Suppl 6):S48–S52.

109. Hackett R, Iype T. Malnutrition and childhood epilepsy in developing countries. Seizure 2001;10:554–558.

110. Meldrum BS. Glutamate as a neurotransmitter in the brain: review of physiology and pathology. J Nutr 2000;130:1007S–1015S.

111. Chapman AG. Glutamate and epilepsy. J Nutr 2000;130:1043S–1045S.

112. Shovic A, Bart RD, Stalcup AM. "We think your son has Lennox–Gastaut syndrome"—a case study of monosodium glutamate's possible effect on a child. J Am Diet Assoc 1997;97:793–794.

113. Dzhala V, Desfreres L, Melyan Z, Ben-Ari Y, Khazipov R. Epileptogenic action of caffeine during anoxia in the neonatal rat hippocampus. Ann Neurol 1999;46:95–102.

114. Zagnoni PG, Albano C. Psychostimulants and epilepsy. Epilepsia 2002;43 (Suppl 2):28–31.

115. Gordon E, Devinsky O. Alcohol and marijuana: effects on epilepsy and use by patients with epilepsy. Epilepsia 2001;42:1266–1272.

116. Huang Z, Xiao B, Wang X, Li Y, Deng H. Betel nut indulgence as a cause of epilepsy. Seizure 2003;12:406–408.

117. Spinella M. Herbal medicines and epilepsy: the potential for benefit and adverse effects. Epilepsy Behav 2001;2:524–532.

III BASIC SCIENCE PERSPECTIVES

14 Effects of the Ketogenic Diet on Cerebral Energy Metabolism

Douglas R. Nordli, Jr. and Darryl C. De Vivo

1. INTRODUCTION

In vivo and in vitro studies show that the ketogenic diet (KD) has effects on cerebral metabolism. These changes act in concert to raise brain energy reserves and may contribute to the anticonvulsant action of the diet. In contrast to the sedative effects of many antiepileptic medications, the biochemical changes induced by the KD serve to enhance brain function. However, the precise mechanisms through which higher cerebral energy reserves reduce seizure activity are unknown. We speculate that failure to meet energy needs contributes to the cellular processes involved in the generation, spread, and maintenance of epileptic activity. We further speculate that the KD ameliorates these deficiencies by bypassing less efficient cytosolic glycolytic pathways and maximizing tricarboxylic acid (TCA) cycle function.

2. BIOCHEMICAL STEPS NECESSARY FOR USE OF KETONE BODIES BY THE BRAIN

2.1. Commitment of Fatty Acids to Ketone Body Production

The major precursors of ketone bodies are nonesterified fatty acids. During the fasting state, the fall in blood glucose reduces plasma insulin production, stimulates lipolysis in fatty tissues, and increases the flux of nonesterified fatty acids to the liver. Nonesterified fatty acids can be esterified or metabolized to ketone bodies. The fate of fatty acids in the liver is determined, at least in part, by the carbohydrate status of the host *(1)*. A critical component of this regulation is malonyl-coenzyme A (malonyl-CoA), an intermediate in the pathway of lipogenesis *(2,3)*. Malonyl-CoA inhibits carnitine acyltransferase I, which is needed to shuttle long-chain fatty acyl-CoA into the mitochondria for oxidation. The production of glucose from glycogen provides the carbon source for lipogenesis and, in particular, malonyl-CoA. If glucose is reduced, so is malonyl-CoA. The reduction in malonyl-CoA decreases the inhibition on (or increases the net activity of) carnitine acyltransferase. This allows more movement of fatty acids into the mitochondria, where fatty acyl-CoA is converted to acetyl-CoA, and later to

From: *Epilepsy and the Ketogenic Diet*
Edited by: C. E. Stafstrom and J. M. Rho © Humana Press Inc., Totowa, NJ

acetoacetate (AcAc), which is in equilibrium with β-hydroxybutyrate, the major ketone body utilized by the brain.

2.2. β-Hydroxybutyrate Gets into the Brain

Passage of ketone bodies into the brain may be the critical factor limiting the rate of brain utilization of ketone bodies. Movement of ketone bodies into the brain relies on the monocarboxylic transport system, MCT-1. This is upregulated during fasting in adults and during milk feeding in neonates *(4,5)*. Fasting studies in humans demonstrated that the brain's ability to extract ketone bodies is inversely related to the age of the subject *(6)*. In contrast to glucose, ketone bodies can pass directly into mitochondria without being processed in the cytosol. Also, in contrast to glucose, ketone bodies may be used directly by neurons for metabolism *(7)*.

2.3. Ketone Bodies Are Incorporated into the TCA Cycle

Once inside the mitochondria, β-hydroxybutyrate is converted to AcAc, and then to AcAc-CoA. The enzyme that facilitates this conversion is 3-oxoacid-CoA transferase or succinyl-CoA-acetoacetate-CoA transferase. As the name implies, this conversion requires commensurate conversion of succinyl-CoA to succinate. Reduced blood glucose and increased blood ketones may be needed to induce the activity of this enzyme *(8)*.

3. EFFECT OF THE KD ON BRAIN METABOLISM AS MEASURED IN ANIMALS

Scientific studies of the KD have revealed important biochemical and metabolic observations. Appleton and De Vivo developed an animal model to permit study of the effect of the KD on cerebral metabolism *(9)*. Adult male albino rats were placed on either a high-fat diet containing (by weight) 38% corn oil, 38% lard, 11% vitamin-free casein, 6.8% glucose, 4% US Pharmacopeia (USP) salt mixture, and 2.2 % vitamin diet fortification mixture, or a high-carbohydrate diet containing (by weight) 50% glucose, 28.8% vitamin-free casein, 7.5 % corn oil, 7.5 % lard, 4% USP salt mixture, and 2.2 % vitamin diet fortification mixture. Parallel studies were conducted to evaluate electro-convulsive shock responses and biochemical alterations. These studies revealed that the mean voltage necessary to produce a minimal convulsion remained constant for 12 d before the high-fat diet was started and for about 10 d after beginning the feedings (69.75 ± 1.88 V). After 10–12 d on the high-fat diet, the intensity of the convulsive response to the established voltage decreased, necessitating an increase in voltage to reestablish a minimal convulsive response. Approximately 20 d after beginning the high-fat diet, a new convulsive threshold was achieved (81.25 ± 2.39 V) $(p < 0.01)$. When the high-fat diet was replaced by a high-carbohydrate diet, a rapid change in response to the voltage was observed. Within 48 h the animal exhibited a maximal convulsion to the electrical stimulus that had previously produced only a minimal convulsion, and the mean voltage to produce a minimal convulsion returned to the prestudy value (70.75 ± 1.37 V).

Blood concentrations of β-hydroxybutyrate, AcAc, chloride, esterified fatty acids, triglycerides, cholesterol, and total lipids increased in the rats fed on the high-fat diet. Brain levels of β-hydroxybutyrate and sodium were also significantly increased in the fat-fed rats.

De Vivo et al. reported the change in cerebral metabolites in chronically ketotic rats *(10)*, and found no changes in brain water content, electrolytes, or pH. As expected, fat-fed rats had significantly lower blood glucose concentrations and higher blood β-hydroxybutyrate and AcAc concentrations. More importantly, brain concentrations of adenosine triphosphate (ATP), glycogen, glucose 6-phosphate, pyruvate, lactate, β-hydroxybutyrate, citrate, α-ketoglutarate, and alanine were higher, and the brain concentrations of fructose 1,6-diphosphate, aspartate, adenosine diphosphate (ADP) creatine, cyclic nucleotides, acid-insoluble CoA, and total CoA were lower in the fat-fed group.

The biochemical implications of these results can be grouped into three major categories, discussed in Sections 3.1–3.3.

3.1. Glycolysis and Glucose Flux Are Reduced During Ketosis

Hexokinase converts glucose into glucose 6-phosphate, which may then either be used to synthesize glycogen or enter glycolysis. Glucose 6-phosphate is in equilibrium with fructose 1,6-diphosphate through the action of phosphofructokinase. The findings of reduced fructose 1,6-diphosphate (decreased 27%), and increased glucose 6-phosphate (increased 12%) can be best explained by a reduction in the activity of phosphofructokinase. This enzyme is negatively modified by ATP and citrate, both of which were elevated in the fat-fed animals. As a consequence, the increased glucose 6-phosphate is converted into glycogen (increased 22%) instead of entering into glycolysis.

As Wilder originally postulated, the effects of eating a high-fat, low-carbohydrate diet are similar to the biochemical consequences of starvation *(11)*. In this regard, the reduction in glycolysis makes physiologic sense, since the starving organism would want to make every attempt to preserve the rather meager stores of glycogen and to provide the brain with an alternate, more substantial fuel for metabolism, i.e., ketone bodies from fats. Measurements of glucose flux in children and adults during ketosis have confirmed the reduced utilization of glucose. Haymond et al. used tagged glucose to perform sequential glucose flux studies in 11 children (5 control, 6 with epilepsy) and 10 adult volunteers *(12)*. All subjects were studied after a fast while consuming either a normal diet or the KD. The authors found that glucose flux and ketonemia were inversely related, particularly when corrected for estimated brain mass. This was consistent with the replacement of glucose by ketone bodies for cerebral metabolism.

Since glycolysis is not increased, the increased pyruvate (by 23%) seen in the fat-fed animals must be explained by another mechanism. The most likely explanation is reduction of the activity of pyruvate dehydrogenase. This multienzymatic complex is also inhibited by higher ATP/ADP ratios. The higher amount of pyruvate causes an increase in lactate (by 28%) through the action of lactate dehydrogenase. This conversion is influenced by the ratio of nicotinic acid dehydrogenase to reduced nicotinamide adenine dinucleotide (NAD/NADH). Since the lactate/pyruvate ratio was similar in the control and fat-fed groups, it is likely that the cytoplasmic oxidation–reduction potential is not substantially altered by chronic ketosis.

3.2. TCA Cycle Flux Is Increased by Chronic Ketosis

The enzyme α-ketoglutarate dehydrogenase is the rate-limiting enzyme in TCA cycle function. The major inhibitor of this enzyme is the concentration of the product of the reaction, succinyl-CoA. This product is relatively reduced in the fat-fed group (down 26%), implying that the enzyme α-ketoglutarate dehydrogenase should be functioning at maximal capacity. Yet, concentrations of α-ketoglutarate, the substrate for this enzyme, were found to be elevated 11% in the fat-fed group. The only reasonable explanation is that the TCA cycle is driven to its maximal capacity and is overwhelming the ability of this rate-limiting enzyme to deal with substrate.

3.3. Cerebral Energy Reserves Are Increased by Chronic Ketosis

An increase in TCA cycle activity should logically lead to increased energy production. Indeed, this was supported by analysis of the data: ATP/ADP ratios in the control were 3.63 ± 0.10 and 4.08 ± 0.10 in the high-fat diet group ($p < 0.005$). Cerebral energy reserves were calculated from these measurements using the following equation *(13)*.

$$energy\ reserve = (PCr + ADP) + 2(ATP + glucose) + 2.9(glycogen)$$

Applying the values determined for PCr (phosphocreatine), ADP, ATP, glucose, and glycogen enabled the calculation of the reserves. Energy reserves were significantly higher in the fat-fed rats (26.4 ± 0.6) than for the controls (23.6 ± 0.2) ($p < 0.005$).

Because ketone bodies avoid the less efficient glycolytic pathway, they are thermodynamically more efficient fuels than glucose. Animals fed an equivalent amount of calories in the form of high-fat diets would therefore be expected to have more efficient energy production. Assuming energy demands do not substantially change during fasting, the increased efficiency of ketone body utilization most likely contributes to higher energy reserves.

4. MEASUREMENTS OF BRAIN METABOLITES DURING KETOSIS IN MAN

Pan et al. used ^{31}P spectroscopic imaging at 4.1T to demonstrate an elevated ratio of PCr to inorganic phosphorus in patients on the KD and concluded that there was improvement of energy metabolism with use of the diet *(14)*. Seven patients with intractable epilepsy (four with Lennox–Gastaut syndrome, one with absence seizures, one with primary generalized tonic–clonic seizures, and one with partial complex seizures) were studied before and after institution of the KD. Coronal ^1H anatomic imaging was performed to provide a correlate to the ^{31}P data. Ratios of PCr to ATP were measured at baseline and compared with those obtained after the KD. These showed a small but significant increase from 0.61 ± 0.08 to 0.69 ± 0.08 ($p < 0.05$). The ratio of PCr to inorganic phosphorus also changed from 2.45 ± 0.27 at baseline to 2.99 ± 0.44 during the diet ($p < 0.05$). The authors made several assumptions to calculate the potential gain in energy by these changes: (1) that the creatine kinase reactions stayed at equilibrium; (2) that the measured values did not change simply as a function of age; and (3) that the levels of creatine decrease proportionately to the PCr increase. Doing this, they calculated an increase in the ΔG of ATP hydrolysis from 12.5 kcal/mol to 12.85 kcal/mol, or an increase of 2.5%.

5. HOW ARE BRAIN METABOLISM AND EPILEPSY RELATED?

Disorders that deprive the brain of essential fuel can cause a common presentation: brain energy failure syndrome *(15)*. Energy failure may be caused by a variety of hypoglycemic syndromes, hypoketonemic syndromes, glycolytic enzymopathies, and mitochondrial defects, but some of these disorders can produce prominent epilepsy. A proto-typic disorder of this class is glucose transporter 1 (GLUT1) deficiency syndrome. GLUT1 deficiency syndrome causes an infantile-onset epileptic encephalopathy. The electroencephalogram (EEG) correlate of this syndrome is distinctive and emerges in early childhood as bursts of generalized 2.5- to 4-Hz spike-wave discharges *(16)*. A characteristic "footprint" is seen on positron emission tomography (PET): hypometabo-lism of the thalamus *(17)*. Because thalamic circuits are critically involved in the gener-ation of spike-wave discharges, it is understandable that this region shows marked changes on PET imaging. Why this region shows such selective vulnerability is not clear, but the effect indicates that the diffuse failure to provide energy can result in regional changes in brain function. Another remarkable feature of this disorder is that the seizures are notoriously refractory to antiepileptic drugs but respond remarkably well to treatment with the KD. This makes a compelling argument that enhancement of energy production is an important mechanism of the KD, in at least some patients with medically intractable epilepsy.

Is deficient energy metabolism an important mechanism causing intractable seizures in other patients? Certainly, seizures themselves exert a great metabolic demand on the brain. One might expect epileptogenic focal structural lesions to be hypermetabolic, but it is well known that the exact opposite is found: hypometabolic neocortical areas revealed on PET scan are associated with focal epileptogenic lesions causing intractable partial epilepsy. Careful coregistration of implanted electrodes in children with intractable epilepsy has recently revealed that the most active ictal regions are those lying within border-zone areas, not within the hypometabolic areas themselves *(18)*. Indeed, a frequent finding during electrocorticography is slow-wave activity with reduced complexity over the lesion, with a surround of interictal epileptiform dis-charges in the border between the lesion and the normal brain. Is the adjacent tissue hypometabolic on PET because the cerebral energy demands in that tissue have not been met? We speculate that this is the case and that this failure contributes to the epileptogenic process in these lesions.

How does an enhancement in cerebral energy reserves help to fend off seizures? This is not precisely known. Possibilities include increased ability to power ion pumps, lead-ing to alteration in the resting membrane potential, increased capacity to produce inhibitory neurotransmitters, and better ability to buffer the extracellular milieu.

6. CONCLUSION

The available biochemical data suggest that the KD favorably influences cerebral energetics by increasing cerebral energy reserves. This may be an important mechanism behind the increased resistance to seizures in ketotic brain tissue and the favorable cog-nitive effect sometimes seen with the ketogenic diet *(19)*.

REFERENCES

1. Robinson AM, Williamson DH. Physiological roles of ketone bodies as substrates and signals in mam-malian tissues. Physiol Rev 1980;60:143–187.
2. McGarry JD, Mannaerts GP, Foster DW. A possible role for malonyl CoA in the regulation of hepatic fatty acid oxidation and ketogenesis. J Clin Invest 1977;60:265–270.
3. McGarry JD, Leatherman GF, Foster DW. Carnitine palmitoyltransferase: I. The site of inhibition of hepatic fatty acid oxidation by malonyl-CoA. J Biol Chem 1978;253:4128–4136.

4. Pan JW, Telang FW, Lee JH, de Graff RA, Rothma DL, Stein DT, Hetherington HP. Measurement of beta-hydroxybutyrate in acute hyperketonemia in human brain. J Neurochem 2001;79:539–544.

5. Cremer JE, Braun LD, Oldendorf WH. Changes during development in transport processes of the blood–brain barrier. Biochim Biophys Acta 1976;448:633–637.

6. Owen OE, Morgan AP, Kemp HG, Sullivan JM, Herrera MG, Cahill GF. Brain metabolism during fasting. J Clin Invest 1967;46:1589–1595.

7. Pan JW, de Graff RA, Rothman DL, Hetherington HP. ^{13}C-[2,4]-β-hydroxybutyrate metabolism in human brain. J Neurochem 2002;81:45.

8. Fredericks M, Ramsey RB. 3-Oxo acid coenzyme A transferase activity in brain and tumors of the nervous stystem. J Neurochem 1978;31:1529–1531.

9. Appleton DB, De Vivo DC. An animal model for the ketogenic diet. Epilepsia 1974;15:211–227.

10. DeVivo DC, Leckie MP, Ferrendelli JS, McDougal DB. Chronic ketosis and cerebral metabolism. Ann Neurol 1978;3:331–337.

11. Wilder RM. Effects of ketonuria on the course of epilepsy. Mayo Clin Bull 1921;2:307–314.

12. Haymond MW, Howard C, Ben-Galim E, De Vivo DC. Effects of ketosis on glucose flux in children and adults. Am J Physiol 1983;245:E373–E378.

13. Lowry OH, Passonneau JV, Hasselberger FX, et al. Effect of ischemia on known substrate and co-factors of the glycolytic pathway in brain. J Biol Chem 1964;239:18–30.

14. Pan JW, Bebin EM, Chu WJ, Hetherington HP. Ketosis and epilepsy: ^{31}P spectroscopic imaging at 4.1 T. Epilepsia 1999;40:703–707.

15. De Vivo DC, Leary L, Wang D. Glucose transporter 1 deficiency syndrome and other glycolytic defects. J Child Neurol 2002;17:3S15–S23.

16. Leary LD, Wang D, Nordli DR, Engelstad K, De Vivo DC. Seizure characterization and electroencephalographic features in glut-1 deficiency syndrome. Epilepsia. 2003 44:701–707.

17. Pascual JM, Van Heertum RL, Wang D, Engelstad K, De Vivo DC. Imaging the metabolic footprint of Glut1 deficiency on the brain. Ann Neurol 2002;52:458–464.

18. Juhasz C, Chugani DC, Muzik O, Watson C, Shah J, Shah A, Chugani HT. Is epileptogenic cortex truly hypometabolic on interictal positron emission tomography? Ann Neurol 2000;48:88–96.

19. Nordli DR, De Vivo DC. The ketogenic diet revisited: back to the future. Epilepsia 1997;38:743–749.

15 The Ketogenic Diet
Interactions With Brain Amino Acid Handling

Marc Yudkoff, Yevgeny Daikhin, Ilana Nissim, and Itzhak Nissim

1. BRAIN GLUCOSE METABOLISM: A SYNOPSIS

The energy requirements of the human brain are enormous. Cerebral oxygen consumption is 35 mL/min/kg or approx 50 mL/min in the adult brain. The rate of whole-body O_2 consumption is 250 mL/min, indicating that approx 20% of oxygen utilization is directed toward the needs of the brain, which occupies only 2% of body weight. Virtually no oxygen is stored in the brain, implying that to maintain the integrity of this vital organ, cerebral blood flow (approx 800 mL/min), which constitutes about 15% of cardiac output, must proceed in an uninterrupted manner. If flow is completely shut down, a state of unconsciousness would ensue within 10 s.

Virtually the sole metabolic substrate of the adult brain is glucose, which is consumed at a rate of 310 µmol/min per kilogram of brain tissue. The stoichiometry of glucose oxidation ($C_6H_{12}O_6 + 6O_2 \rightarrow 6CO_2 + 6H_2O$) implies a rate of oxygen consumption that would be six times that of glucose utilization, or 1860 µmol/min/kg. In fact, brain oxygen consumption is only five times that of glucose utilization (1560 µmol/min/kg) because a fraction of glucose is not oxidized completely but is converted to lactate, a portion of which is released from brain to blood. In addition, a relatively minor fraction of brain glucose utilization is given over to the synthesis of macromolecules and other cellular constituents [1,2].

Both neurons and astrocytes process glucose via the glycolytic pathway. However, glycolysis may be relatively more active in glia, which release lactate to neurons, where this intermediate serves as an important metabolic substrate [3]. The rate of glial lactate production is coupled to neuronal activity because neuronal depolarization favors release of glutamate and K^+, both of which are taken up by astrocytes in an energy-dependent manner. To fuel these processes, astrocytic glycolysis increases in intensity.

The metabolism of glucose does not proceed in a straightforward manner through glycolysis and the tricarboxylic acid cycle to yield CO_2 and H_2O. This is because two essential intermediates of the tricarboxylic acid cycle, oxaloacetate and 2-ketoglutarate, are in very rapid equilibrium with the large aspartate and glutamate pools of the brain (Fig. 1) [4,5]. Such equilibrium is sustained by highly efficient transamination reactions

From: *Epilepsy and the Ketogenic Diet*
Edited by: C. E. Stafstrom and J. M. Rho © Humana Press Inc., Totowa, NJ

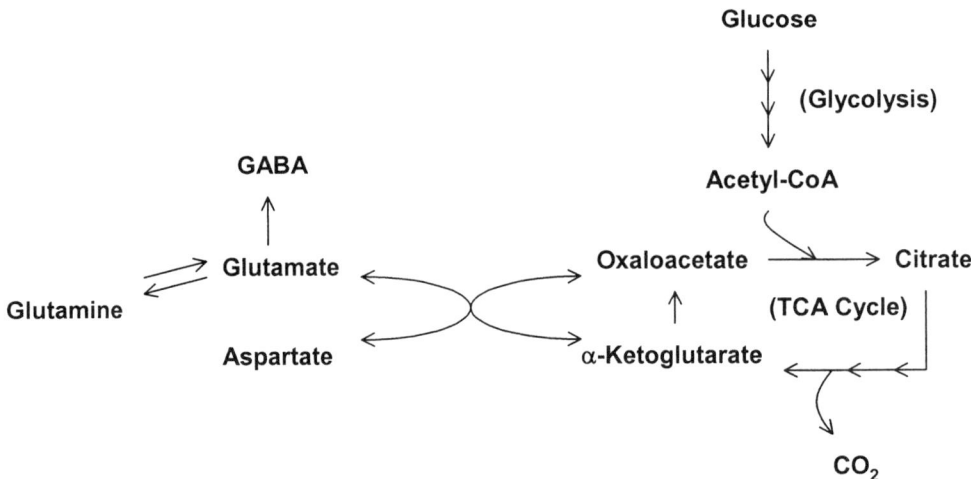

Fig. 1. Schema of interaction of metabolism in brain of glucose and glutamate. The crucial site of intersection occurs via the aspartate aminotransferase reaction, which, in effect, couples the glutamate–aspartate interchange via transamination to the metabolism of glucose through the tricarboxylic acid (TCA) cycle. Glutamate is converted to aspartate by reacting with oxaloacetate. The other major routes of glutamate disposition consist of the synthesis of either glutamine or GABA.

that effectively link brain metabolism of these amino acids with that of glucose *(6)*. If there is an apparent "delay" in the production of CO_2 from glucose carbon, the primary reason is that this carbon flows virtually seamlessly not only through the tricarboxylic acid cycle, but through large pools of amino acids such as aspartate, glutamate, glutamine, and γ-aminobutyric acid (GABA).

As we shall discuss, in the ketotic brain, there may occur a significant change in the interrelationship of metabolism through the tricarboxylic acid cycle and through the brain glutamate pools. We have hypothesized that the net effect of these changes is to favor the flow of glutamate carbon into GABA and to glutamine, which the brain readily converts to GABA *(7–9)*. This chapter explains the details of these putative adaptations. To better understand the relevant biochemistry and physiology, we must first consider the handling by brain of glutamate, the most important excitatory neurotransmitter.

2. BRAIN GLUTAMATE HANDLING: AN OVERVIEW

Glutamic acid is the major excitatory neurotransmitter of the mammalian nervous system. This amino acid must be quickly cleared from the extracellular fluid following its release from nerve endings. A persistently high glutamate concentration in the synaptic cleft would obscure the high signal-to-noise ratio that is essential to effective neurotransmission. By efficiently removing glutamate from the extracellular space, the system is repoised to detect the release of additional glutamate from presynaptic neurons. In addition, an untoward external glutamate level would favor the development of excitotoxicity because of excessive stimulation of vulnerable neurons. Considerable evidence now points to astrocytes as the major site of brain glutamate uptake (Fig. 2) *(10–12)*. Glial cells are favored with a plenitude of excitatory amino acid transporters that abet the rapid and efficient removal of glutamate from the synapse. They also have

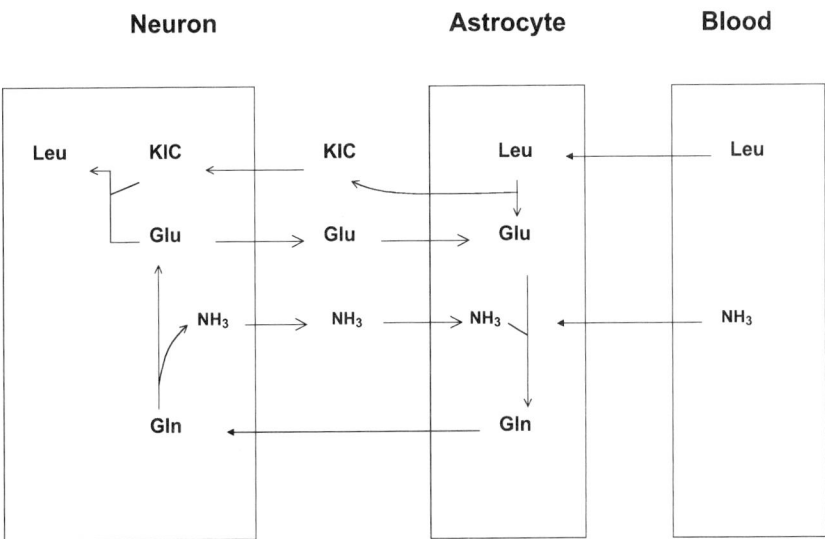

Fig. 2. The glutamine–glutamate cycle of brain. Glutamate released from neurons is preferentially taken up into astrocytes, which then convert glutamate to glutamine. It is as glutamine, a nonneuroactive amino acid, that glutamate is restored to the neurons. Astrocytes release glutamine, which is accumulated by neurons and enzymatically converted back to glutamate via phosphate-dependent glutaminase.

a relatively high membrane potential, an important consideration in enabling the action of sodium-dependent transport systems for excitatory amino acids *(13)*.

Following the uptake of glutamate by the glia, the system must somehow restore this amino acid to the neuronal pools from which it originated. Releasing glutamate directly into the extracellular fluid would not be a workable solution because the extracellular "trafficking" of this excitatory neurotransmitter would expose the system to the risk of depolarization. Instead, astrocytes convert glutamate to glutamine via the glutamine synthetase reaction, a pathway that in brain is dependent on adenosine triphosphate (ATP) and is almost exclusively localized to the astrocytes *(14,15)*. The ammonia that is a coreactant for the glutamine synthetase reaction is derived either from internal sources or from the blood *(16)*. Glia then release glutamine to neurons, where this non-neuroactive amino acid is enzymatically cleaved back to glutamate via phosphate-dependent glutaminase, a mitochondrial enzyme *(17)*.

The series of reactions that begins with the release of glutamate from nerve endings and finishes with the cleavage of glutamine to glutamate is called the "glutamate–glutamine cycle". First propounded more than 20 yr ago, the cycle remains the centerpiece of our thinking regarding brain amino acid metabolism *(18)*. This model provides an excellent framework with which to develop concepts of brain nitrogen metabolism, but, like all models, it necessarily oversimplifies important details.

One aspect of the system that the glutamate–glutamine cycle ignores is the question of the external sources of $-NH_2$ groups that the brain, like any other organ, must import to replace inevitable losses from the system. Virtually no glutamate or glutamine is directly taken up from blood to brain *(19,20)*, and alternate sources of nitrogen must become available. One likely nitrogen donor is leucine, which is actively transported into the central nervous system and is which readily transaminated by brain to glutamate and ketoleucine *(20–24)*. Indeed, studies performed with [^{15}N]leucine have suggested that at least one-third of all brain nitrogen may have derived from leucine alone, with significant contributions also coming form valine and isoleucine, the other branched-chain amino acids *(25)*. There may be an intricate cycling of leucine between astrocytes and neurons such that 2-oxoisocaproate, the ketoacid of leucine, is released to neurons, where it can be converted back to leucine, in the process "buffering" glutamate *(24)*.

The model implicit in the glutamate–glutamine cycle ignores a second pivotal aspect of brain nitrogen handling, namely, that amino acids such as glutamate, glutamine, and aspartate not only are critical to neurotransmission but also function as essential metabolic intermediates. As noted earlier, an appreciable fraction of glucose carbon flows through relatively large pools of these amino acids before final combustion to CO_2. If the brain respires on a fuel other than glucose—and the ketone bodies are the most important alternate source—then we might anticipate that this fundamental shift in the metabolic "set" of the system would significantly affect brain glutamate handling. This appears to be the case.

3. BRAIN METABOLISM OF THE KETONE BODIES: RELATIONSHIP TO GLUTAMATE METABOLISM

Although glucose ordinarily is the sole fuel of the brain, when the plasma concentration of the ketone bodies rises into the range of 2–4m*M,* these organic acids can satisfy as much as 70% of the metabolic requirements of the brain *(26)*. Such intense ketonemia occurs most commonly during starvation, when hepatic glycogen stores become depleted and the breakdown of triglycerides in adipose tissue favors the delivery of fatty acids to the liver. The liver first oxidizes these lipids to acetyl-coenzyme A (acetyl-CoA), and from this intermediate the liver synthesizes the major ketone bodies 3-hydroxybutyrate and acetoacetate. Liver does not utilize ketone bodies to satisfy its own metabolic needs. This requirement is met primarily by the large influx of fatty acids from adipose tissue. Instead, the liver releases the ketone bodies into the bloodstream, where they are taken up by a number of tissues, primarily skeletal muscle, kidney, and the brain.

A series of monocarboxylate transporters mediates the uptake of ketone bodies into and through the central nervous system *(27–30)*. The rate of uptake appears to follow closely the concentration of the ketone bodies in the blood. It is likely that intracerebral metabolism of the ketone bodies occurs in both neurons and glia, although the relative contributions of either cell type to this process are uncertain. Furthermore, the avidity with which individual cells utilize ketone bodies varies during brain development. The relatively immature brain, which must form copious amounts of myelin, appears to draw heavily on the ketone bodies as a source of the acetyl-CoA units that are the fundamental precursors to myelin lipid *(31–33)*. Ketosis is favored in the suckling animal by the high fat content of maternal milk *(34,35)*.

Figure 3 shows the metabolic pathways that mediate the utilization of ketone bodies. The initial step is the conversion of 3-hydroxybutyrate to acetoacetate in a mitochondrial reaction for which nicotinamide adenine dinucleotide (NAD) serves as an electron acceptor. Acetoacetate then is converted to acetoacetyl-CoA in the succinyl-CoA transferase reaction, a pathway that is especially active in the nervous system *(36)*. Succinate, the other product of this reaction, is further oxidized in the tricarboxylic acid

$$\text{3-OH-Butyrate + NAD} \longrightarrow \text{Acetoacetate + NADH}$$

$$\text{Acetoacetate + Succinyl-CoA} \longrightarrow \text{Acetoacetyl-CoA + Succinate}$$

$$\text{Acetoacetyl-CoA + CoA} \longrightarrow \text{2 Acetyl-CoA}$$

Fig. 3. Metabolic pathways of ketone body degradation. The primary circulating compound is 3-hydroxybutyrate (3-OH-butyrate), which is converted to acetoacetate in a NAD-dependent reaction. Acetoacetyl-CoA then is formed in the succinyl-CoA transferase reaction. A specific thiolase then converts acetoacetyl-CoA to acetyl-CoA, and in this form the ketone bodies enter the tricarboxylic acid cycle.

cycle. Acetoacetyl-CoA is cleaved via the action of a specific thiolase to yield acetyl-CoA, which enters the tricarboxylic acid cycle via the citrate synthetase reaction.

The consumption of either glucose or ketone bodies provides the energy that is necessary to fuel brain function, most importantly the maintenance of the ionic gradients that are essential to all neurotransmission. In this sense, the choice of either glucose or ketone bodies as a metabolic substrate is essentially transparent to the brain. However, as shown in Fig. 4, it is evident that distinctive biochemical pathways mediate the consumption of these respective fuels. In the cytosol, the glycolytic pathway converts glucose to pyruvate, which is transported into mitochondria and further metabolized to acetyl-CoA via the pyruvate dehydrogenase reaction. The cytosolic glycolytic pathway also yields reduced NAD (NADH), which is indirectly transported into mitochondria via the malate–aspartate shuttle, as shown in Fig. 4. In mitochondria the NADH becomes oxidized in the electron transport chain, in the process yielding ATP.

In contrast to the cellular metabolism of glucose, which yields NADH in both the cytoplasmic and mitochondrial compartments, the metabolism of ketone bodies occurs exclusively in the mitochondria, according to the sequence of reactions shown in Fig. 3. Thus, the metabolism of the ketone bodies occurs *only* through mitochondrial formation of acetyl-CoA, whereas the consumption of glucose includes a cytoplasmic component (glycolysis) that allows the derivation of energy without the necessity of funneling all glucose carbon through a pool of mitochondrial acetyl-CoA. Indeed, as noted earlier, in the nonketotic state glycolysis may be the predominant pathway of glucose metabolism in astrocytes, which may furnish lactate to neurons that use this intermediate as a fuel.

In addition to enhanced internal production of acetyl-CoA, it also may be that in ketosis external acetate, which likely is present at a higher concentration in the blood of the ketotic individual, is readily consumed in the brain (Fig. 4). It is thought that the astrocytes are the favored site of cerebral acetate consumption *(37,38)*, primarily because acetate uptake into glia is faster *(39)*. An expected consequence would be greater acetyl-CoA levels as well as glutamine production in ketotic brain, conclusions we have recently confirmed (unpublished data).

The utilization of acetyl-CoA as an energy source occurs via the citrate synthetase reaction, which constitutes the "entry" point for acetyl-CoA into the tricarboxylic acid cycle (Fig. 4). Citrate synthetase is a very active pathway in brain. Maximal velocity of this reaction (>25 μmol/min/g tissue) may be 10 times greater than that of pyruvate dehydrogenase *(40,41)*. Indeed, basal flux through pyruvate dehydrogenase barely

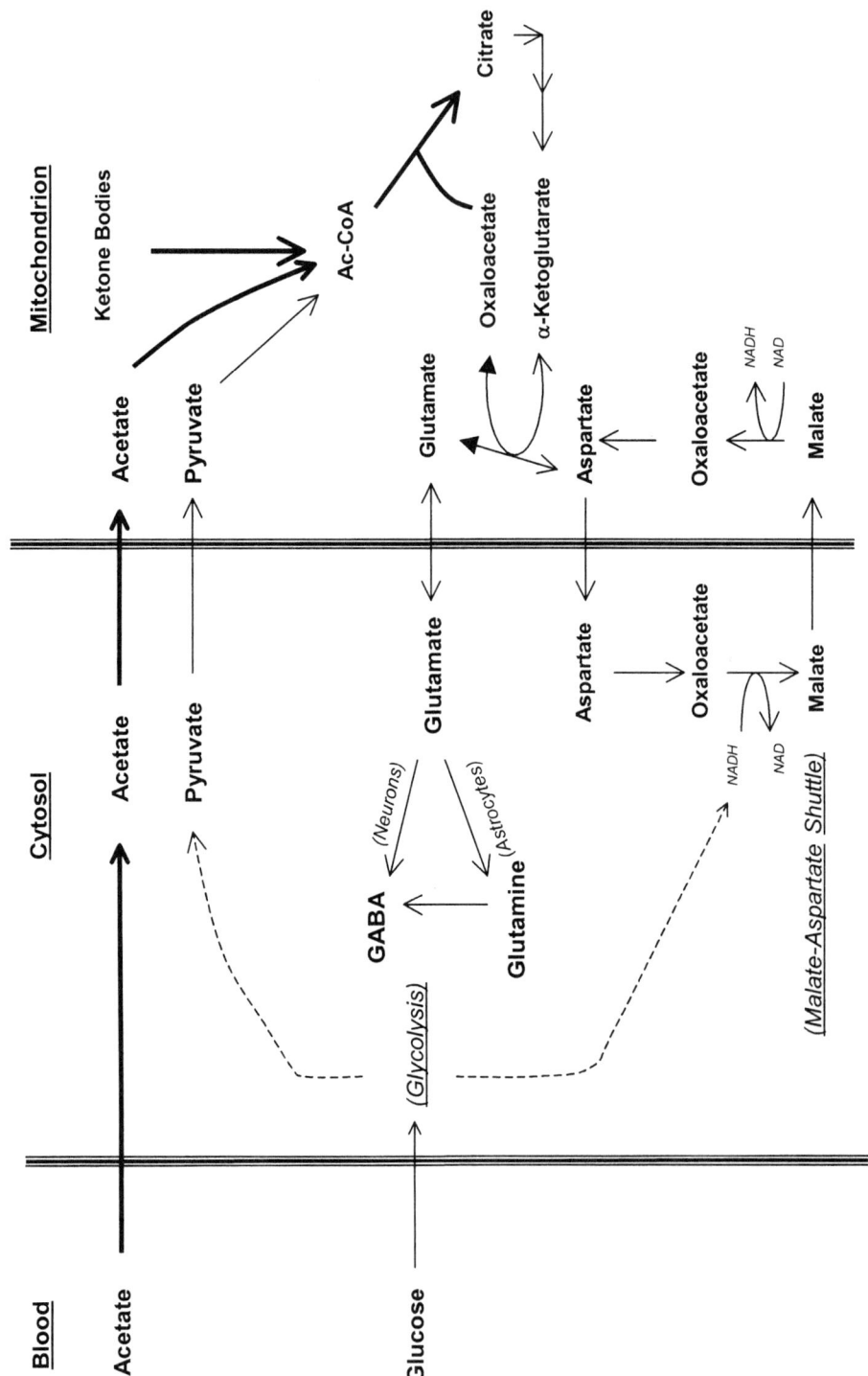

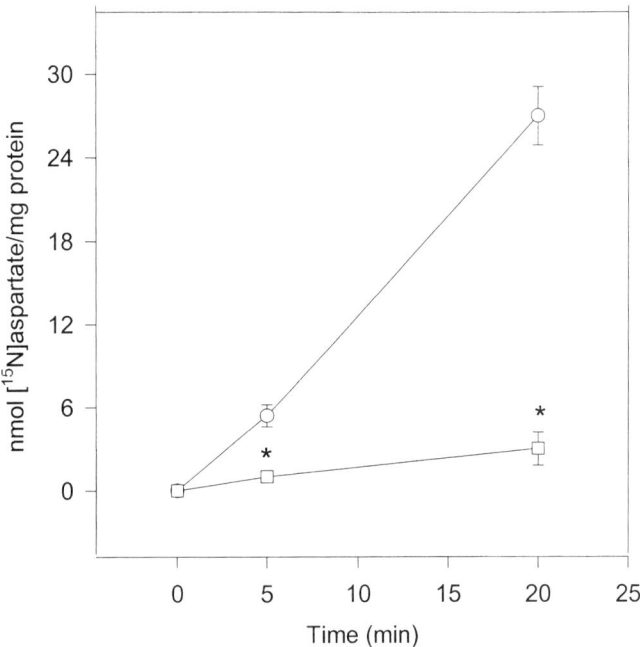

Fig. 5. Formation of [^{15}N]aspartate from [^{15}N]glutamate in cultured astrocytes. Cells were incubated in the presence of [^{15}N]glutamate for the indicated times. Gas chromatography–mass spectrometry was used to measure the appearance of label in [^{15}N]aspartate: circles, control; squares, acetoacetate (5mM); *, $p < 0.05$ relative to control. Data from ref. 7.

equals the rate of synaptosomal respiration *(42)*. Formation of citrate involves the condensation of acetyl-CoA with oxaloacetate, and, as flux through citrate synthetase becomes intensified, the concentration of oxaloacetate in brain is diminished. As already noted, transamination to aspartate is a major route of brain glutamate metabolism *(6,7,23,43,44)*. Furthermore, flux through aspartate aminotransferase, an equilibrium enzyme, will be closely linked to the size of the oxaloacetate pool. The relative diminution of the latter in ketosis would be expected to lead to a reduced rate of transamination of glutamate to aspartate because oxaloacetate serves as the acceptor of the amino group of glutamate in this reaction (Fig. 1) *(4,45)*.

The data in Fig. 5 are consistent with this formulation *(7)*. Cultured astrocytes were incubated in the presence of [^{15}N]glutamate to trace the appearance of this label in

Fig. 4. Schema of putative effects of brain ketone body metabolism on glutamate metabolism. As brain respires to a relatively greater extent on ketone bodies, it must form relatively more ATP from acetyl-CoA; this is because the diminution of glucose flux through brain lessens the importance of glycolysis as a source of energy. In addition, it is likely that during ketosis the brain utilizes external acetate as a major fuel. Increased combustion of acetyl-CoA implies greater flux through the citrate synthetase reaction and a corresponding reduction in the availability of oxaloacetate to the aspartate aminotransferase pathway. A consequence is less conversion of glutamate to aspartate and a more efficient conversion of glutamate to both glutamine and GABA. The anticonvulsant effect of the ketogenic diet may be a salutary effect of augmented GABA-ergic "tone" in the brain.

[^{15}N]aspartate. Gas chromatography—mass spectrometry was used to measure the ^{15}N enrichment in amino acids. When the incubation medium also contained acetoacetate (5mM), there occurred a significant reduction in the rate of glutamate transamination to aspartate. At 5 min, the concentration of intra-astrocytic aspartate, in nanomoles of [^{15}N]aspartate per milligram of protein, was ($\pm$ SD) 5.4 $\pm$ 0.8 (control) and 1.0 $\pm$ 0.1 (acetoacetate) ($p < 0.05$). After 20 min the difference was 27 $\pm$ 2.1 (control) and 3 $\pm$ 1.2 (acetoacetate) ($p < 0.05$). Internal [^{15}N]glutamate was similar in control and experimental incubations, indicating that ketone bodies affected glutamate transamination rather than uptake. A similar response to ketosis had been observed previously. Thus, reductions of brain aspartate concentration have been observed in suckling mice injected with ketone bodies *(46)* and in rats fed a high-fat diet *(45)*.

As less glutamate is transaminated to yield aspartate, more glutamate becomes available to the glutamate decarboxylase reaction (glutamate $\rightarrow$ GABA + CO$_2$; Figs 1 and 4) to yield GABA, the primary inhibitory neurotransmitter and a probable anticonvulsant factor *(47–55)*. The rate of brain GABA synthesis is not always considered to be sensitive to the ambient brain glutamate concentration, which is present at a level (8–10mM) that should saturate the glutamate decarboxylase pathway (K_m 0.2–1.2mM). However, glutamate concentration in the brain is not uniform in all cell types, and levels in GABA-forming neurons are especially low *(56,57)*. Furthermore, the pool of glutamate that serves as a precursor to GABA probably is less than 5% of total brain glutamate *(58,59)*, even though GABA-ergic neurons constitute 20% of all neurons. In addition, it should be emphasized that the glutamate decarboxylase pathway is tightly controlled, with flux through it (approx 0.5 nmol/min/mg protein) *(44,60)* far less than overall enzymatic activity *(60)*. Relatively slight changes of glutamate concentration in GABA-ergic neurons can alter flux through the pathway *(61)*. Metabolic regulators of glutamate decarboxylase include Cl$^-$ and aspartate, which, by increasing the affinity of the enzyme for glutamate *(62,63)*, may render GABA formation even more responsive to the ambient glutamate concentration.

The experiments shown in Fig. 6 illustrate this process *(43)*. When synaptosomes were incubated in the presence of acetoacetate (5mM), the internal glutamate concentration was consistently greater than control values and the internal aspartate concentration was significantly reduced (Fig. 6, left). A very rapid and significant increase of intrasynaptosomal GABA concentration was noted (Fig. 6, right). We documented that the increase of GABA concentration reflected increased synthesis by incubating the synaptosomes with either L-[^{2}H$_5$-2,3,3,4,4]glutamine or L-[^{15}N]glutamine (0.5 mM each) and following the appearance of label in [^{2}H$_4$]GABA or [^{15}N]GABA. This work confirmed that inclusion of acetoacetate in the incubation medium significantly enhances the rate of GABA synthesis from glutamine *(43)*.

The synaptosomal studies just cited utilized glutamine as a precursor to GABA. Neurons would derive GABA from glutamine after enzymatically hydrolyzing the latter through the action of phosphate-dependent glutaminase *(64)*. It is well established that glutamine is a highly efficient GABA precursor, perhaps even more effective than external glutamate, because glutamine is rapidly taken up by GABA-ergic neurons. Brain glutamine is formed almost entirely in astrocytes from glutamate and ammonia (*see* Fig. 2). During ketosis, when less glutamate becomes transaminated in glia to aspartate, relatively more enters the glutamine synthetase pathway, and the availability of glutamine to GABA-ergic neurons is correspondingly increased. In studies of ketotic mice

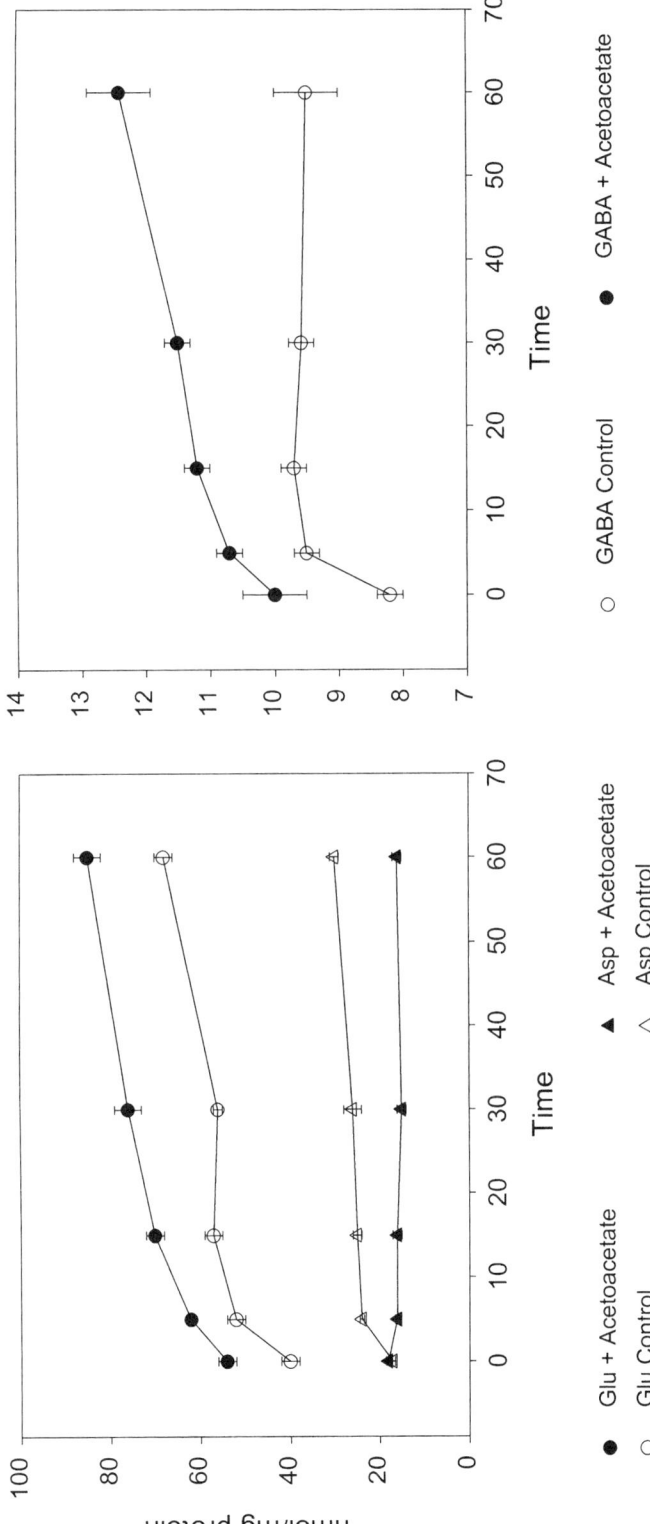

Fig. 6. Metabolism of glutamate in synaptosomes in presence of acetoacetate. Synaptosomes incubated for the indicated times in the presence of glutamate with or without acetoacetate (5m*M*). Presence of acetoacetate inhibited the transamination of glutamate to aspartate, thereby increasing the internal concentration of glutamate, lowering that of aspartate, and increasing that of GABA. Data from ref. *43*.

193

(Yudkoff et al., unpublished data), we have found that the administration of acetate, which brain metabolizes primarily in astrocytes, is associated with an increased rate of synthesis of both glutamine and GABA.

4. POSSIBLE RELATIONSHIP OF METABOLIC CHANGES TO ANTICONVULSANT EFFECT

Previous investigators have speculated that the ketogenic diet improves overall brain metabolism and that this might be the basis for the antiepileptic effect. Certainly the diet appears to favorably influence energy charge of the brain in selected groups of subjects (65,66). An outstanding issue is whether the improvement in overall energy metabolism is the cause or the consequence of reduced seizure frequency. It also has been postulated that the diet imposes a mild cerebral acidosis that diminishes the responsiveness of brain NMDA receptors, although efforts to document an accumulation of brain H+ have yielded a negative result (67,68).

We have identified an alteration of amino acid metabolism that entails reduced transamination of glutamate to aspartate in ketogenic brain and greater availability of glutamate for GABA synthesis. As noted earlier, an increase of cerebral GABA-ergic activity would be expected to result in an anticonvulsant effect. In addition, it is plausible that a diminution of brain aspartate concentration could help to attenuate the frequency or severity of seizures. Glutamate transamination to aspartate is essential to normative brain glutamate metabolism (5,10,69), particularly after depolarization (70–72). The "product" of glutamate transamination is aspartate, the extracellular level of which increases following a seizure (73,74), moreover, aspartate may have have a primary epileptogenic role (75,76). A pathogenic role has been postulated for aspartate in hippocampal epilepsy (77–80).

By lowering the rate of transamination of glutamate to aspartate, the ketogenic diet would attenuate the production of the latter excitatory neurotransmitter. Relatively more glutamate then would be available for conversion to GABA, thereby abetting an anticonvulsant effect, and for the production of glutamine, which is an effective GABA precursor.

5. KETOGENIC DIET AND AMINO ACID TRANSPORT

The foregoing discussion involved changes in the metabolism of glutamate and related compounds that appear to occur consequent to ketosis. It also appears that significant alterations of amino acid transport occur in the ketotic brain and that these adaptations may contribute to the anticonvulsant effect. We have found, for example, that the entry of leucine into brain is greatly increased in ketotic mice (8). The uptake from blood to brain of leucine and other large neutral amino acids is mediated via the L-transporter system, which functions primarily as an amino acid exchanger (81,82). Although the affinity of the transporter for glutamine is not especially high (83), the abundance of glutamine in brain favors the utilization of glutamine for facilitating neutral amino acid uptake (84). Glutamine would be formed in astrocytes from glutamate that had been transported from the synaptic cleft (see Fig. 7).

In ketosis the brain/blood ratio for leucine is increased and that for glutamine is unchanged relative to control (Yudkoff et al., unpublished data), a factor that would favor leucine entry into brain via exchange for glutamine. An important consequence of

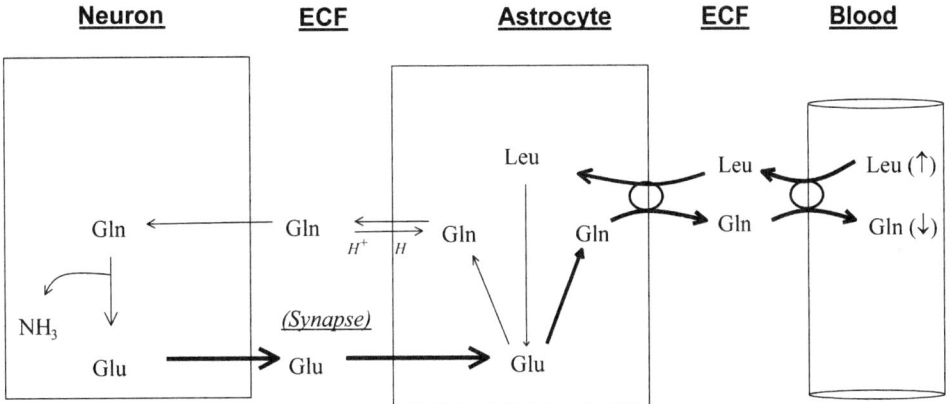

Fig. 7. Putative effects of ketosis on brain amino acid transport. The uptake of leucine into brain, which is increased in the ketotic mouse, may occur via exchange for internal glutamine. Glutamine, in turn, is formed from intrasynaptic glutamate that is taken up by astrocytes, the major site in brain of the glutamine synthetase pathway. Release of glutamate by epileptic brain is probably increased, and the development of more rapid large neutral amino acid–glutamine exchange affords the system with a more efficient capacity for the removal of glutamate from the extracellular fluid (ECF).

this adaptation might be an enhanced capacity to dispose of glutamate that had been released into the synaptic cleft. In effect, the brain would "detoxify" extracellular glutamate not simply by swiftly removing it from the synapse into astrocytes and then converting it to glutamine, but by exporting the latter into the blood rather than exporting it back to neurons (Fig. 2). This "loss" of glutamine would quickly be compensated by the transamination of the newly imported leucine (Fig. 7). However, during periods of enhanced glutamate release from neurons, a phenomenon that characterizes seizure activity, the system would have at its disposal a new mechanism for the removal of external glutamate.

A highly ordered array of amino acid transporters mediate the exchange of glutamate, glutamine, and related compounds between neurons, astrocytes, and capillaries *(82)*. It is likely that the ketogenic diet, which, as we have seen, induces fundamental alterations in the metabolism of brain amino acids, and also changes the function of these tissue-specific amino acid transport systems. We cannot know *a priori* that these presumed adaptations will give rise to an anticonvulsant effect, although the accepted clinical efficacy of the ketogenic diet affords a rationale for future experimentation to test the hypothesis that ketosis-induced changes in the function of amino acid transporters enable the ability of the brain to contain seizures by favoring novel mechanisms for the removal of glutamic acid.

6. CONCLUSION

The ketogenic diet appears to evoke numerous changes in brain metabolism of the amino acids. These adaptations alter the metabolism of glutamic acid, which is the most important excitatory neurotransmitter and the central element of brain amino acid handling. Thus, ketosis is associated with a diminution in the rate of glutamate transamination to aspartate and, possibly, an enhancement in the rate of glutamate decarboxylation to GABA. Furthermore, ketosis may alter brain amino acid transport systems in such manner that uptake of glutamate from the synaptic cleft becomes much more efficient. To the extent that the epileptic state is associated with increased glutamatergic activity, an increased glutamate clearance from the extracellular fluid would be expected to attenuate and even abolish convulsive activity. An enhancement of GABA-ergic activity would favor inhibitory influences and diminish the seizure diathesis.

ACKNOWLEDGMENTS

This work was supported by grants HD26979, NS37915, and NS007413 from the National Institutes of Health.

REFERENCES

1. Siesjo BK. Brain Energy Metabolism. Wiley, New York, 1997.
2. Clarke DD, Sokoloff L. Circulation and energy metabolism of the brain. In: Siegel GJ, Agranoff BW, Albers RW, Fisher SK, Uhler MD (eds.). Basic Neurochemistry: Molecular, Cellular and Medical Aspects, 6th ed. Lippincott-Raven, Philadelphia, 1999, pp. 637–669.
3. Magistretti PJ, Pellerin L, Rothman DL, Shulman RG. Energy on demand. Science 1999;283:496–497.
4. McKenna MC, Tildon JT, Stevenson JH, Boatright R, Huang S. Regulation of energy metabolism in synaptic terminals and cultured rat brain astrocytes: differences revealed using aminooxyacetate. Dev Neurosci 1994;15:320–322.
5. Yudkoff M, Nelson D, Daikhin Y, Erecinska M. Tricarboxylic acid cycle in rat brain synaptosomes. Fluxes and interactions with aspartate aminotransferase and malate/aspartate shuttle. J Biol Chem 1994;269:27414–27420.
6. Fitzpatrick SM, Cooper AJL, Duffy TE. Use of β-methylene-DL-aspartate to assess the role of aspartate aminotransferase in cerebral oxidative metabolism. J Neurochem 1983;41:1370–1383.
7. Yudkoff M, Daikhin Y, Nissim I, Grunstein R, Nissim I. Effect of ketone bodies on astrocyte amino acid metabolism. J Neurochem 1997;69:682–692.
8. Yudkoff M, Daikhin M, Nissim I, Lazarow A, Nissim I. Brain amino acid metabolism and ketosis. J Neurosci Res 2001;66:272–281.
9. Yudkoff M, Daikhin Y, Nissim I, Lazarow A, Nissim I. Ketogenic diet, amino acid metabolism and seizure control. J Neurosci Res 2001;66:931–940.
10. Hertz L, Peng L, Westergaard N, Yudkoff M, Schousboe A. Neuronal–astrocytic interactions in metabolism of transmitter amino acids of the glutamate family. In: Schousboe A, Diemer NH, Kofod H (eds.). Drug Research Related to Neuroactive Amino Acids, Alfred Benzon Symposium 32. Munksgaard, Copenhagen, 1992, pp. 30–48.
11. Gegelashvili G, Schousboe A. Cellular distribution and kinetic properties of high-affinity glutamate transporters. Brain Res Bull 1998;45:233–238.
12. Takahashi M, Billups B, Rossi D, Sarantis M, Hamann M, Attwell D. The role of glutamate transporters in glutamate homeostasis in the brain. J Exp Biol 1997;200:401–409.
13. Erecinska M, Silver IA. Metabolism and role of glutamate in mammalian brain. Prog Neurobiol 1990;35:245–296.
14. Martinez-Hernandez A, Bell KP, Norenberg MD. Glutamine synthetase: glial localization in brain. Science 1997;195:1356–1358.
15. Norenberg MD, Martinez-Hernandez A. Fine structural localization of glutamine synthetase in astrocytes of rat brain. Brain Res 1979;161:303–310.
16. Cooper AJL, McDonald JM, Gelbard AS, Gledhill RF, Duffy TE. The metabolic fate of ^{13}N-labelled ammonia in rat brain. J Biol Chem 1979;254:4982–4992.
17. Erecinska M, Zaleska MM, Nelson D, Nissim I, Yudkoff M. Neuronal glutamine utilization: glutamine/glutamate homeostasis in synaptosomes. J Neurochem 1990;54:2057–2069.
18. Shank RP and Aprison MH. Present status and significance of the glutamine cycle in neural tissues. Life Sci 1977;28:837–842.

19. Grill V, Björkhem M, Gutniak M, Lindqvist M. Brain uptake and release of amino acids in nondiabetic and insulin-dependent diabetic subjects: important role of glutamine release for nitrogen balance. Metabolism 1992;41:28–32.

20. Smith QR, Momma S, Aoyagi M, Rapoport SI. Kinetics of neutral amino acid transport across the blood–brain barrier. J Neurochem 1987;49:1651–1658.

21. Bixel MG, Hutson SM, Hamprecht B. Cellular distribution of branched-chain amino acid aminotransferase isoenzymes among rat brain glial cells in culture. J Histochem Cytochem 1997;45:685–694.

22. Hutson SM, Wallin R, Hall TR. Identification of mitochondrial branched chain aminotransferase and its isoforms in rat tissues. J Biol Chem 1992;267:15681–15686.

23. Yudkoff M, Daikhin Y, Lin Z-P, Nissim I, Stern J, Pleasure D, Nissim I. Interrelationships of leucine and glutamate in cultured astrocytes. J Neurochem 1994;62:1192–1202.

24. Yudkoff M, Daikhin Y. Nelson D, Nissim I, Erecinska M. Neuronal metabolism of branched-chain amino acids: flux through the aminotransferase pathway in synaptosomes. J Neurochem 1996;66:2136–2145.

25. Kanamori K. Ross BD. Kondrat RW. Rate of glutamate synthesis from leucine in rat brain measured in vivo by ^{15}N NMR. J Neurochem 1998;70:1304–1315.

26. Owen OE, Morgan AP, Kemp HG, Sullivan JM, Herrera MG, Cahill GF. Brain metabolism during fasting. J Clin Invest 1967;46:1589–1595.

27. Gjedde A, Crone C. Induction processes in blood–brain transfer of ketone bodies during starvation. Am J Physiol 1975;229:1165–1169.

28. Tildon JT, Roeder LM. Transport of 3-hydroxy[3-^{14}C]butyrate by dissociated cells from rat brain. Am J Physiol 1998;255:C133–C139.

29. Leino RL, Gerhart DZ, Duelli R, Enerson BE, Drewes LR. Diet-induced ketosis increases monocarboxylate transporter (MCT1) levels in rat brain. Neurochem Int 2001;38:519–527.

30. Pierre K, Magistretti PJ, Pellerin L. MCT2 is a major neuronal monocarboxylate transporter in the adult mouse brain. J Cereb Blood Flow Metab 2002;22:586–595.

31. Koper JW, Lopes-Cardozo M, Van Golde LM. Preferential utilization of ketone bodies for the synthesis of myelin cholesterol in vivo. Biochim Biophys Acta 1981;666:411–417.

32. Lopes-Cardozo M, Koper JW, Klein W, Van Golde LM. Acetoacetate is a cholesterogenic precursor for myelinating rat brain and spinal cord. Incorporation of label from [3-^{14}C]acetoacetate, [^{14}C]glucose and ^{3}H$_2$O. Biochim Biophys Acta 1984;794:350–352.

33. Gerhart DZ, Enerson BE, Zhdankina OY, Leino RL, Drewes LR. Expression of monocarboxylate transporter MCT1 by brain endothelium and glia in adult and suckling rats. Am J Physiol 1997;273:E207–E213.

34. Dombrowski GJ Jr, Swiatek KR, Chao K-L. Lactate, 3-hydroxybutyrate and glucose as substrates for early postnatal rat brain. Neurochem Res 1989;14:667–675.

35. Nehlig A, Pereira de Vasconcelos A. Glucose and ketone body utilization by the brain of neonatal rats. Prog Neurobiol 1993;40:163–221.

36. Fukao T, Song XQ, Mitchell GA, Yamaguchi S, Sukegawa K, Orii T, Kondo N. Enzymes of ketone body utilization in human tissues: protein and messenger RNA levels of succinyl-coenzyme A (CoA):3-ketoacid CoA transferase and mitochondrial and cytosolic acetoacetyl-CoA thiolases. Pediatr Res 1997;42:498–502.

37. Berl S, Takagaki G, Clarke DD, Waelsch H. Metabolic compartments in vivo. Ammonia and glutamic acid metabolism in brain and liver. J Biol Chem 1962;237:2562–2569.

38. Cerdan S, Kunnecke B, Seelig J. Cerebral metabolism of [1,2-^{13}C$_2$]acetate as detected by in vivo and in vitro ^{13}C NMR. J Biol Chem 1990;265:12916–12926.

39. Waniewski RA, Martin DL. Preferential utilization of acetate by astrocytes is attributable to transport. J Neurosci 1998;18:5225–5233.

40. Booth RFG, Clark JB. A rapid method for the preparation of relatively pure, metabolically competent synaptosomes from rat brain. Biochem J 1978;176:365–370.

41. Ratnakumari L, Murthy CRK. Activities of pyruvate dehydrogenase, enzymes of citric acid cycle, and aminotransferases in the subcellular fractions of cerebral cortex in normal and hyperammonemic rats. Neurochem Res 1989;14:221–228.

42. Erecinska M, Dagani F. Relationships between the neuronal sodium/potassium pump and energy metabolism. Effects of K$^+$, Na$^+$ and adenosine triphosphate in isolated brain synaptosomes. J Gen Physiol 1990;95:591–616.

43. Erecinska M, Nelson D, Daikhin Y, Yudkoff M. Regulation of GABA level in rat brain synaptosomes: fluxes through enzymes of the GABA shunt and effects of glutamate, calcium, and ketone bodies. J Neurochem 1996;67:2325–2334.

44. Mason GF, Gruetter R, Rothman DL, Behar KL, Shulman RG, Novotny EJ. Simultaneous determination of the rates of the TCA cycle, glucose utilization, alpha-ketoglutarate/glutamate exchange, and glutamine synthesis in human brain by NMR. J Cereb Blood Flow Metab 1995;15:12–25.

45. DeVivo DC, Leckie MP, Ferrendelli JS, McDougal DB Jr. Chronic ketosis and cerebral metabolism. Ann Neurol 1978;3:331–337.

46. Thurston JH, Hauhart RE, Schiro JA. Beta-hydroxybutyrate reverses insulin-induced hypoglycemic coma in suckling–weanling mice despite low blood and brain glucose levels. Metab Brain Dis 1986;1:63–82.

47. DeDeyn PP, Marescau B, MacDonald RL. Epilepsy and the GABA-hypothesis: a brief review and some samples. Acta Neurol Belg 1990;90:65–81.

48. Olsen RW, Avoli M. GABA and epileptogenesis. Epilepsia 1997;38:399–407.

49. Loscher W, Swark WS. Evidence for impaired GABAergic activity in the substantia nigra of amygdaloid kindled rats. Brain Res 1985;339:146–150.

50. Lasley SM, Yan QS. Diminished potassium-stimulated GABA release in vivo in genetically epilepsy-prone rats. Neurosci Lett 1994;175:145–148.

51. Gould EM, Curto KA, Craig CR, Fleming WW, Taylor DA. The role of GABA-A receptors in the subsensitivity of Purkinje neurons to GABA in genetic epilepsy prone rats. Brain Res 1995;698:62–68.

52. Hovanics GE, DeLorey TM, Firestone LL, Quinlan JJ, Handforth A, Harrison NL, Krasowski MD, Rick CE, Korpi ER, Makela R, Brilliant MH, Hagiwara N, Ferguson C, Snyder K, Olsen RW. Mice devoid of gamma-aminobutyrate type A receptor beta$_3$ subunit have epilepsy, cleft palate, and hypersensitive behavior. Proc Natl Acad Sci U S A 1997;94:4143–4148.

53. White HS. Clinical significance of animal seizure models and mechanism of action studies of potential antiepileptic drugs. Epilepsia 1997;38 (Suppl 1):S9–S17.

54. Meldrum BS. Update on the mechanism of action of antiepileptic drugs. Epilepsia 1996;37 (Suppl 6):S4–S11.

55. Petroff OA, Rothman D, Behar KL, Mattson RH. Low brain GABA level is associated with poor seizure control. Ann Neurol 1996;40:908–911.

56. Storm-Mathisen J, Leknes AK, Bore AT, Vaaland JL, Edminson P, Haug FM, Ottersen OP. First visualization of glutamate and GABA in neurones by immunocytochemistry. Nature 1983;301:517–520.

57. Storm-Mathisen J, Ottersen OP. Antibodies against amino acid neurotrnasmitters. In: Paunula P, Paivarinta H, Soinila S (eds.). Neurohistochemistry: Modern Methods and Applications. Liss, New York, 1986, pp. 107–136.

58. Patel AJ. Balazs R, Richter D. Contribution of the GABA bypath to glucose oxidation, and the development of compartmentation in the brain. Nature 1970;226:1160–1161.

59. Patel AJ, Johnson AL, Balazs R. Metabolic compartmentation of glutamate associated with the formation of γ-aminobutyrate. J Neurochem 1974;23:1271–1279.

60. Battaglioli G, Martin DL. Stimulation of synaptosomal γ-aminobutyric acid synthesis by glutamate and glutamine. J Neurochem 1990;54:1179–1187.

61. Paulsen RE, Fonnum F. Role of glial cells for the basal and Ca^{2+}-dependent K^+-evoked release of transmitter amino acids investigated by microdialysis. J Neurochem 1989;52:1823–1829.

62. Wu J-Y. Purification, characterization and kinetic studies of GAD and GABA-T from mouse brain. In: Roberts E, Chase TN, Tower DB (eds.). GABA in Nervous System Function. Raven, New York, 1976, pp. 7–55.

63. Porter TG, Martin DL. Stability and activation of glutamate apodecarboxylase from pig brain. J Neurochem 1988;51:1886–1891.

64. Sonnewald U, Westergaard N, Schousboe A, Svendsen JS, Unsgard G, Petersen SB. Direct demonstration by [^{13}C]NMR spectroscopy that glutamine from astrocytes is a precursor for GABA synthesis in neurons. Neurochem Int 1993;22:19–29.

65. DeVivo DC, Malas KL, Leckie MP. Starvation and seizures: observations on the electroconvulsive threshold and cerebral metabolism of the starved adult rat. Arch Neurol 1975;32:755–760.

66. Pan JW, Bebin EM, Chu WJ, Hetherington HP. Ketosis and epilepsy: ^{31}P spectroscopic imaging at 4.1T. Epilepsia 1999;40:703–707.

67. Al-Mudallal AS, LaManna JC, Lust WD, Harik SI. Diet-induced ketosis does not cause cerebral acidosis. Epilepsia 1996;37:258–261.

68. Novotny EJ Jr, Chen J, Rothman DL. Alterations in cerebral metabolism with the ketogenic diet. Epilepsia 1997;38 (Suppl 8):S147.

69. Erecinska M, Zaleska MM, Nissim I, Nelson D, Dagani F, Yudkoff M. Glucose and synaptosomal glucose metabolism: studies with [^{15}N]glutamate. J Neurochem 1988;51:892–902.

70. McKenna MC, Tildon JT, Stevenson JH, Boatright R, Huang S. Regulation of energy metabolism in synaptic terminals and cultured rat brain astrocytes: differences revealed using aminooxyacetate. Dev Neurosci 1993;15:320–329.

71. Peng L, Hertz L. Potassium-induced stimulation of oxidative metabolism of glucose in cultures of intact cerebellar granule cells but not in corresponding cells with dendritic degeneration. Brain Res 1993;629:331–334.

72. Waagepetersen HS, Sonnewald U, Larsson OM, Schousboe A. Compartmentation of TCA cycle metabolism in cultured neocortical neurons revealed by ^{13}C MR spectroscopy. Neurochem Int 2000;36:349–358.

73. Do KQ, Klancnik J, Gahwiler BH, et al. Release of EAA: animal studies and epileptic foci studies in humans. In: Meldrum BS, Moroni F, Simon RP (eds.). Excitatory Amino Acids. Press, New York, 1991, pp. 677–685.

74. Carlson H, Ronne-Engstrum E, Ungerstedt U, Hillered L. Seizure-related elevations of extracellular amino acids in human focal epilepsy. Neurosci Lett 1992;140:30–32.

75. Flavin HJ, Wieraszko A, Seyfried TN. Enhanced aspartate release from hippocampal slices of epileptic (EL) mice. J Neurochem 1991;56:1007–1001.

76. Millan MH, Chapman AG, Meldrum BS. Extracellular amino acid levels in hippocampus during pilocarpine-induced seizures. Epilepsy Res 1993;14:139–148.

77. Raiteri M, Marchi M, Costi A, Volpe G. Endogenous aspartate release in the rat hippocampus inhibited by M2 "cardiac" muscarinic receptors. Eur J Pharmacol 1990;177:181–187.

78. Martin D, Bustos GA, Bowe MA, Bray SD, Nadler JV. Autoreceptor regulation of glutamate and aspartate release from slices of the hippocampal CA1 area. J Neurochem 1991;56:1647–1655.

79. Fleck MW, Henze DA, Barrionuevo G, Palmer AM. Aspartate and glutamate mediate excitatory synaptic transmission in area CA1 of the hippocampus. J Neurosci 1993;13:3944–3955.

80. Meldrum BS. The role of glutamate in epilepsy and other CNS disorders. Neurology 1994;44:S14–S23.

81. Boado RJ, Li JY, Nagaya M, Zhang C, Pardridge WM. Selective expression of the large neutral amino acid transporter at the blood–brain barrier. Proc Natl Acad Sci U S A 1999;96:12079–12084.

82. Broer S, Brookes N. Transfer of glutamine between astrocytes and neurons. J Neurochem 2001;77:705–719.

83. Yanagida O, Kanai Y, Chairoungdua A, Kim DK, Segawa H, Nii T, Cha SH, Matsuo H, Fukushima J, Fukasawa Y, Tani Y, Taketani Y, Uchino H, Kim, JY, Inatomi J, Okayasu I, Miyamoto K, Takeda E, Goya T, Endou H. Human L-type amino acid transporter 1 (LAT1): characterization of function and expression in tumor cell lines. Biochim Biophys Acta 2001;1514:291–302.

84. Huang Y, Zielke HR, Tildon JT, Zielke CL, Baab PJ. Elevation of amino acids in the interstitial space of the rat brain following infusion of large neutral amino and keto acids by microdialysis: leucine infusion. Dev Neurosci 1996;18:415–419.

16 Molecular Regulation of Ketogenesis

Tim E. Cullingford

1. INTRODUCTION

In this chapter I discuss the molecular effects of changes in the diet on liver and brain metabolic fuel adaptation, with special reference to ketogenesis and the anticonvulsant ketogenic diet (KD). I examine metabolic adaptation in terms of the effects of diet-imposed blood hormone and fuel switches on metabolism of fatty acids, amino acids, and sugars, with special attention to the regulation of activity of multiple enzymes of intermediary metabolic pathways by metabolic sensor proteins. As an example of the effect of dietary change on genetic programming, I examine the regulation of a gene encoding the key enzyme of the ketogenic pathway. In the context of the antiepileptic action of the KD and the structural organization of brain cells, I discuss recent work indicating that the brain possesses both functional fuel sensors and the capacity for localized ketogenesis. Finally, I examine the implications for the anticonvulsant mechanism of the KD of changes in liver and brain ketogenesis and fuel adaptation.

2. METABOLIC FUEL ADAPTATION

The sugar glucose is an essential blood fuel for all the cells in the body (1). It is derived from the breakdown of carbohydrate provided by the typical low-fat/high-carbohydrate diet. Although glucose is the major cellular fuel, many cell types can also use alternative fuels such as fatty acids (derived from dietary fats and body fat stores), ketone bodies (derived from fatty acid breakdown by the liver), and amino acids (derived from dietary protein and muscle protein stores) (1). The brain can use such alternative fuels for part of its energy requirements; however, unlike liver, it has an absolute requirement for a continuous supply of blood glucose fuel. The liver is the major organ responsible for the maintenance of stable blood glucose concentrations under differing dietary conditions. At the cellular level, hepatocytes can detect and flexibly respond to changes in blood fuel concentrations resulting from alterations in the quality or quantity of the diet (1). Diet quantity ranges from "well fed" through varying degrees of calorie restriction to, ultimately, starvation; diet quality ranges, for example, from low fat to high fat. Thus, the liver of a child who switches from consuming a normal diet to the KD (2) must detect and respond to both quantitative (calorie unrestricted to calorie restricted), and qualitative (low fat, high carbohydrate and protein to high fat, low carbohydrate and protein) changes in blood fuel supply.

From: *Epilepsy and the Ketogenic Diet*
Edited by: C. E. Stafstrom and J. M. Rho © Humana Press Inc., Totowa, NJ

Thus, when blood glucose concentrations begin to decrease, during starvation or the conditions imposed by the KD, liver hepatocytes respond by switching from using blood glucose as a fuel to using blood fatty acids. Furthermore, they use the energy derived from the catabolism ("burning") of fatty acid fuel to synthesize glucose from blood amino acid carbon skeletons. Such glucose is then exported back to the blood, thus compensating for the initial diet-imposed decreases in blood glucose concentrations. This process of generating blood glucose from the liver is known as gluconeogenesis and serves to maintain a steady supply of blood glucose fuel for the brain. The liver therefore acts as a "thermostat" for the maintenance of a steady concentration of blood glucose. A consequence of switching from using glucose to using fatty acids for fuel is that hepatocytes also return to the blood high concentrations of the ketone bodies acetoacetate and 3-hydroxybutyrate, partial breakdown products of such fatty acids. This is because under conditions of low blood glucose, hepatocytes cannot fully oxidize fatty acids to carbon dioxide *(1)*. This process of converting fatty acids to ketone bodies by hepatocytes is termed ketogenesis, and a diet, i.e., the KD, a fuel, or a drug that stimulates ketogenesis is described as ketogenic.

Although liver hepatocytes are considered to be the major cell type that regulates fuel supply in blood, it is becoming clear that certain other cell types may have a similar role in regulating fuel supply in an organ *(3)*. An emerging example of such a cell type, particularly relevant to the anticonvulsant action of the KD, is the brain astrocyte. Astrocytes are juxtaposed between the blood fuel supply and the neuronal cells, which are critical to conducting the electrical impulses involved in neurotransmission in brain. Moreover, astrocytes exhibit metabolic adaptations to dietary changes and, as such, may be regarded as a "dialysis machine" for neurons, acting as a fuel filter between neurons and the blood supply. Later in this chapter, I examine the growing body of evidence indicating that astrocytes perform ketogenesis under certain conditions, with implications for the supply of ketone body fuels on behalf of surrounding neurons.

3. ENZYMES OF FATTY ACID OXIDATION AND KETOGENESIS

Fatty acids, the precursors of ketone bodies, exist in a variety of chain lengths, from long-chain fatty acids, e.g., palmitate, through medium-chain fatty acids, e.g., octanoate, to short-chain fatty acids, e.g., butanoate. All such fatty acids can be catabolized in the mitochondria of hepatocytes by β-oxidation (1) (Fig. 1), whereby 2-carbon units are progressively removed from the fatty acid chain. The 2-carbon units generated are in the form of the ubiquitous cellular molecule, acetyl-coenzyme A (CoA) (Fig. 1). The ketone body acetoacetate is then formed by the condensation of acetyl-CoA, followed by the removal of the CoA moiety. Subsequently the ketone body 3-hydroxybutyrate is formed on reduction of acetoacetate, which in turn is dependent on reduced nicotinamide adenine dinucleotide (NADH). In addition, under conditions of high rates of ketogenesis, the ketone body acetone is formed spontaneously. A series of enzymes, upstream of acetyl-CoA, is responsible for catalyzing the breakdown of fatty acids of differing chain lengths. Subsequently, two enzymes downstream of acetyl-CoA are responsible for the formation of the first ketone body, acetoacetate. All such enzymes must be present for fatty acid oxidation and ketogenesis (FAOK) to be executed, as evidenced by the potentially lethal effects of inborn errors of FAOK *(4)*. However, only certain enzymes appear to have a major regulatory role in the flux of fatty acids to ketone bodies *(3)*. This is because such enzymes catalyze key branch-

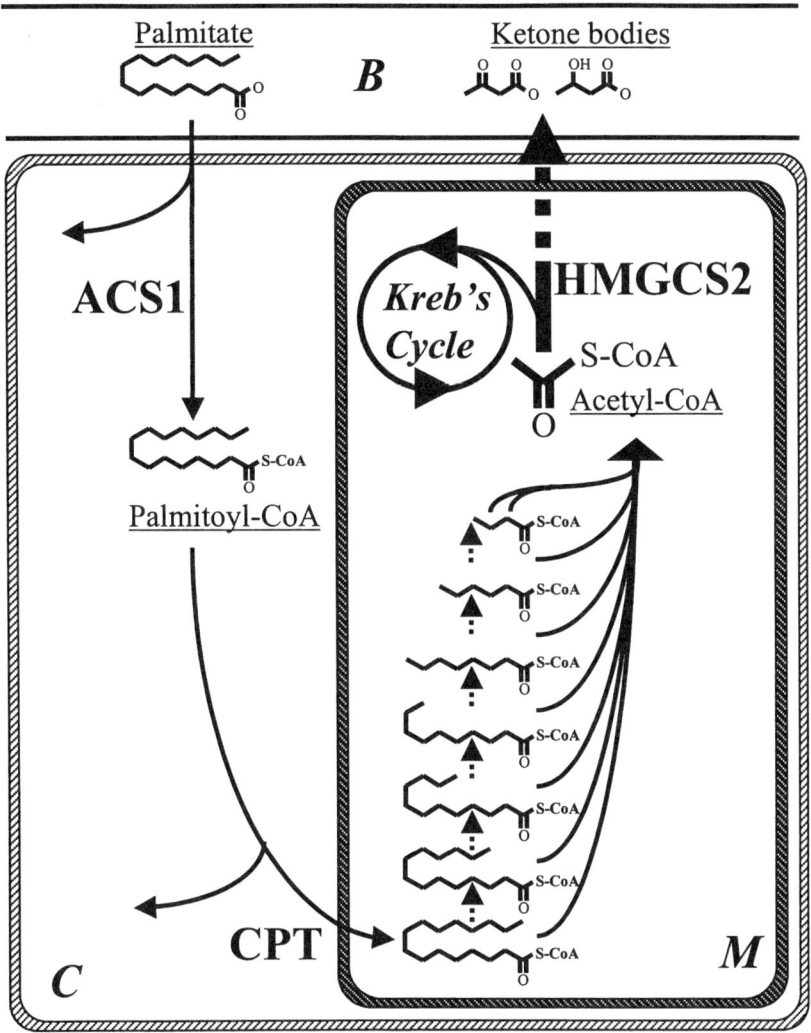

Fig. 1. Oxidation and ketogenesis of the 16-carbon fatty acid palmitate in the hepatocyte: B, blood; C, cytosol of hepatocyte; M, mitochondria of hepatocyte. Key branch-point steps of FAOK are catalyzed by the following enzymes: ACS1, entrapping palmitate in the hepatocyte for the oxidation pathway; CPT, committing palmitate to entry into the mitochondria, away from metabolism in the cytosol; and HMGCS2, committing acetyl-CoA to ketogenesis, away from complete oxidation to CO_2 by the Krebs cycle.

point steps in the commitment toward FAOK, at the expense of other competing pathways (Fig. 1). Such enzymes include long-chain fatty acyl-CoA synthetase 1 (ACS1), carnitine palmitoyl transferase (CPT) and mitochondrial 3-hydroxy-3-methylglutaryl-CoA synthetase (HMGCS2), the critical enzyme of ketogenesis from acetyl-CoA.

4. METABOLIC SENSOR PROTEINS

Hepatocytes respond to dietary change by adjusting the activities of a spectrum of enzymes of intermediary metabolism—i.e., enzymes that interconvert fatty acids, sugars, and amino acids. For example, a hepatocyte may potentially adjust the activities of at least 50 different enzymes *(1)*, catalyzing reactions of intermediary metabolism to respond to alterations in blood fuel concentrations resulting from the transition from the well-fed state to starvation. This can be achieved at the molecular level through metabolic sensor proteins whose activity is changed according to diet-induced changes in blood metabolites. Upon receiving a signal from the blood indicating a dietary change in metabolite supply, such sensors can target several enzymes to simultaneously alter their activities in an appropriate manner. Such enzyme activities can be altered in a number of ways: e.g., by direct phosphorylation of the enzyme or by altering the cellular levels of the enzyme through changes in expression of the gene encoding the enzyme. I examine two examples of such metabolite sensors in hepatocytes, namely metabolic hormone receptors and fuel sensors.

4.1. Metabolic Hormone Sensors

A variety of blood hormones, subject to changes in concentration in response to the quality and quantity of the diet, exert actions on hepatic metabolism. These include the pancreatic-secreted hormones insulin and glucagon, and the adrenal glucocorticoids. Thus, blood insulin concentrations decrease, while glucagon concentrations increase, in response to the switch from the well-fed state to starvation *(1)*. This results in an appropriate dietary response because glucagon and insulin, respectively, stimulate and repress liver gluconeogenesis and ketogenesis *(5)*. Blood glucocorticoid concentrations tend to rise during periods of stress such as starvation. Thus, appropriately, they also stimulate liver ketogenesis *(5)*. Hepatocytes sense changes in such blood hormone concentrations via cellular hormone receptors. Glucocorticoids bind and activate glucocorticoid receptor (GR) protein sensors located in the nucleus of hepatocytes. GRs are transcription factors and, when activated, GRs alter the expression levels of many genes encoding metabolic enzymes *(6)*. In contrast, insulin and glucagon bind receptor sensors in the cell membrane of the hepatocyte *(7)*. Subsequently, the insulin or glucagon signal is transduced via a pathway of signal proteins, ultimately resulting again in regulation of expression of genes encoding metabolic enzymes. Thus, for example, glucocorticoids and glucagon act to upregulate expression of the gene encoding the key ketogenic enzyme HMGCS2; in contrast, insulin acts to downregulate its expression *(8)*.

4.2. Fuel Sensors

4.2.1. Fatty Acids

As described in Section 2., fatty acids in blood are an important alternative fuel to glucose but, in addition, they have a role as a messenger or "hormone" indicating changes in dietary conditions. For example, fatty acid levels in blood will rise during starvation, as fat reserves in the body are released into blood. Similarly, fatty acid levels may rise under KD-induced conditions of calorie restriction (semistarvation) and high-fat intake. The major sensor of fatty acids in hepatocytes is the peroxisome proliferator-activated receptor alpha (PPARα) protein. PPARα is a fatty acid-activated transcription factor that is critical to the genetic reprogramming of hepatocyte metabolism in response to starvation *(9)*. It possesses a broad binding specificity for such fatty acid activators, ranging from long-chain to medium-chain fatty acids *(10)*. Similar to glucocorticoid receptors, PPARα is located in the nucleus of hepatocytes. Thus, fatty acids entering the hepatocyte bind and activate PPARα, resulting in alterations in the expres-

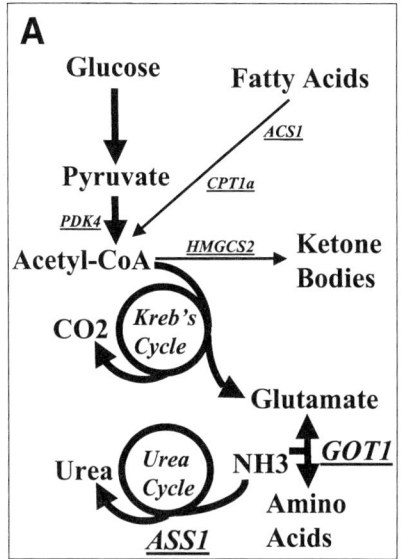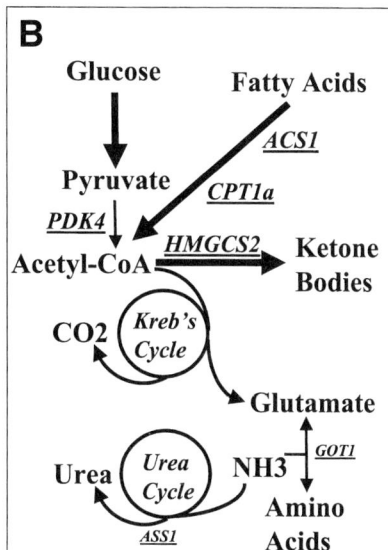

Fig. 2. Fed-to-starved switch alters expression of a battery of PPARα-regulated genes encoding key enzymes of intermediary metabolism. **(A)** Fed state. **(B)** Starved state. Selected (*see* ref. *11*) PPARα-regulated genes are italicized and underscored, with font size used to indicate up- or downregulation of gene expression between the fed and starved states. Abbreviations: ACS1, acyl-CoA synthetase 1; CPT1a, carnitine palmitoyl transferase 1a; PDK4, pyruvate dehydrogenase kinase 4; HMGCS2, mitochondrial 3-hydroxy-3-methylglutaryl-CoA synthetase; GOT1, cytosolic glutamate-oxaloacetate transaminase; ASS1, arginosuccinate synthetase.

sion of many genes encoding enzymes of intermediary metabolism (Fig. 2). This results in changes in cellular concentrations of such enzymes and, therefore, changes in the flow of fatty acids, glucose, and amino acids through the hepatocyte. For example, when PPARα is activated in the mouse liver by starvation, it causes an increase in fatty acid oxidation, an increase in ketogenesis, a decrease in glucose oxidation, and a decrease in amino acid transamination and deamination (*11*) (Fig. 2). In addition, blood levels of insulin and glucocorticoids alter the expression of the *PPARα* gene, hence the concentration of PPARα protein available for fatty acid activation (*12*). It can be seen, therefore, that activation of PPARα by a variety of blood-borne dietary signals results in an integrated metabolic response through reprogramming expression of genes encoding enzymes of hepatocyte intermediary metabolism. Three such genes regulated by PPARα, in human hepatocyte-derived cell lines, encode the key branch-point enzymes of FAOK described earlier, namely ACS1, CPT1a, and HMGCS2 (*13*). In the next section, I examine the regulation of HMGCS2 in more detail, with reference to its regulation by the KD.

4.2.2. Amino Acids and Sugars

Considerably less is known about the existence of molecular sensors in hepatocytes for changes in blood amino acid or sugar fuels. However, there is recent evidence to suggest that certain amino acids, and sugars such as glucose, may have specific cellular receptors that can affect genetic reprogramming, as already described for PPARα and fatty acids. For example, the proto-oncogene transcription factor *c-myc* may be important in mediating appropriate increases in glycolysis and decreases in gluconeogenesis and ketogenesis in response to increases in blood glucose fuel. Thus, glucose acts indirectly to decrease hepatocyte *HMGCS2* expression via increases in *c-myc* expression that in turn decrease *PPARα* expression and hence PPARα activity *(14)*. However, the details of such pathways, and the sensors that directly interact with glucose and various amino acids remain to be established.

5. REGULATION OF HMGCS2 ACTIVITY IN LIVER

HMGCS2 catalyzes the following interconversion in the mitochondria:

Acetyl-CoA + Acetoacetyl-CoA ↔ 3-Hydroxy-3-methylglutaryl-CoA + CoA – SH

As with all enzymes, the active site of the HMGCS2 protein provides the intricate surface on which either acetyl-CoA and acetoacetyl-CoA molecules can form 3-hydroxy-3-methylglutaryl-CoA (HMG-CoA), or HMG-CoA and CoA-sulfhydryl (SH) molecules can form acetyl-CoA and acetoacetyl-CoA. The rate at which both the forward and reverse reactions proceed is entirely dependent on the number of active molecules of HMGCS2 enzyme. If no molecules of HMGCS2 exist in the mitochondria, then the spontaneous rate of both the forward and reverse reaction is so low as to be negligible, thus the reaction just illustrated is effectively blocked. Equally, if all such molecules are inactivated, e.g., by an inhibitor molecule, in spite of high concentrations of HMGCS2 molecules in the mitochondria, the reaction will again effectively not take place. Thus, the concentrations of active HMGCS2 in mitochondria strictly dictate the rate of formation of HMG-CoA. HMG-CoA gives rise to the first ketone body, acetoacetate:

HMG-CoA ↔ Acetoacetate + Acetyl-CoA

and acetoacetate gives rise to the remaining ketone bodies 3-hydroxybutyrate and acetone. Thus, the concentrations of active HMGCS2 in mitochondria also strictly dictate the rate of ketogenesis. I now examine the means by which HMGCS2 concentration and active-to-inactive ratio in mitochondria is regulated in the liver.

5.1. Regulation by Changes in Active/Inactive HMGCS2 Enzyme Ratio

Liver HMGCS2 enzyme activity is very low during the fed state, whereas during starvation it rises substantially. HMGCS2 enzyme activity is directly regulated by succinylation of the protein *(15)*. Thus, the Krebs cycle intermediate succinyl-CoA directly binds the active site of HMGCS2, resulting in its inactivation. As we have noted, blood concentrations of the pancreatic hormone glucagon increase during starvation, resulting in stimulation of hepatic ketogenesis. Appropriately, glucagon acts in the hepatocyte to decrease the number of succinylated HMGCS2 molecules, thus increasing the ratio of active to inactive HMGCS2 enzyme *(15)*. Acute regulation of HMGCS2 activity by succinylation/desuccinylation according to the concentrations of the Krebs cycle intermediate succinyl-CoA may be linked to the need for rapid changes in the routing of acetyl-CoA between Krebs cycle and ketogenesis.

5.2. Regulation by Absolute Changes in Protein HMGCS2 Concentration

At the genetic level *HMGCS2* gene expression is upregulated by glucocorticoids, fatty acids, and cyclic adenosine monophosphate (cAMP) and downregulated by insulin

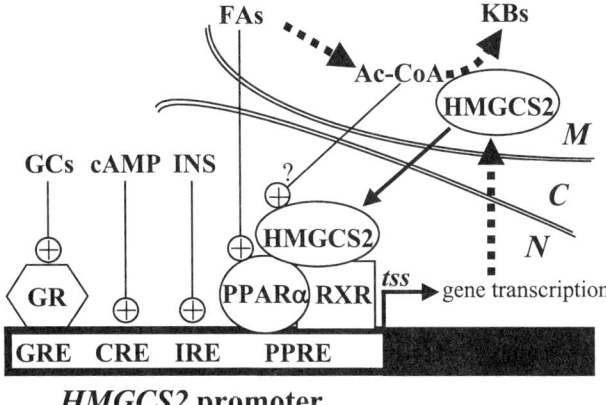

HMGCS2 promoter

Fig. 3. The *HMGCS2* gene promoter. The promoter region is depicted by an open box for the DNA sequence upstream of the transcription start site tss and a solid box for the transcribed region downstream of the transcription start site. Abbreviations for DNA sequence elements and receptors: GRE, glucocorticoid response element; CRE, cAMP response element; IRE, insulin response element; PPRE, peroxisome proliferator response element; GR, glucocorticoid receptor; RXR, retinoid X receptor. Abbreviations for signals that regulate *HMGCS2* gene expression: GCs, glucocorticoids; cAMP, cyclic AMP; INS, insulin; FAs, fatty acids. Also depicted is the relationship between the nucleus (N), cytosol (C), and mitochondria (M), in terms of the dual actions of HMGCS2 as an enzyme generating ketone bodies (KBs) from acetyl-CoA (Ac-CoA) and as a transcription cofactor (*see* text).

(8). Thus, the promoter region of the HMGCS2 gene (Fig. 3) contains DNA response elements *(8)* mediating the action of fatty acids (peroxisome proliferator response element, PPRE), insulin (insulin response element, IRE), glucagon (cAMP response element, CRE) and glucocorticoids (glucocorticoid response element, GRE). The HMGCS2 PRRE binds PPARα, always in combination with another nuclear receptor, the retinoid X receptor (RXR) (Fig. 3), which is activated by retinoids *(8,16)*. Furthermore, in a superb demonstration of nature's ingenuity, Meertens and others have shown that HMGCS2 protein has a second role as a transcription factor coactivator of PPARα that selectively activates expression of the *HMGCS2* gene itself (Fig. 3) *(17)*. This may occur via the acetyltransferase activity of HMGCS2, resulting in changes in the ratio of acetylated/deacetylated nuclear histone proteins that regulate access of transcription factors such as PPARα to the *HMGCS2* gene promoter *(17,18)*. Thus, changes in cellular concentrations of acetyl-CoA resulting from fatty acid oxidation will alter the ratio of acetylated to deacetylated HMGCS2. Upon translocation to the nucleus, the ratio of acetylated to deacetylated HMGCS2 molecules would then determine their capacity to acetylate/deacetylate histone proteins bound to the promoter of the *HMGCS2* gene. In its dual role as an enzyme and PPARα transcription cofactor, HMGCS2 protein may thus act as a messenger in the cellular dialog between the nucleus and the mitochondrion, critical to controlling intracellular acetyl-CoA concentrations *(17)*.

In terms of its importance in regulation of FAOK, of the three FAOK regulatory enzymes, i.e., ACS1, CPT1a, and HMGCS2, only HMGCS2 lies downstream of acetyl-CoA, the critical moiety for the formation of ketone bodies (Fig. 1). Moreover, the critical regulatory role of HMGCS2 in FAOK is reflected in the observation that fatty acid oxidation can be inhibited, by end-product inhibition at several enzyme steps if acetyl-CoA concentrations are allowed to build up in the mitochondrion. Thus, the intimate formation of a PPARα/HMGCS2 transcription complex, which selectively activates transcription of *HMGCS2* at the expense of other PPARα-activated genes *(17)*, suggests that upregulation of *HMGCS2* expression is of paramount importance in the fatty acid "hormone" regulation of the FAOK pathway.

5.3. Regulation of HMGCS2 by the KD

As we have stated, switching from a normal diet to the KD imposes several changes in blood hormone and fatty acid balance that would be predicted to increase *HMGCS2* expression, hence HMGCS2 activity. This is borne out in an experimental model of the KD in which rats are fed a custom-made diet high in fat and low in carbohydrate and protein that is calorie restricted to 90% of the recommended daily allowance for a rat *(19)*. Such a KD is protective against pentylenetetrazole-induced seizures in rats *(19)*. Thus, we have shown that such rats exhibit significant increases in hepatic *HMGCS2* expression compared to rats fed a control diet *ad libitum (20)*. This suggests that the rise in blood ketone bodies in response to the KD is a direct result of its molecular action on the liver. Furthermore, we have shown that the hypolipidemic drug ciprofibrate also results in increases in hepatic *HMGCS2* expression *(21)*. Ciprofibrate is one of a number of artificial compounds that, similar to the naturally occurring fatty acids already described, is capable of activating PPARα *(22)*. Moreover, ciprofibrate is highly selective for activating PPARα compared with the two remaining members of the PPAR family, PPARγ and PPARδ *(22)*. Thus, at the molecular level, it is likely that the effects of the KD on blood ketone body levels result from fatty acid-dependent activation of the PPARα/HMGCS2 transcription complex hence *HMGCS2* gene expression, together with switches in hormones such as insulin, glucagon, and glucocorticoids.

6. REGULATION OF HMGCS2 IN BRAIN

I mentioned in Section 2. that astrocytes in brain may have many of the characteristics of hepatocytes in terms of exhibiting a flexible response to blood fuel availability. In this regard, we have shown that whole-brain *(23)* and primary cultures of neonatal cortical astrocytes *(23,24)* express *HMGCS2*, together with other enzymes of FAOK *(20,21,23,24)*. Furthermore, we have shown that, similar to liver, rats fed the experimental KD described above exhibit significant increases in whole-brain *HMGCS2* expression *(20)* in comparison to rats fed the control diet. Again, part of this effect is likely to be mediated by a functional brain PPARα; this is because rats treated with the PPARα-selective drug ciprofibrate exhibit major increases in brain *HMGCS2* gene expression *(21)*. Astrocytes are likely to be the site of action of ciprofibrate and the KD on brain PPARα: we have demonstrated expression of *PPARα* in primary cultures of neonatal cortical astrocytes *(25)*. Furthermore, *PPARα* expression has been demonstrated in astrocyte cells in brain slices *(26)* and in astrocyte-like cells in reaggregated brain cell cultures *(27)*. In addition, we have shown that the glucocorticoid hydrocortisone increases *HMGCS2* expression in primary cultures of neonatal cortical astrocytes *(24)*, which suggests that KD-induced changes in glucocorticoids could contribute to increases in brain *HMGCS2* expression.

7. REGULATION OF FAOK FLUX IN BRAIN
AND CULTURED ASTROCYTES

From the foregoing discussion, it appears that the presence and activation of PPARα/HMGCS2 in brain indicates the capacity of brain to conduct ketogenesis. This has been corroborated by studies examining FAOK in whole-brain and astrocyte cultures. Thus, in vivo, brain homogenates derived from ciprofibrate-treated rats exhibit potently increased capacities to oxidize radiolabeled fatty acids *(28)*. Moreover, regarding the calorie-restriction aspect of the KD, brain preparations derived from suckling rat pups fed a normal diet that is 50% calorie restricted compared with controls exhibit a threefold increase in fatty acid oxidation *(29)*. In vitro, several studies have shown that primary cultures of neonatal cortical astrocytes are capable of tightly regulated ketogenesis from the long-chain fatty acid palmitate. Thus, Auestad et al. *(30)* were the first to demonstrate that cultured astrocytes convert palmitate to the ketone bodies acetoacetate and 3-hydroxybutyrate. Furthermore, subsequent studies have demonstrated that FAOK in cultured astrocytes is regulated by a variety of physiologically relevant stimuli, including cannabinoids *(31)*, forskolin *(32)*, and activators of cAMP-activated protein kinase *(33)*. In addition, it has been shown that astrocytes can generate ketone bodies from the ketogenic amino acid leucine, which may constitute an important blood-derived brain fuel *(34)*.

Overall, such studies indicate that the brain has the capacity to perform ketogenesis, most likely localized to astrocytes, and that brain ketogenesis is intricately regulated by multiple physiological stimuli. In the next section, I examine the structural role of astrocytes in brain and the possible functions of astrocyte-generated ketone bodies.

8. REGULATION OF KETOGENESIS AND CELL ORGANIZATION

Insofar as the liver is considered to be the prototype organ responsible for ketone body production, hepatocyte cells provide the paradigm for the molecular regulation of ketogenesis *(3)*. Thus, because it contains the complete enzyme complement necessary for the FAOK pathway, an individual hepatocyte performs the complete FAOK pathway. Moreover, as noted earlier, the proposed HMGCS2-mediated dialog between the nucleus and the mitochondrion that regulates cellular acetyl-CoA concentrations can occur in individual hepatocytes.

The structural and metabolic organization of brain cells provides an intriguing contrast to that of hepatocytes (Fig. **4A**). The functional cell unit of electrical impulse transmission in brain is the neuron (Fig. **4A**), and it can be seen that in contrast to hepatocytes, the locations of the neuronal cell body nucleus and, for example, the mitochondria of the neuronal presynaptic knob may be separated by the considerable length of the neuronal axon. This potentially rules out an intracellular HMGCS2-mediated dialog between the nucleus and the mitochondria of an individual neuron, as described for individual hepatocytes. Moreover, the studies of our group and others suggest that neurons may not express the *PPARα* and *HMGCS2* genes to any significant degree, thus potentially ruling out their capacity to perform ketogenesis *(24–27)*. In contrast, astrocytes may be similar to hepatocytes insofar as they actively express the *PPARα* and *HMGCS2* genes *(23–25)*. Furthermore, astrocytes are juxtaposed between neurons and the blood environment (Fig. 4A) and are therefore ideally situated to integrate detection of diet-induced changes in blood metabolites with a response that results in appropriate

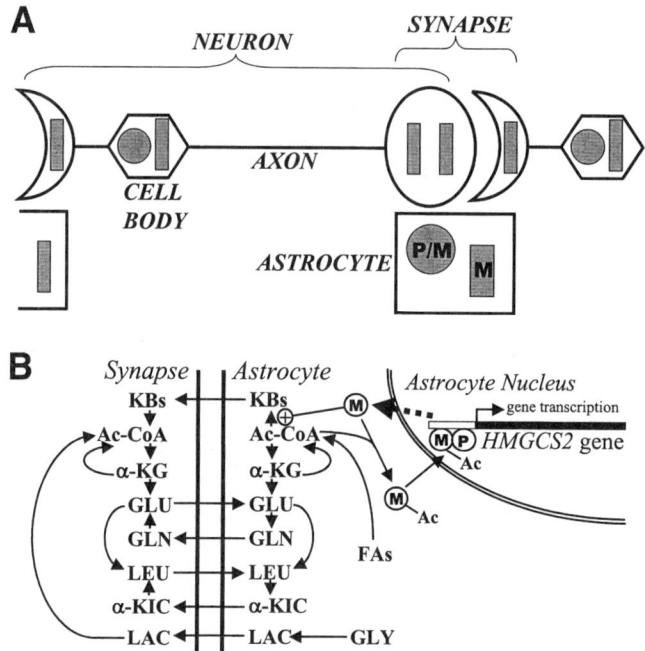

Fig. 4. (A) Interrelationship between astrocytes and neurons in the central nervous system. Shaded rectangles depict the locations of mitochondria, the site of action of HMGCS2 (M) in its role as an enzyme. Shaded circles depict the location of the cell nucleus, the site of action of PPARα (P) and HMGCS2 (M), in its role as a cotranscription factor for PPARα. **(B)** How dietary genetic programming of gene expression in the astrocyte nucleus may influence levels, and neuron–astrocyte cycles, of metabolites in the nucleus-free neuronal synapse. Abbreviations: KBs, ketone bodies; FAs, fatty acids; Ac-CoA, acetyl-CoA; α-KG, α-ketoglutarate; GLU, glutamate; GLN, glutamine; LEU, leucine; α-KIC, α-ketoisocaproate; LAC, lacate; GLY, glycogen. Changes in acetyl-CoA level can alter the ratio of unacetylated to acetylated (-Ac) HMGCS2 (M), influencing the level of expression of the PPARα (P)-regulated *HMGCS2* gene.

changes in synaptic neurotransmission. Indeed, the astrocyte may be regarded as a cellular "diode" whose "output," i.e., metabolic response, is determined by its capacity to integrate the "input" of blood fuel/hormone signals with that of synaptic neurotransmitter signals.

On the foregoing basis, it has been proposed that neurons and astrocytes engage in an ongoing "metabolic dialog." Thus, for example, the excitatory neurotransmitter glutamate participates in both a glutamate–glutamine cycle *(35)* and a leucine–glutamate cycle *(36)* (Fig. 4B), to form a continuous and dynamic means by which the astrocyte responds to changes in synaptic activity. Moreover, astrocytes have a role in the provision of fuel to the neuronal synapse. Thus, similar to hepatocytes, astrocytes store blood glucose in the form of glycogen *(37)*. According to need, such astrocytic glycogen stores can be broken down and fed to the neuron in the form of lactate *(37)* (Fig. 4B). Furthermore, our work together with that of the groups of John Edmond and Manuel Guzman indicates a similar role for ketone bodies, whereby fatty acids from the blood or from within brain can be broken down by astrocyte FAOK pathways to generate ketone bodies that are likewise fed to neurons *(38–40)* (Fig. 4B). Thus, many research groups are currently establishing the existence of a network of dialogs between astrocytes and neurons.

Future research in this area will expand to examine the exciting possibility of astrocytic genetic programming of synaptic acetyl-CoA/neurotransmitter/fuel concentrations, via intercellular synaptic mitochondria–astrocytic nucleus dialogs (Fig. 4B).

9. PPARα, HMGCS2, KETOGENESIS, AND THE MECHANISM OF THE KD

Thus far, our studies indicate a functional PPARα/HMGCS2 ketogenic "system" in brain, predominantly localized to astrocytes. Furthermore, we have demonstrated that the KD has clear effects on the molecular regulation of ketogenesis, not only in liver, the classical ketogenic organ, but also in brain. In turn, this points to several potential anticonvulsant mechanisms for the KD that could be explored in the future.

9.1. Neurotransmitter Perturbations Via PPARα Activation

The KD may be anticonvulsant via its ability to correct disturbances in neurotransmitter concentrations associated with epilepsy. These include alterations in excitatory neurotransmitters such as glutamate and aspartate, inhibitory neurotransmitters such as γ-aminobutyric acid (GABA), and taurine, and/or neurotransmitters such as glycine that may adopt either excitatory or inhibitory roles *(41)*. Thus, for example, the KD decreases aspartate *(42)* and enhances synthesis of GABA from glutamate *(42)*. Furthermore, changes in a variety of other neurotransmitters, including dopamine, norepinephrine, and serotonin, may be implicated in epilepsy *(41)*. Also, polyamines such as putrescine, spermine, and spermidine are implicated in disturbed glutamatergic neurotransmission in actively epileptogenic human brain *(41)*. In addition, levels of neuroinactive amino acids such as glutamine and leucine play important roles in brain nitrogen balance and thus are implicated in epilepsy *(42)*.

Such neurotransmitters either are amino acids or are readily derived from amino acids, especially glutamate, and thus their metabolic pathways of synthesis substantially overlap with those of classical intermediary metabolism. Thus, the concentrations of several neurotransmitters may be simultaneously perturbed through changes in activity of key enzymes of amino acid metabolism and interconversion. For example, epileptic human brain exhibits raised activities of glutamate oxaloacetate transaminase (GOT) (also known as aspartate aminotransferase) *(43)*. GOT exhibits a high intrinsic activity in normal brain, and the KD may alter glutamate neurotransmitter concentrations through inhibition of GOT activity *(42)*. Because GOT may also catalyze other transamination reactions, e.g., tyrosine and tryptophan, this finding has implications in the synthesis of the neurotransmitters dopamine, norepinephrine, taurine, and serotonin. As mentioned previously, PPARα in liver regulates expression not only of genes encoding enzymes of FAOK, but also many genes encoding enzymes of amino acid metabolism *(11)*. Such genes include *GOT1,* encoding the cytosolic form of GOT and genes encoding enzymes that metabolize tyrosine, tryptophan, glycine, polyamine, glutamine, and leucine. Thus, it is reasonable to hypothesize that in addition to regulating brain *HMGCS2* gene expression, KD-activated brain PPARα may alter expression of enzymes of amino acid metabolism in brain. This would then result in changes in the brain concentrations of amino acid and amino acid-derived neurotransmitters. It follows that profound consequences on seizure propagation in the epileptic brain would be predicted following a KD-induced change in the balance of such neurotransmitters. The role of astrocytic PPARα in mediating dietary programming of expression of *HMGCS2* and many other PPARα-regulated genes is under investigation.

9.2. Neurotransmitter Perturbations by Ketone Bodies

There are changes in the balance of amino acid neurotransmitters when high concentrations of ketone bodies are directly applied to astrocyte cell cultures *(44)* or to synaptosomes derived from the whole brain *(45)*. Thus, ketone bodies entering brain from the blood as a result of KD-induced hepatic ketogenesis may directly perturb brain neurotransmitter levels. However, it is not known whether blood ketone body concentrations are high enough to cause the effects observed in astrocyte cell cultures and synaptosomes. Nevertheless, such concentrations could be achievable within brain in vivo, if KD-induced astrocytic ketogenesis indeed results in high local ketone body concentrations on behalf of adjacent neurons, as discussed in Section 7. Future studies, for example using microdialysis probes, will be required to establish the concentrations of ketone bodies produced by KD-induced astrocytes in vivo.

9.3. Link Between FAOK and Electrostatic Membrane Potential

KD-related increases in expression of FAOK enzyme encoding genes imply increases in the rate of FAOK. It has been proposed that changes in dietary status, e.g., fed/fasting and low fat/high fat, that alter the rate of hepatic FAOK can modulate food-intake behavior through alterations in hepatic stimulation of vagus nerve afferents to the brain *(46)*. This is hypothesized to occur through increased oxidation of fatty acids by hepatocytes, resulting in increases in hepatocyte membrane potential and, therefore, increased stimulation of the hepatic vagus nerve *(46)*. A novel epilepsy therapy called vagus nerve stimulation involves exogenous electrical stimulation of the left cervical vagus nerve sheath *(47)*, through which hepatic vagus nerve afferents run. Thus it is intriguing to speculate whether an element of the antiepileptic effect of the KD lies in its ability to endogenously alter hepatic vagus nerve stimulation through changes in hepatic FAOK rate. Experiments such as the effect of vagotomy on KD antiseizure efficacy will be required to test this hypothesis. Another factor in epilepsy is astrocyte cell membrane potential, which would be anticipated to affect neuron depolarization thresholds. Thus, another site of action of the KD may be via increases in FAOK in astrocytes, resulting in increased astrocyte membrane potential.

10. CONCLUSION

The switch from a normal diet to the KD, by mimicking the conditions of starvation, imposes many profound adaptations on body metabolism. Such adaptations are mediated at the molecular level by metabolic sensor proteins that detect changes in the incoming fuel and hormonal environment of the blood. Cells throughout the body possess such molecular systems to adapt to this dietary change. In particular, the responses of liver hepatocytes and brain astrocytes may be particularly relevant to the antiepileptic effects of AEDs, fibrates, fatty acids and the KD through PPARα-mediated changes in amino acid neurotransmitter concentrations, electropotential properties and gap–junction intercellular exchange. Modern molecular biology techniques will be important in establishing the precise mechanisms of the KD and will open up novel therapeutic approaches to improve the KD as well as develop KD-mimicking drugs.

11. FUTURE PERSPECTIVES

In addition to the possible links between PPARα and the action of the KD, recent intriguing evidence is emerging that PPARα may be involved in the action of certain antiepileptic drugs (AEDs) and could therefore, potentially, provide a novel convergence point for a number of antiepileptic treatments. Thus, in addition to naturally occurring fatty acids, PPARα is activated by a variety of fatty acid-like drugs, including the AEDs phenytoin, valproate, and several antiepileptic valproate analogs *(48,49)*. For example, the proconvulsant pentylenetetrazol has been administered to rodents as a test of the anticonvulsant potency of a series of valproate analogs *(48)*. From this it has been shown that the anticonvulsant potency of a given valproate analog in vivo, may correlate with its PPARα activation potency in vitro. Although activation of PPARα by the KD is associated with increases in ketogenesis, valproate exhibits an antiketogenic effect, possibly through independent inhibitory actions on fatty acid oxidation. Therefore, if part of the action of the KD and valproate is mediated by brain PPARα, this is unlikely to be via alterations in ketogenesis. Instead, PPARα may mediate such common effects via its regulation of amino acid and neurotransmitter metabolism, as described earlier. Studies using normal mice and mice deficient in PPARα *(50)* will allow determination of the effects of the KD, valproate, and PPARα-selective drugs such as ciprofibrate on brain neurotransmitter metabolism and ketogenesis via PPARα.

REFERENCES

1. Berg JM, Tymoczko JL, Stryer L. Biochemistry, 5th ed. Freeman, New York, 2002.
2. Freeman JM, Kelly MT, Freeman JB. The Epilepsy Diet Treatment. Demos, New York, 1994.
3. Quant PA. The role of mitochondrial HMG-CoA synthase in regulation of ketogenesis. Essays Biochem 1994;28:13–25.
4. Rinaldo P, Matern D, Bennett MJ. Fatty acid oxidation disorders. Annu Rev Physiol 2002;64:477–502.
5. Nandi J, Meguid MM, Inui A, et al. Central mechanisms involved with catabolism. Curr Opin Clin Nutr Metab Care 2002;5:407–418.
6. Mangelsdorf DJ, Thummel C, Beato M, et al. The nuclear receptor superfamily: the second decade. Cell 1995;83:835–839.
7. Foufelle F, Ferre P. New perspectives in the regulation of hepatic glycolytic and lipogenic genes by insulin and glucose: a role for the transcription factor sterol regulatory element binding protein-1c. Biochem J 2002;366:377–391.
8. Hegardt FG. Mitochondrial 3-hydroxy-3-methylglutaryl-CoA synthase: a control enzyme in ketogenesis. Biochem J 1999;338:569–582.
9. Leone TC, Weinheimer CJ, Kelly DP. A critical role for the peroxisome proliferator-activated receptor alpha (PPARalpha) in the cellular fasting response: the PPARalpha-null mouse as a model of fatty acid oxidation disorders. Proc Natl Acad Sci U S A 1999;96:7473–7478.
10. Kliewer SA, Sundseth SS, Jones SA, et al. Fatty acids and eicosanoids regulate gene expression through direct interactions with peroxisome proliferator-activated receptors alpha and gamma. Proc Natl Acad Sci U S A 1997;94:4318–4323.
11. Kersten S, Mandard S, Escher P, et al. The peroxisome proliferator activated receptor α regulates amino acid metabolism. FASEB J 2001;15:1971–1978.
12. Steineger HH, Sorensen HN, Tugwood JD, Skrede S, Spydevold O, Gautvik KM. Dexamethasone and insulin demonstrate marked and opposite regulation of the steady-state mRNA level of the peroxisomal proliferator-activated receptor (PPAR) in hepatic cells. Hormonal modulation of fatty-acid-induced transcription Eur J Biochem 1994;225:967–974.
13. Hsu MH, Savas U, Griffin KJ, Johnson EF. Identification of peroxisome proliferator-responsive human genes by elevated expression of the peroxisome proliferator-activated receptor alpha in HepG2 Cells. J Biol Chem 2001;276:27950–27958.

14. Riu E, Ferre T, Mas A, Hidalgo A, Franckhauser S, Bosch F. Overexpression of c-*myc* in diabetic mice restores altered expression of the transcription factor genes that regulate liver metabolism. Biochem J 2002;368:931–937.

15. Quant PA, Tubbs PK, Brand MD. Glucagon activates mitochondrial 3-hydroxy-3-methylglutaryl-CoA synthase in vivo by decreasing the extent of succinylation of the enzyme. Eur J Biochem 1990;187:169–174.

16. Rodriguez JC, Gil-Gomez G, Hegardt FG, Haro D. Peroxisome proliferator-activated receptor mediates induction of the mitochondrial 3-hydroxy-3-methylglutaryl-CoA synthase gene by fatty acids. J Biol Chem 1994;269:18767–18772.

17. Meertens LM, Miyata KS, Cechetto JD, Rachubinski RA, Capone JP. A mitochondrial ketogenic enzyme regulates its gene expression by association with the nuclear hormone receptor PPARalpha. EMBO J 1998;17:6972–6978.

18. Kuo MH, Allis CD. Roles of histone acetyltransferases and deacetylases in gene regulation. BioEssays 1998;20:615–626.

19. Bough KJ and Eagles DA. A ketogenic diet increases the resistance to pentylenetetrazole-induced seizures in the rat. Epilepsia 1999;40:138–143.

20. Cullingford TE, Eagles DA, Sato H. The anti-epileptic ketogenic diet upregulates expression of the gene encoding the ketogenic enzyme mitochondrial 3-hydroxy-3-methylglutaryl-CoA synthase in rat brain. Epilepsy Res 2002;49:99–107.

21. Cullingford TE, Dolphin CT, Sato H. The peroxisome proliferator-activated receptor α-selective activator ciprofibrate upregulates expression of genes encoding fatty acid oxidation and ketogenesis enzymes in rat brain. Neuropharmacology 2002;42:724–730.

22. Takada I, Yu RT, Xu HE, et al. Alteration of a single amino acid in peroxisome proliferator-activated receptor-alpha (PPAR alpha) generates a PPAR delta phenotype. Mol Endocrinol 2000;14:733–740.

23. Cullingford TE, Dolphin CT, Bhakoo K, Peuchen S, Canevari L, Clark JB. Molecular cloning of rat mitochondrial 3-hydroxy-3-methylglutaryl CoA lyase and detection of the corresponding mRNA and of those encoding the remaining enzymes comprising the ketogenic HMG-CoA cycle in CNS of suckling rat. Biochem J 1998;329:373–381.

24. Cullingford TE, Bhakoo KK, Clark JB. Hormonal regulation of the mRNA encoding the ketogenic enzyme mitochondrial 3-hydroxy-3-methylglutaryl-CoA synthase in neonatal primary cultures of cortical astrocytes and meningeal fibroblasts. J Neurochem 1998;71:1804–1812.

25. Cullingford TE, Bhakoo KK, Peuchen S, Dolphin CT, Patel R, Clark JB, Distribution of mRNAs encoding the peroxisome proliferator-activated receptor (PPAR) -α, -β, and -γ and the retinoid X receptor (RXR) -α, -β, and -γ in rat central nervous system. J Neurochem 1998;70:1366–1375.

26. Braissant O, Foufelle F, Scotto C, Dauca M, Wahli W. Differential expression of peroxisome proliferator-activated receptors (PPARs): Tissue distribution of PPAR-α, -β, and -γ in the adult rat. Endocrinology 1996;137:354–366.

27. Basu-Modak S, Braissant O, Escher P, Desvergne B, Honegger P, Wahli W, Peroxisome proliferator-activated receptor beta regulates acyl-CoA synthetase 2 in reaggregated rat brain cell cultures. J Biol Chem 1999;274:35881–35888.

28. Singh I, Lazo O. Peroxisomal enzyme activities in brain and liver of pups of lactating mothers treated with ciprofibrate. Neurosci Lett 1992;138:283–286.

29. Padmini S and Rao PS. Enhanced beta-oxidative utilization of [1-^{14}C]palmitate during active myelinogenesis in developing rat brain under nutritional stress. Lipids 1991;26:83–85.

30. Auestad N, Korsak RA, Morrow JW, Edmond J. Fatty acid oxidation and ketogenesis by astrocytes in primary culture J. Neurochem 1991;56:1376–1386.

31. Blazquez C, Sanchez C, Daza A, Galve-Roperh I, Guzman M. The stimulation of ketogenesis by cannabinoids in cultured astrocytes defines carnitine palmitoyltransferase I as a new ceramide-activated enzyme. J Neurochem 1999;72:1759–1768.

32. Blazquez C, Sanchez C, Velasco G, Guzman M. Role of carnitine palmitoyltransferase I in the control of ketogenesis in primary cultures of rat astrocytes. J Neurochem 1998;71:1597–1606.

33. Blazquez C, Woods A, de Ceballos ML, Carling D, Guzman M. The AMP-activated protein kinase is involved in the regulation of ketone body production by astrocytes. J Neurochem 1999;73:1674–1682.

34. Bixel MG, Hamprecht B. Generation of ketone bodies from leucine by cultured astroglial cells. J Neurochem 1995;65:2450–2461.

35. Daikhin Y, Yudkoff M. Compartmentation of brain glutamate metabolism in neurons and glia. J Nutr 2000;130 (4S Suppl):1026S–1031S.
36. Yudkoff M. Brain metabolism of branched-chain amino acids. Glia 1997;21:92–98.
37. Dringen R, Gebhardt R, Hamprecht B. Glycogen in astrocytes: possible function as lactate supply for neighboring cells Brain Res 1993;623:208–214.
38. Cullingford TE, Bhakoo KK, Peuchen S, Dolphin CT, Clark JB. Regulation of the ketogenic enzyme mitochondrial 3-hydroxy-3-methylglutaryl-CoA synthase in astrocytes and meningeal fibroblasts; implications in normal brain development and seizure neuropathologies. In: Quant PA, Eaton S (eds.). Current Views of Fatty Acid Oxidation and Ketogenesis—From Organelles to Point Mutations, Advances in Experimental Medicine and Biology. Kluwer/Plenum, New York, 1999, pp. 241–252.
39. Guzman M, Blazquez C. Is there an astrocyte–neuron ketone body shuttle? Trends Endocrinol Metab 2001;12:169–173.
40. Edmond J. Energy metabolism in developing brain cells. Can J Physiol Pharmacol 1992;70 (Suppl):S118–S129.
41. Sherwin AL. Neuroactive amino acids in focally epileptic human brain: a review. Neurochem Res 1999;24:1387–1395.
42. Yudkoff M, Daikhin Y, Nissim I, Lazarow, A, Nissim I. Ketogenic diet, amino acid metabolism, and seizure control. J Neurosci Res 2001;66:931–940.
43. Kish SJ, Dixon LM, Sherwin AL. Aspartic acid aminotransferase activity is increased in actively spiking compared with non-spiking human epileptic cortex. J Neurol Neurosurg Psychiatr 1988;51:552–556.
44. Yudkoff M, Daikhin Y, Nissim I, Grunstein R, Nissim I. Effects of ketone bodies on astrocyte amino acid metabolism J Neurochem 1997;69:682–692.
45. Erecinska M, Nelson D, Daikhin Y, Yudkoff M. Regulation of GABA level in rat brain synaptosomes: fluxes through enzymes of the GABA shunt and effects of glutamate, calcium, and ketone bodies. J Neurochem 1996;67:2325–2334.
46. Scharrer E. Control of food intake by fatty acid oxidation and ketogenesis. Nutrition 1999;15:704–714.
47. DeGiorgio CM, Schachter SC, Handforth A, et al. Prospective long-term study of vagus nerve stimulation for the treatment of refractory seizures. Epilepsia 2000;41:1195–1200.
48. Lampen A, Carlberg C, Nau H. Peroxisome proliferator-activated receptor delta is a specific sensor for teratogenic valproic acid derivatives. Eur J Pharmacol 2001;431:25–33.
49. Maguire JH, Murthy AR, Hall IH. Hypolipidemic activity of antiepileptic 5-phenylhydantoins in mice. Eur J Pharmacol 1985;117:135–138.
50. Lee SS, Pineau T, Drago J, et al. Targeted disruption of the alpha isoform of the peroxisome proliferator-activated receptor gene in mice results in abolishment of the pleiotropic effects of peroxisome proliferators. Mol Cell Biol 1995;15:3012–3022.

17 The Effects of Ketone Bodies on Neuronal Excitability

Sergei S. Likhodii and W. McIntyre Burnham

1. THE KETOGENIC DIET, KETOSIS, AND SEIZURE CONTROL

1.1. The Ketogenic Diet: Induction of Ketosis

In the early 1900s, medical practitioners recognized fasting as an effective method for controlling seizures *(1,2)*. The mechanism by which fasting suppressed seizures was initially explained as an alleviation of "intestinal intoxication," which in turn was thought to be the cause of epilepsy *(1)*.

The history of the ketogenic diet began with the realization that the metabolic changes induced by starvation—not the alleviation of "intoxication"—could result in seizure control *(3)*. This innovative hypothesis led Wilder in 1921, to propose a high-fat, low-carbohydrate diet that came to be known as the "ketogenic diet" *(3)*. The ketogenic diet induced metabolic changes similar to those caused by fasting, and it was equally effective at suppressing epileptic seizures *(4)*.

Ketosis, i.e., the systemic elevation of the three "ketone bodies," β-hydroxybutyrate, acetoacetate, and acetone—is central to the metabolic changes induced by the diet (*see* Fig. 1). The ketosis induced by fasting, and mimicked by the ketogenic diet, is a critical adaptative mechanism for the brain. The human brain contributes only about 2% of the body's total weight, yet its energy requirements are disproportionately high: approx 20% of the body's total energy needs at rest *(5)*. During fasting (in the absence of glucose), ketone bodies, derived from adipose fat, are the main source of energy for the human brain. After 5–6 wk of starvation, ketone bodies account for about 60% of the brain's energy supply in adults *(6)*.

The young brain is characterized by an even greater capacity for the uptake and utilization of ketone bodies, especially during the first 2 yr of life. This capacity is believed to allow the developing brain the greatest chance of survival within a diverse range of nutritional states *(7)*. Overall, ketosis appears to have been instrumental in the survival of early man as a species and, perhaps, essential for the evolution of human brain *(8)*.

1.2. Ketone Bodies: Levels and Metabolic Roles

Figure 2 outlines the biochemical pathways by which ketone bodies are generated. β-Hydroxybutyrate is the most frequently measured ketone body. The concentration of

From: *Epilepsy and the Ketogenic Diet*
Edited by: C. E. Stafstrom and J. M. Rho © Humana Press Inc., Totowa, NJ

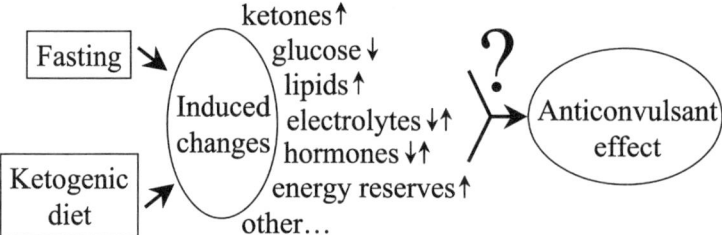

Fig. 1. Both fasting and the ketogenic diet induce a number of common changes in the body. These include an elevation of ketone bodies in the blood and brain, a decrease in glucose utilization, and a shift in electrolytes and hormones. The identification of specific changes resulting in anticonvulsant effects has been challenging.

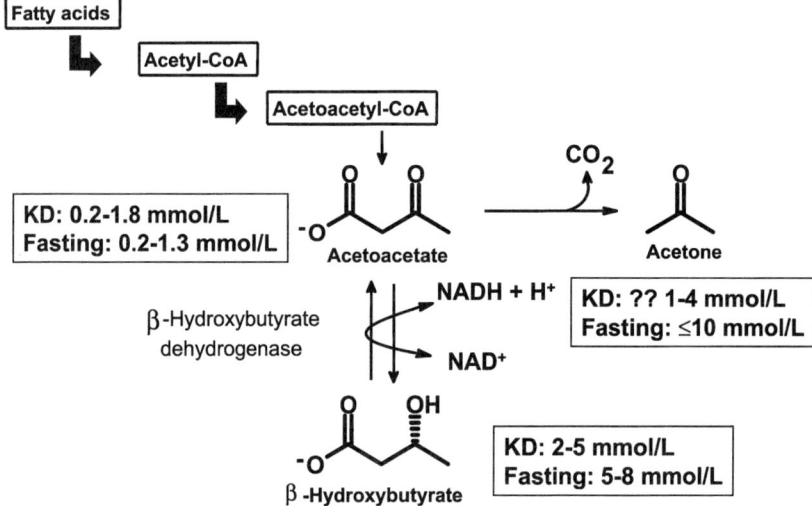

Fig. 2. Biochemical pathways that generate "ketone bodies and approximate concentrations of 'ketones' in blood, plasma, or serum." (In chemical terms, acetone is the only ketone among the three ketone bodies; *see* text.) Acetoacetate is the key molecule from which both β-hydroxybutyrate and acetone are derived. β-Hydroxybutyrate, however, is the most commonly measured ketone body. The blood and brain concentrations of acetone in patients on the ketogenic diet are imperfectly known.

β-hydroxybutyrate varies over a wide range in plasma of patients on the ketogenic diet, reaching values of 2–5 mmol/L *(9)*. β-Hydroxybutyrate blood concentrations of 5–8 mmol/L have been reported in humans undergoing prolonged fasting *(6,8)*.

β-Hydroxybutyrate is in equilibrium with acetoacetate owing to a reaction catalyzed by the enzyme β-hydroxybutyrate dehydrogenase (Fig. 2). In the "fed" state, the ratio of β-hydroxybutyrate to acetoacetate is close to 1:1. As ketosis increases, however, the ratio of β-hydroxybutyrate to acetoacetate increases as well. After 28–42 d of starvation, it may be as high as 4.5:1 *(6,10,11)*.

Acetoacetate plays a central role in the biochemistry of the ketone bodies. It is the only ketone body that can be directly used for the generation of energy. Acetoacetate is maintained within a relatively narrow range of concentrations (0.2–0.5 mmol/L during short-term fasting). β-Hydroxybutyrate's probable metabolic role is to buffer the acetoacetate pool, replenishing it during periods of peak demand. In adults undergoing prolonged fasting, acetoacetate in the blood rises to a maximum of about 1.3 mmol/L *(6)*. In children aged 2–9 yr, Huttenlocher, in 1976, reported fasting plasma levels of acetoacetate of 1.66 mmol/L; ketogenic diets—classic or medium chain triglyceride (MCT)—subsequently maintained acetoacetate levels in these children in the range of 0.95–1.84 mmol/L *(9)*.

It is worth noting that when applied to β-hydroxybutyrate or acetoacetate, the term "ketone body" is not quite accurate. Defined from a strict chemical basis, β-hydroxybutyrate is not a ketone. It is an organic acid containing an additional alcohol group. Acetoacetate is also an organic acid, one that contains an additional ketone group. It is traditional practice, however, to refer to both compounds as "ketone bodies," or "ketones" for short.

Acetone is the only "true" ketone among the three ketone bodies. Acetone is formed from acetoacetate by an irreversible reaction involving the spontaneous loss of a carbon as CO_2 (Fig. 2). This reaction is not in equilibrium. It may therefore lead to the accumulation of acetone in the body. Some data suggest that the serum concentration of acetone during fasting can be as high or higher than 10 mmol/L *(12)*.

Very little is known about the blood/serum/plasma or brain acetone concentrations induced by the ketogenic diet. Acetone has long been considered to be a minor ketone body, with little biological significance. An early study, however, found that in children treated with 2:1 to 5:1 ketogenic diets, blood acetone concentrations were in the range of 0.071–0.935 g/L *(4)*. These concentrations correspond to concentrations of 1.2–16.1 mmol/L. These data should be viewed cautiously, however: the authors provide few details about the specificity of their analytical methods or the conditions under which blood samples were stored before analysis. More recently, nuclear magnetic resonance (NMR) spectroscopic measurements in patients on the ketogenic diet have suggested that the concentration of acetone in the brain is about 1 mmol per kilogram of brain weight *(13)*. Our own measurements, utilizing the NMR and high-performance liquid chromatography techniques on plasma samples from patients on the ketogenic diet, suggest a large range of acetone concentrations, in one instance exceeding 8 mmol/L (*see* Fig. 3, unpublished data, derived from samples provided by K. Musa-Veloso and Drs. S.C. Cunanne, R. Curtis, and R. Wennberg).

1.3. Ketosis and Seizure Control: Correlational Studies

The suggestion by Wilder in 1921 that the anticonvulsant effects of fasting and the ketogenic diet were owing to the "sedative" effects of acetoacetate *(3)* reflected the belief at the time that a drug must have sedative properties to be anticonvulsant *(14)*. It implied, however, that the ketone bodies have direct anticonvulsant effects. Not surprisingly, many studies since the time of Wilder have attempted to establish a correlation between the level of ketosis and seizure control.

Overall, the clinical data derived from these studies have been somewhat conflicting. Many of the early reports suggested a significant relationship between ketosis and seizure control *(3,4,15)*. Later reports, however, have sometimes supported *(9,16–18)* and sometimes disputed the existence of such a relationship *(19,20)*.

Results from animal studies, although allowing for better control over experimental factors, are also inconclusive or conflicting *(21–25)*. In particular, a study of Bough and Eagles in 1999 reported a positive correlation between plasma β-hydroxybutyrate con-

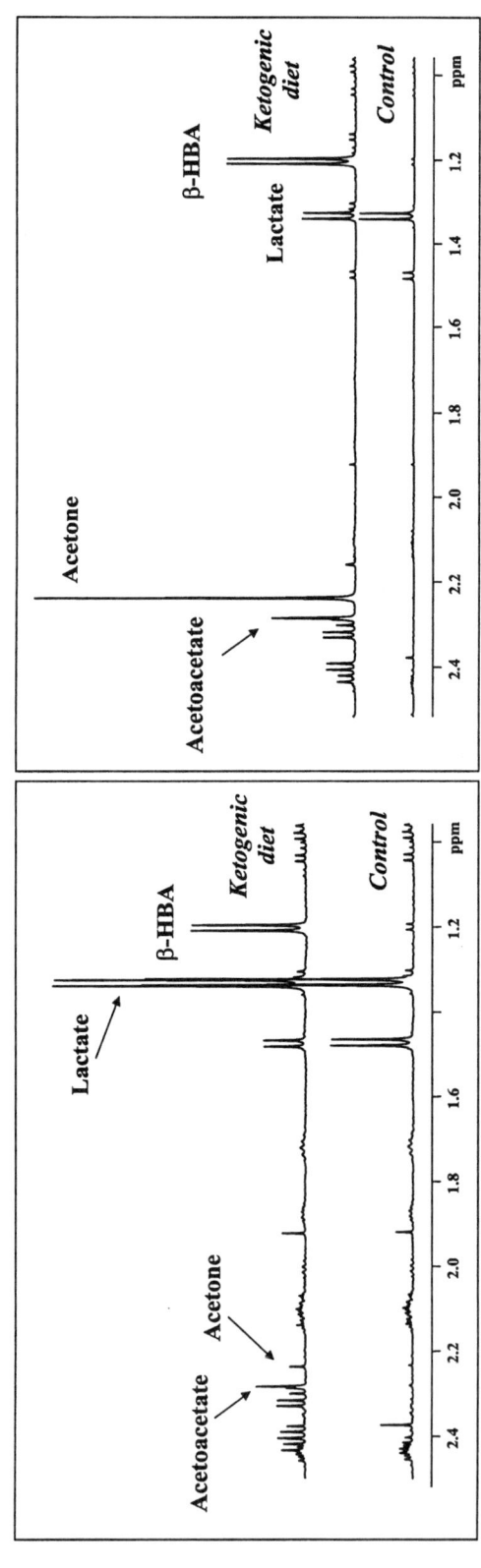

Fig. 3. Left: ¹H-NMR spectra from plasma of a rat fed control diet (bottom trace) and from plasma of a rat fed the classic ketogenic diet (top trace). Right: ¹H-NMR spectra from control plasma of a human volunteer (bottom trace), and from the plasma of a patient with epilepsy receiving the classic ketogenic diet (top trace). The spectra were obtained after filtering off the plasma proteins. Ketogenic diets with similar ratios of fat to protein plus carbohydrate appear to produce higher acetone concentrations in humans than in rats. Acetone concentrations in human patients can be 1.0–3.0 mmol/L or higher.

centration and seizure suppression in rats *(23)*. Other studies, however, have found that seizure suppression does not correlate with plasma levels of β-hydroxybutyrate *(24,25)*.

One of the strongest arguments *for* a causal relationship between ketosis and anticonvulsant effects is the demonstration of Huttenlocher that infusion of glucose into a patient on the ketogenic diet led to a rapid (within 45 min) decrease in plasma concentrations of the ketones, accompanied by a return of seizure activity *(9)*.

In contrast, one of the strongest arguments *against* a causal relationship between ketosis and anticonvulsant effects has been the observation that seizure control in animals may take several days *(21)*, despite elevations in plasma ketone levels within hours of fasting *(25)*. Clinical studies cast some doubt on the animal experiments, however. These results suggest that seizure control in children—like ketosis—*does* occur rapidly. Seizures in children may stop even during introductory fasting or in the very early stages of the ketogenic diet *(26)*.

A possible explanation for the conflicting data from studies of ketosis and seizure suppression is the use by most of these studies of blood/plasma β-hydroxybutyrate concentrations as the only index of ketosis. (Urinary ketones poorly represent blood/plasma concentrations and are less informative.) Acetoacetate and acetone, the other two ketones, have rarely been measured. How these other ketone bodies rise in patients on the diet, and whether they correlate with seizure control, is not known. Interestingly, the early clinical studies that found a correlation between ketosis and the efficacy of the ketogenic diet used "total acetone bodies" as their measure of ketosis. It appears that "total acetone bodies" included acetoacetate and acetone, but not β-hydroxybutyrate *(4,15)*. Measurements of ketosis in future studies, should include not only β-hydroxybutyrate, but acetoacetate and acetone as well.

Examining the relationship between ketosis and efficacy of the ketogenic diet continues to be a principal goal of many clinical studies. The correlational approach by itself, however, cannot provide proof of the *causal* involvement of ketones in the mechanism of the ketogenic diet *(27)*. Direct experimental manipulation is needed.

1.4. Animal Models of Ketosis

Animal models and in vitro preparations afford a number of advantages for the study of the ketogenic diet and the effects of ketosis. In animal models, blood, brain, and cerebrospinal fluid samples may be ethically obtained. Likewise, individual ketone bodies can be injected in isolation to permit the assessment of their effects on seizure threshold in the absence of the other ketone bodies. In *in vitro* models, voltage- or patch-clamp techniques may help to establish the molecular and cellular mechanisms associated with ketosis.

Animal models, however, are useful research tools only if they parallel the effects observed in humans. For example, Fig. 3 shows proton NMR spectra obtained in our laboratory from the plasma of a rat fed the classic ketogenic diet and from a human patient undergoing treatment with the classic ketogenic diet. NMR spectroscopy can simultaneously measure the concentrations of all three ketone bodies.

Two observations can be made from the NMR spectra in Fig. 3. First, although rats do develop ketosis, the concentrations of all three ketone bodies appear to be far lower than those in humans. This observation is in agreement with the observations of other investigators. Their work includes studies suggesting that ketone bodies provide a significantly higher proportion of brain energy in fasted humans than in fasted rats. After a few days of starvation, for example, ketone bodies account for approx 25% of total brain energy requirements in humans *(28),* whereas in fasted rats they only account for 3–4% *(29).*

The second observation is that acetone plays a smaller role in rat ketosis than in human ketosis. The NMR spectra show concentrations of acetone in human plasma of 3.5 mmol/L or higher. These concentrations are comparable to, or higher than, the concentrations of β-hydroxybutyrate and acetoacetate (Fig. 3). Thus, in humans, acetone significantly contributes to ketosis. In rats fed the ketogenic diet, however, the NMR spectra show acetone concentrations of approx 0.1–0.2 mmol/L, values far lower than those seen with either β-hydroxybutyrate or acetoacetate (Fig. 3).

Rodents (rats) provide a model for studying the effects of the ketogenic diet, but it must be kept in mind that they may not perfectly replicate effects seen in humans.

2. DIRECT ANTICONVULSANT EFFECTS OF KETONE BODIES

2.1. Problems in Interpretation

Ketone bodies can be injected into experimental animals and seizure suppression can be assessed using the standard seizure tests. This approach can provide *direct* evidence of the anticonvulsant effects of ketones.

This direct approach avoids many of the problems that arise in correlational studies. Even a direct approach, however, leads to certain interpretational problems. The first of these is that β-hydroxybutyrate and acetoacetate rely on the monocarboxylic acid transporter to cross the blood–brain barrier. The monocarboxylic acid transporter has a limited capacity in nonfasted animals *(30)* and may not be sufficient to elevate brain concentrations of exogenously injected ketone bodies to anticonvulsant levels in the brain. These problems do not arise with acetone. Acetone easily crosses the blood–brain barrier—without the need for a transporter—and, when injected intraperitoneally into a rat, appears in the brain within 1 min *(31).*

In addition, acetoacetate is taken up by the brain at a significantly higher rate than β-hydroxybutyrate. In studies involving infants, children, and adults, investigators found that the uptake of acetoacetate by brain is twice that of β-hydroxybutyrate at any given blood concentration *(32–34).* Thus, injection of equal amounts of different ketones may not produce equivalent brain concentrations.

Fasting, the ketogenic diet, and (possibly) the chronic administration of β-hydroxybutyrate or acetoacetate may upregulate the monocarboxylic acid transporter and enhance the transport of these ketones into the brain *(30).* This postulated sequence may explain the anticonvulsant effects of chronic β-hydroxybutyrate intake provided chronically in drinking water *(35).*

A second problem with direct administration is that β-hydroxybutyrate and acetoacetate are in equilibrium in the body and are rapidly interconverted. Acetoacetate is also converted into acetone. Administration of β-hydroxybutyrate or acetoacetate, therefore, will lead to elevation of all three ketones (Fig. 2). Attributing anticonvulsant effects to any specific ketone in experiments with β-hydroxybutyrate or acetoacetate, therefore, is difficult. Anticonvulsant effects, if any, may relate to any one of the three ketones, or to all of them in combination. Once again, this problem does not arise with acetone, which is not converted to acetoacetate or β-hydroxybutyrate (Fig. 2).

Even the interpretation of experimental data involving acetone is not without difficulties, however. The hepatic metabolism of acetone can result in brain accumulation of intermediary products, such as isopropanol *(31,36)*. Isopropanol has been shown to possess anticonvulsant properties *(37–39)*. Isopropanol has also been found in the breath of patients on the ketogenic diet (Musa-Veloso, personal communication), although its potential role in the anticonvulsant mechanisms of the diet has not yet been explored.

2.2. Classic Studies

Investigations of the possible direct anticonvulsant effects of the ketone bodies began shortly after the introduction of the diet. In 1931–1933, Keith produced a series of pioneering reports suggesting that acetone and acetoacetate had anticonvulsant effects in a rabbit model of experimental seizures *(40–42)*. Keith also tested the effects of some compounds structurally related to the ketone bodies and found that ethylacetoacetate and diacetone alcohol were anticonvulsant *(40)*. According to Keith, sodium acetoacetate had the most marked anticonvulsant effects *(42)*. Interestingly, β-hydroxybutyrate was not found to have anticonvulsant properties in these experiments *(41)*.

Unfortunately, Keith's results were largely ignored by the scientific community. Shortly after Keith's reports, Merritt and Putnam discovered the anticonvulsant effects of diphenylhydantoin (phenytoin, or Dilantin®) in 1938, a "monumental landmark" in the history of epilepsy therapy *(43)*. Interest in the ketogenic diet, and subsequently its mechanisms, began to decline. Friedlander *(14)*, in his historical overview entitled "Putnam, Merritt, and the discovery of Dilantin," notes that "as late as 1945, Merritt and Putnam had evaluated only one of the ketone bodies tested by Keith, and that this was one of the least promising—ethylacetoacetate."

In 1947 Driver returned to the study of the ketone bodies. He tested the anticonvulsant activity of a number of compounds structurally related to the "products of fat and carbohydrate metabolism," contrasting the effects of these "ketogens" to the effects of phenytoin *(37)*. Driver found that acetone, ethyl acetoacetate, diacetone alcohol, isopropanol, and several other compounds significantly raised the threshold for electrically induced seizures. From these data, Driver suggested that the activity of acetone and its related compounds might explain the anticonvulsant activity of the ketogenic diet *(37)*. Interestingly, Driver found that acetone and isopropyl alcohol raised convulsive thresholds to a greater extent than phenytoin. He characterized isopropyl alcohol as having "a tremendous anticonvulsant effect without ataxia or narcosis" and suggested that its activity might be explained by partial transformation into acetone in the body *(37)*. Curiously, however, Driver did not cite the work of Keith on acetone *(40)*. It is not clear whether he was even aware of Keith's work.

Following the reports of Driver and his colleagues *(37–39)*, there were no animal studies assessing the anticonvulsant properties of ketone bodies or their possible role in the ketogenic diet for 35 yr. In 1983 Mahoney et al. performed a study in which they gavage-fed rats with β-hydroxybutyrate, using a model of magnesium deficiency. In agreement with Keith's earlier study *(41)*, β-hydroxybutyrate was not found to be anticonvulsant *(44)*.

2.3. Anticonvulsant Effects of β-Hydroxybutyrate and Acetoacetate

The recent rebirth of clinical interest in the ketogenic diet has led to a renewed interest in its mechanism(s) of action. Recently, the effects of both β-hydroxybutyrate and acetoacetate have been studied in rat hippocampal slices. Neither compound was found to alter excitatory or inhibitory synaptic transmission *(45)*.

Several other recent preliminary reports, however, have suggested that β-hydroxy-butyrate does have anticonvulsant activity in hippocampal slice models of epilepsy *(46)*. These stand in contrast to several reports suggesting that β-hydroxybutyrate is not anticonvulsant *(41,44,45,47)*. Rho et al. have suggested that impurities, such as dibenzylamine in commercial supplies of β-hydroxybutyrate, may be responsible for an anticonvulsant effect *(47)*.

In our own laboratory, we have assessed the anticonvulsant properties of acutely administered β-hydroxybutyrate and acetoacetate using maximal electroshock seizures in mice. When injected intraperitoneally 30 min before the seizure test, neither of these two ketone bodies was active, even at the highest doses of 12 mmol/kg (S. Likhodii et al., unpublished data).

A recent study by Rho et al., however, reported anticonvulsant effects of acetoacetate in a mouse model of audiogenic seizures *(47)*. This report is in agreement with the classical study by Keith *(42)*. The source of the discrepancy between these results and our own data requires further investigation.

2.4. Anticonvulsant Effects of Acetone

In contrast to the paucity of reports on the anticonvulsant effects of β-hydroxybu-tyrate and acetoacetate, reports on the anticonvulsant effects of acetone have appeared regularly from the 1940s to the present. Altogether, including the classic work of Keith and Driver, there have been over a dozen articles reporting anticonvulsant properties of acetone *(31,37–40,47–56,58)*.

As noted earlier, Keith (1931) was the first to provide experimental evidence of acetone's anticonvulsant activity, utilizing the chemical convulsant thujone *(40)*. In 1947 Driver showed that acetone increased the threshold for electrically induced seizures in rats *(37)*. A subsequent series of studies showed that acetone was also effective in suppressing repeated maximal seizures produced by the powerful chemical convulsant semicarbazide *(48,49,52)*. It was noted in these studies that acetone was more efficacious than phenytoin or pentobarbital *(48)*. Later, acetone was shown to provide protection against the convulsions induced by isonicotinic acid and electroshock *(50)*. In a recent series of neurotoxicity studies related to the volatile solvents, short-term inhalation of acetone vapors suppressed both audiogenic *(53)* and electrically induced seizures in rats *(54,55)*. Given such reports of acetone's anticonvulsant effects, it is surprising that it has received little attention in discussions of the anticonvulsant mechanisms of the ketogenic diet.

In 1999 Seymour et al. showed an elevation of brain acetone in epileptic children on the ketogenic diet *(13)*. The authors suggested a possible role for acetone in the effects of the diet, although they did not link their findings to those of Talbot et al. *(4)*, who in 1927 reported elevated blood acetone in patients on the ketogenic diet, or to Keith's *(40)* report of the anticonvulsant properties of acetone.

Subsequent animal studies have demonstrated an elevation in breath acetone in rats fed the ketogenic diet *(57)* and have documented the anticonvulsant effects of acute and chronic acetone against pentylenetetrazole (PTZ) seizures in rats *(31,56)* and audiogenic seizures in mice *(47)*.

Our own group has undertaken an investigation designed to show that acetone, like the ketogenic diet, has a broad spectrum of anticonvulsant activity at subtoxic doses. Our results indicate that acetone is effective in the maximal electroshock model, in the subcu-

Table 1
Dose–Response Effects for Anticonvulsant and Ataxia Effects of Acetone in Rats

Type of test	ED_{50} (mmol/kg, 95% confidence interval)	TD_{50} (mmol/kg, 95% confidence interval)	Therapeutic index
MES	6.6 (4.2–10.2)	28.4 (26.8–30.1)	4.3
PTZ	9.7 (7.6–12.3)	27.5 (25.6–29.7)	2.8
Kindled			
Generalized	13.1 (7.9–21.8)	30.5 (28.6–32.5)	2.3
Focal	26.5 (21.3–32.8)		1.2
AY-9944	4.0 (3.7–4.4)	24.0 (21.5–26.9)	6.0

Note: Rats were injected with acetone intraperitoneally 30 min before the tests. Dose–response effects were measured by means of four different models: (1) the maximal electroshock (MES) test, which models human tonic–clonic seizures, (2) the subcutaneous pentylenetetrazole (PTZ) test, which models human typical absence seizures, (3) the amygdala kindling test, which models human complex partial seizures with secondary generalization, and (4) the AY-9944 test, which models chronic atypical absence seizures, a component of the Lennox–Gastaut syndrome. Median effective doses (ED_{50} s) for these tests are provided. Ataxia was scored in the open field in the following six categories: 0, no ataxia; 1, a slight ataxia in the hind limbs, with no decrease in abdominal muscle tone; 2, a more pronounced ataxia, with a slight decrease in abdominal muscle tone; 3, a further increase in ataxia with a more marked decrease in abdominal muscle tone; 4, marked ataxia, where animals lose balance during forward locomotion and there is a loss of abdominal muscle tone; and 5, very marked ataxia with frequent losses of balance during forward locomotion and a loss of abdominal muscle tone. Median toxic doses (TD_{50}s) for these tests are provided. Therapeutic indices were calculated as TD_{50}/ED_{50}.

taneous PTZ model, in the amygdala kindling model, and in the AY-9944 model of atypical absence seizures (*58;* also *see* Table 1). These results suggest that acetone and related compounds might be developed as anticonvulsants for the treatment of clinical seizures. Like the ketogenic diet, acetone and its congeners might be effective against a wide range of seizures, including those that do not respond to the standard anticonvulsants.

While it is now clear that acetone is anticonvulsant, it cannot yet be concluded that the elevation of brain acetone accounts for the anticonvulsant effects of the ketogenic diet. Demonstrations of the anticonvulsant effects of acetone are a necessary, but not *sufficient,* proof of acetone's involvement in the actions of the diet. We have recently proposed a series of studies that could provide crucial evidence linking acetone to the anticonvulsant effects of the ketogenic diet *(31).* Among these were experiments designed to show that the ketogenic diet elevates acetone to anticonvulsant concentrations in the brain, that acetone, like the ketogenic diet, possesses a broad spectrum of anticonvulsant effects, that the time course of acetone's elevation in the brain correlates with that of the ketogenic diet's anticonvulsant effects, and that the ketogenic diet loses its anticonvulsant effects if acetone does not rise in blood and brain.

3. CONCLUSION

The hypothesis that the ketone bodies are anticonvulsant has been one of the major hypotheses concerning the anticonvulsant effects of the ketogenic diet. Unfortunately, only a few experiments have examined the anticonvulsant properties of the ketones.

The existing reports on the anticonvulsant effects of β-hydroxybutyrate and acetoacetate are somewhat conflicting. Most studies have suggested that β-hydroxybutyrate is not directly anticonvulsant. There is greater support for the idea that acetoacetate has anticonvulsant effects. It must be established, however, that these effects are not the result of transformation of acetoacetate to acetone.

It is clear that acetone itself *does* exhibit anticonvulsant properties. These have now been observed at nontoxic doses in a large number of animal seizure models. This suggests that acetone—or similar compounds—could be developed as broad-spectrum anticonvulsants. The blood and brain concentrations of acetone in human patients on the ketogenic diet require further research. Nevertheless, acetone is present in millimolar concentrations and might, therefore, contribute significantly to the anticonvulsant effects of the diet. More research will be required to determine whether the elevation of acetone can explain all the anticonvulsant effects of the ketogenic diet.

REFERENCES

1. Guelpa G, Marie A. La lutte contre l'épilepsie par la désintoxication et par la rééducation alimentaire [The fight against epilepsy by detoxification and by food reeducation]. Rev Ther Med Chir [Paris] 1911;78:8–13.
2. Geyelin HR. Fasting as a method for treating epilepsy. Med Rec 1921;99:1037–1039.
3. Wilder RM. The effects of ketonemia on the course of epilepsy. Mayo Clin Proc 1921;2:307–308.
4. Talbot FB, Metcalf KM, Moriarty ME. Epilepsy: chemical investigations of rational treatment by production of ketosis. Am J Dis Child 1927;33:218–225.
5. Kety SS. The general metabolism of the brain in vivo. In: Richter D (ed.). Metabolism of the Nervous System. Pergamon, London, 1957, pp. 221–237.
6. Owen OE, Morgan AP, Kemp HG, Sullivan JM, Herrera MG, Cahill GF Jr. Brain metabolism during fasting. J Clin Invest 1967;46:1589–1595.
7. Edmond J. Energy metabolism in developing brain cells. Can J Physiol Pharmacol 1992;70 (Suppl):S118–S129.
8. Cahill GF Jr. Starvation in man. N Engl J Med 1970;282:668–675.
9. Huttenlocher PR. Ketonemia and seizures: metabolic and anticonvulsant effects of two ketogenic diets in childhood epilepsy. Pediatr Res 1976;10:536–540.
10. Cahill GF Jr, Herrera MG, Morgan AP, Soeldner JS, Steinke J, Levy PL, Reichard GA Jr, Kipnis DM. Hormone-fuel interrelationships during fasting. J Clin Invest 1966;45:1751–1769.
11. Williamson DH, Whitelaw E. Physiological aspects of the regulation of ketogenesis. Biochem Soc Symp 1978;43:137–161.
12. Freund G. The calorie deficiency hypothesis of ketogenesis tested in man. Metabolism 1965;14:985–990.
13. Seymour KJ, Bluml S, Sutherling J, Sutherling W, Ross BD. Identification of cerebral acetone by ^{1}H-MRS in patients with epilepsy controlled by ketogenic diet. MAGMA 1999;8:33–42.
14. Friedlander WJ. Putnam, Merritt, and the discovery of Dilantin. Epilepsia 1986;27 (Suppl 3):S1–S20.
15. McQuarrie I, Keith HM. Relationship of variations in the degree of ketonuria to occurrence of convulsions in epileptic children on ketogenic diets. Am J Dis Child 1927;34:1013–1029.
16. Helmholz HF, Keith HM. Eight years' experience with the ketogenic diet in the treatment of epilepsy. JAMA 1930;95:707–709.
17. Gilbert DL, Pyzik PL, Freeman JM. The ketogenic diet: seizure control correlates better with serum beta-hydroxybutyrate than with urine ketones. J Child Neurol 2000;15:787–790.
18. Ross DL, Swaiman KF, Torres F, Hansen J. Early biochemical and EEG correlates of the ketogenic diet in children with atypical absence epilepsy. Pediatr Neurol 1985;1:104–108.
19. Millichap JG, Jones JD, Rudis BP. Mechanism of anti-convulsant action of ketogenic diet. Am J Dis Child 1964;107:593–604.
20. Hassan AM, Keene DL, Whiting SE, Jacob PJ, Champagne JR, Humphreys P. Ketogenic diet in the treatment of refractory epilepsy in childhood. Pediatr Neurol 1999;21:548–552.
21. Appleton DB, DeVivo DC. An animal model for the ketogenic diet. Epilepsia 1974;15:211–227.
22. Uhlemann ER, Neims AH. Anticonvulsant properties of the ketogenic diet in mice. J Pharmacol Exp Ther 1972;180:231–238.

23. Bough KJ, Eagles DA. A ketogenic diet increases the resistance to pentylenetetrazole-induced seizures in the rat. Epilepsia 1999;40:138–143.
24. Bough KJ, Chen RS, Eagles DA. Path analysis shows that increasing ketogenic ratio, but not beta-hydroxybutyrate, elevates seizure threshold in the rat. Dev Neurosci 1999;21:400–406.
25. Likhodii SS, Musa K, Mendonca A, Dell C, Burnham WM, Cunnane SC. Dietary fat, ketosis, and seizure resistance in rats on the ketogenic diet. Epilepsia 2000;41:1400–1410.
26. Freeman JM, Vining EP. Seizures decrease rapidly after fasting: preliminary studies of the ketogenic diet. Arch Pediatr Adolesc Med 1999;153:946–949.
27. Stafstrom CE. Animal models of the ketogenic diet: what have we learned, what can we learn? Epilepsy Res 1999;37:241–259.
28. Hasselbalch SG, Knudsen GM, Jakobsen J, Hageman LP, Holm S, Paulson OB. Brain metabolism during short-term starvation in humans. J Cereb Blood Flow Metab 1994;14:125–131.
29. Hawkins RA, Mans AM, Davis DW. Regional ketone body utilization by rat brain in starvation and diabetes. Am J Physiol 1986;250(2 Pt 1):E169–E178.
30. Leino RL, Gerhart DZ, Duelli R, Enerson BE, Drewes LR. Diet-induced ketosis increases monocarboxylate transporter (MCT1) levels in rat brain. Neurochem Int 2001;38:519–527.
31. Likhodii SS, Burnham WM. Ketogenic diet: does acetone stop seizures? Med Sci Monit 2002;8:HY19–HY24.
32. Persson B, Settergren G, Dahlquist G. Cerebral arterio-venous difference of acetoacetate and D-β-hydroxybutyrate in children. Acta Paediatr Scand 1972;61:273–278.
33. Owen OE, Reichard GA Jr, Boden G, Shuman C. Comparative measurements of glucose, beta-hydroxy-butyrate, acetoacetate, and insulin in blood and cerebrospinal fluid during starvation. Metabolism 1974;23:7–14.
34. Lamers KJ, Doesburg WH, Gabreels FJ, Romsom AC, Lemmens WA, Wevers RA, Renier WO. CSF concentration and CSF/blood ratio of fuel related components in children after prolonged fasting. Clin Chim Acta 1987;167:135–145.
35. Lustig S, Niesen CE. Beta-hydroxybutyrate suppresses pentylenetetrazol (PTZ) induced seizures in young adult rats. Epilepsia 1998;39 (Suppl 6):S36.
36. Bailey DN. Detection of isopropanol in acetonemic patients not exposed to isopropanol. J Toxicol Clin Toxicol 1990;28:459–466.
37. Driver RL. Isopropyl alcohol, other ketogens, and miscellaneous agents on thresholds for electrical convulsions and diphenylhydantoin. Proc Soc Exp Biol Med 1947;64:248–251.
38. Chu N, Driver RL, Hanzlik PJ. Anticonvulsant action of isopropyl alcohol. J Pharmacol Exp Ther 1948;92:291–302.
39. Schaffarzick RW. Anticonvulsant action of isopropanol. Proc Soc Exp Biol Med 1950;74:211–215.
40. Keith HM. The effect of various factors on experimentally produced convulsions. Am J Dis Child 1931;41:532–543.
41. Keith HM. Further studies of the control of experimentally produced convulsions. J Pharmacol Exp Ther 1932;44:449–455.
42. Keith HM. Factors influencing experimentally produced convulsions. Arch Neurol Psych 1933;29:148–154.
43. Rowland LP. Introduction to first annual Merritt–Putnam Symposium, Cambridge. Epilepsia 1982;23 (Suppl 1):S1–S4.
44. Mahoney AW, Hendricks DG, Bernhard N, Sisson DV. Fasting and ketogenic diet effects on audiogenic seizures susceptibility of magnesium deficient rats. Pharmacol Biochem Behav 1983;18:683–687.
45. Thio LL, Wong M, Yamada KA. Ketone bodies do not directly alter excitatory or inhibitory hippocampal synaptic transmission. Neurology 2000;54:325–331.
46. Niesen CE, Ge S. The effect of ketone bodies, β-hydroxybutyrate, and acetoacetate on acute seizure activity in hippocampal CA1 neurons. Epilepsia 1998;39 (Suppl 6):S35.
47. Rho JM, Anderson GD, Donevan SD, White HS. Acetoacetate, acetone, and dibenzylamine (a contaminant in 1-(+)-beta-hydroxybutyrate) exhibit direct anticonvulsant actions in vivo. Epilepsia 2002;43:358–361.
48. Jenney EH, Lee LD. The convulsant effect of semicarbazide. J Pharmacol Exp Ther 1951;103:349.
49. Jenney EH, Pfeiffer CC. The convulsant effect of hydrazides and the antidotal effect of anticonvulsants and metabolites. J Pharmacol Exp Ther 1958;122:110–123.

50. Kohli RP, Kishor K, Dua PR, Saxena RC. Anticonvulsant activity of some carbonyl containing compounds. Indian J Med Res 1967;55:1221–1225.

51. Postolache V, Safta L, Cuparencu B, Steiner L. Die Wirkung von Aceton auf Pentamethylentetrazol-Krämpfe [Effect of acetone upon pentamethylenetetrazole convulsions.] Arch Toxikol 1970;26:273–276.

52. Yamashita J. Convulsive seizure induced by intracerebral injection of semicarbazide (an anti-vitamin B$_6$) in the mouse. J Nutr Sci Vitaminol (Tokyo) 1976;22:1–6.

53. Frantik E, Horvath M, Vodickova L. Effects of solvent mixtures on behaviour and seizure characteristics at the utmost additive. Act Nerv Super (Praha) 1988;30:260–264.

54. Vodickova L, Frantik E, Vodickova A. Neutrotropic effects and blood levels of solvents at combined exposures: binary mixtures of toluene, _o_-xylene and acetone in rats and mice. Cent Eur J Public Health 1995;3:57–64.

55. Frantik E, Vodickova L, Hornychova M, Nosek M. Pattern of inhalation exposure: blood levels and acute subnarcotic effects of toluene and acetone in rats. Cent Eur J Public Health 1996;4:226–232.

56. Likhodii SS, Snead OC, Burnham WM: The ketogenic diet. Does acetone stop seizures? 55th Annual Meeting of the Eastern Association of Electroencephalographers, New York, March 24, 2001. Clin Neurophysiol 2002;113:1365.

57. Likhodii SS, Musa K, Cunnane SC. Breath acetone as a measure of systemic ketosis assessed in a rat model of the ketogenic diet. Clin Chem 2002;48:115–120.

58. Likhodii SS, Serbanescu I, Cortez MA, Murphy P, Snead OC III, Burnham WM. Anticonvulsant properties of acetone, a brain ketone elevated by the ketogenic diet. Ann Neurol 2003;54:219–226.

18

Effects of the Ketogenic Diet on Acute Seizure Models

Douglas A. Eagles and Kristopher J. Bough

1. PERSPECTIVE

The ketogenic diet (KD) is both a therapy and a tool for investigating the mechanisms of seizures and, perhaps, epilepsy. Despite our ignorance of the mechanisms by which the KD acts to alter seizures, the observation that seizure threshold can vary widely depending on what an animal eats suggests that seizure threshold is a (patho)physiological variable. The general hypothesis underlying experimental studies of the KD is that, by understanding the physiological changes consequent to a switch from a carbohydrate-based metabolism to one based on fats, we might gain insight into fundamental processes that affect ictogenesis. If a person whose seizures are controlled by a KD abandons the diet abruptly and suffers a seizure, then we might consider elevated blood glucose (or decreased ketonemia) to be ictogenic. Because central nervous system (CNS) metabolism is normally based entirely on glucose, the success of KDs in treating seizures and epilepsies presents interesting questions and opportunities.

Several experimental tools have been employed to gain an improved understanding of seizures and the epilepsies. These include studies of the mechanisms of action of proconvulsant medications and of antiepileptic drugs (AEDs), determination of genetic pedigrees in human populations, and studies of animal mutants expressing heritable epilepsies. This chapter considers the action of the KD relative to seizures induced by acute application of proconvulsant drugs. A general problem in evaluating animal studies in attempts to identify mechanism(s) of action of the KD is the variety of strains (most studies are of rats or mice), diets, level of calorie restriction, proconvulsant drugs, and doses or routes of administration. Prasad et al. *(1)*, in recognizing this problem, noted that meta-analysis was impossible. We discuss the limitations, constraints, and what we think we have learned from such studies.

2. INTRODUCTION

2.1. Overview

Acute seizure models in animals were introduced by Merritt and Putnam *(2)*, who used maximal electroshock (MES) in cats to identify the anticonvulsant effects of pheny-

From: *Epilepsy and the Ketogenic Diet*
Edited by: C. E. Stafstrom and J. M. Rho © Humana Press Inc., Totowa, NJ

toin, and by Richards and Everett *(3)*, who used pentylenetetrazole (PTZ) and picrotoxin (PTX) in mice and rats to identify a similar role for 3,5,5-trimethyloxazoliidine-2,4-dione. Decades later, Krall et al. *(4)* employed MES and threshold PTZ, plus use of a rotorod to test for neurotoxicity, as a screening strategy for assessing putative anticonvulsant drugs in an attempt to standardize measures and determine the relative effectiveness of drugs being used, or studied for use, against seizures. Recently, Schachter *(5)* revisited the observation that current anticonvulsant drugs are only antiictal and proposed a protocol for evaluating their effectiveness against the underlying epilepsies.

The current fundamental goal of most research and clinical practice directed toward epilepsy is to counter the epileptic substrate, rather than just suppress the symptomatic seizure *(6)*. Two basic, related issues arise. First, the chronic nature of epilepsy, and the variety of forms it takes, mean that testing drugs for effectiveness against epilepsy is likely to be difficult and costly. Second, as Meldrum *(7)* has pointed out, the convenience of seizure testing, most often by PTZ and MES, as a paradigm for selecting AEDs has likely led to the development of families of drugs that share undesirable side effects owing to the central role of γ-aminobutyric acid, type A (GABA$_A$) receptors and voltage-gated sodium channels, respectively, in seizures induced by these two testing protocols.

The development of the earliest anticonvulsant drugs was often indirect, even serendipitous. An attempt to calm epileptic patients led to the discovery of the anticonvulsant properties of phenobarbital, whose structure led to the development of phenytoin and recognition of its anticonvulsant properties by Merritt and Putnam *(2)* through application of MES screening *(8)*. There was no understanding of the mechanism by which either drug acted, other than a sense that the ring structure in the molecules might be related to their anticonvulsant properties. It was not until 45 yr after Merritt and Putnam's *(2)* discovery of the use of phenytoin in epilepsy that the drug was shown to reduce repetitive firing of action potentials *(9)* and, later, to cause a voltage-dependent block of voltage-gated sodium channels *(10)*. Without knowing its mechanism(s), Merritt and Putnam had identified one of the first drugs to be usefully deployed against partial-onset seizures, one of the most common seizure types.

2.2. What Are the Limitations of Acute Studies?

By contrast to the relatively undirected discovery of phenytoin, vigabatrin (GVG) was developed specifically to inhibit GABA-transaminase, the enzyme that degrades GABA; the goal, which was to elevate synaptic GABA levels *(11)*, was rationalized on the basis of the concept that augmentation of inhibitory synaptic transmission would suppress seizures. GVG has been shown *(12,13)* to be an effective anticonvulsant, particularly against partial seizures (but *see* ref. *14*). The validity of the rationale seemed to be confirmed, but it was surprising to find that γ-acetylenic GABA, a closely related compound developed at about the same time as GVG and sharing many of its properties, gave no protection against either PTZ or PTX, even when GABA levels had reached six times normal *(15)*. GVG itself did not prevent seizures evoked by either bicuculline (BIC) or PTX, although it did increase the latency to picrotoxin-induced seizures *(16)*. Gale and Iadorola *(17)* were the first to show that GVG is protective against MES-induced seizures, but that such protection is not seen until 2 d after systemic injection, coincident with the time required for elevation of GABA levels. This finding explains the delays in efficacy but does not explain the failure of γ-acetylenic GABA to give seizure protection. Subsequently, Gale *(18)* reported that direct injection of GVG into substantia nigra produced rapid protection against MES. This observation showed a major limitation of acute seizure tests employing systemic injection of either pro- or anticonvulsant agents; it illustrated that global measures of transmitters may not reflect conditions at relevant synaptic sites such as within the substantia nigra. Acute seizure testing by MES and PTZ would have failed to identify GVG as an anticonvulsant, because this drug is ineffective against PTZ and because systemic injection has such a long latent period for development of protection against MES.

The major limitation of acute studies is that potential therapies are evaluated in a nonepileptic brain, with "normal" gene expression, "normal" channel/receptor function, "normal" transporter function, "normal" populations of neurons and glia, and "normal" circuitry (among a myriad of other factors). AEDs tested in epileptic brains can respond very differently from those tested in normal brains; e.g., actions of benzodiazepines as $GABA_A$ receptor subunits are altered following prolonged seizures. Additionally, the acute nature of the treatment is not likely to reflect what may occur following chronic treatment, as seen, for example, in the GVG studies already cited and studies showing that fasting (short-term) and KD effects (long-term) may be acting similarly or differently (19).

2.3. What Are the Benefits of Acute Studies?

The major benefit of acute studies is the speed with which new agents or treatments may be identified or evaluated. It is time-consuming and costly to test (and generate) a variety of "epileptic" animals, e.g., genetic models, kindled animals, spontaneous seizures generated in animals following status epilepticus induced with either pilocarpine or kainate. As with acute models, there is the question of which model of epilepsy to study. Acquired epilepsies (kindling, pilocarpine, kainate) are only part of the story. Hence, acute testing has led to the identification of nearly all the "classical" drugs used in the treatment of epileptic seizures (phenytoin, carbamazepine, barbiturates, benzodiazepines, valproic acid [VPA], and ethosuximide). Importantly, investigations into the mechanisms by which these drugs exert their effects at therapeutic concentrations have identified three main targets of most of these drugs (20): voltage-gated sodium channels (phenytoin and carbamazepine), binding sites on $GABA_A$ receptors (barbiturates and benzodiazepines), and low-threshold calcium channels (T-type Ca^{2+} channels), first described by Llinás and Yarom (21). Acute models also help to establish important variables, such as dose, in the administration of these drugs.

3. VARIABLES OF DIET ADMINISTRATION

3.1. Role of Diet Type

In general, studies of the effectiveness of KDs against acute seizures have shown that such diets are protective, irrespective of formulation. This is in contrast to a general statement by Swinyard (22) that they were ineffective in all but the hyponatremic test. The only species in which the relationship between high-fat diets and seizures has been studied are mice, rats, and humans. Experimental diets have been varied but generally are of one of two types, either the "classical" long-chain triglyceride (LCT) diet originally formulated by Wilder (23), implemented most often clinically as a 4:1 ratio of fats to carbohydrate + protein (24) or as the medium-chain triglyceride (MCT) diet developed by Huttenlocher et al. (25). The MCT diet was developed in an attempt to achieve higher levels of ketonemia in a diet that had a lower ketogenic ratio, reflecting a long-standing view that seizure protection depends on ketonemia. In addition, the MCT diet was thought to be more palatable. Both diet types have been shown to be effective in humans, although the MCT diet has generally been less well tolerated.

Ketogenic diets fed to rodents generally conform to the classical LCT diet. Thavendiranathan et al. *(26)*, however, fed the MCT diet to rats and found ketonemia equal to, or greater than, that found with the LCT diet, but no seizure protection against minimal electroshock threshold (MET) and no elevation of PTZ threshold. Interestingly, against MES and maximal PTZ seizures they found that the MCT diet was pro-convulsant. That substantial differences exist among such diets is suggested by variations in weight gain and levels of ketonemia attained by different laboratories. For example, Appleton and DeVivo *(19)*, DeVivo et al. *(27)*, and Al-Mudallal et al. *(28)* all reported weight gains in rats fed KDs that were not significantly different from those of animals fed control (rodent chow) diets; by contrast we *(29,30)* have routinely observed lower rates of growth in rats fed an LCT KD, even when it was fed *ad libitum*. Recently, Likhodii et al. *(31)* investigated qualitative differences among KDs but reported little difference in seizure protection among LCT diets differing in fat source. Another important variable in the administration of both ketogenic diets and non-KDs is whether there is calorie restriction and, if so, the degree of restriction imposed. This general issue is addressed elsewhere in this volume *(see* Chapter 19). It is also likely that some of the differences in growth, ketonemia, and seizure protection are attributable to differences in animal strains or in the ages of the animals used.

3.2. Role of Age

Ketone bodies are used preferentially in brain and lung in newborn rats for both energy *(32,33)* and synthesis of phospholipids in myelination *(34)*. β-Hydroxybutyrate (BHB) has also been shown to contribute more to cerebral energy than does glucose in early human fetal brains *(35)*. We have found that age is inversely related to ketonemia *(29,36)* a conclusion that was supported by path analysis *(37)*. Uhlemann and Neims *(38)* showed that young but not old mice fed a KD were protected from MES, where "young" was considered to be postnatal day 16 (P16) and "old" was P40. In children, both age and age-independent factors were found to affect the level of ketonemia when an MCT diet was consumed *(39);* a positive relationship between the level of BHB and the degree of seizure control was determined to exist. The study population consisted of 18 children ranging from 1.5 to 18 yr, but there was no indication of whether age differences contributed to the relationship, a conclusion favored in a recent study of rats *(29)*.

3.3. Role of Ketonemia

3.3.1. β-HYDROXYBUTYRATE

Otani et al. *(40)* showed that an MCT KD gave robust, i.e., 6- to 20-fold, elevation of BHB but did not protect mice from MET and was not correlated with the protection they observed against daily ip injections of PTZ (45 mg/kg). A similar lack of correlation between seizure threshold and BHB was noted in juvenile rats fed either the LCT diet *(37,41)* or the MCT diet *(26)* or in adult rats fed the MCT diet *(31)*. In adult male Wistar rats fed a KD *ad libitum*, Harik et al. *(42)* found only modest ketonemia (0.5m*M*) and several-fold elevation of cerebral BHB but no significant reduction in blood glucose.

Regrettably, the investigators did not test seizure susceptibility. Harney et al. *(43)* found that blockade with mercaptoacetate, an inhibitor of fatty acid oxidation, lowered ketonemia and shortened latency to threshold PTZ-induced seizures but reported no correlation between latency and BHB levels. Ketone bodies do not appear to have direct effects on synaptic transmission in the hippocampus, at least when applied acutely in tissue taken from rats not fed a KD *(44)*. Cullingford et al. *(45)* have shown that the gene for a key ketogenic synthetic enzyme, mitochondrial 3-hydroxy-3-methylglutaryl-CoA synthase, is upregulated in both liver and brain in rats fed a KD. The same gene is downregulated in suckling rats weaned to a low-fat, high-carbohydrate diet *(46)*. BHB uptake by the rat brain is proportional to the arterial blood concentration, and all BHB entering the brain is metabolized *(47)*. Sokoloff *(48)* observed that when BHB completely replaced glucose in the medium used to perfuse a rat brain, brain function deteriorated as rapidly as it did following removal of all energetic substrates, suggesting that BHB cannot substitute fully for glucose or, perhaps, other ketone bodies.

3.3.2. ACETONE

Elevation of brain acetone has been reported by Seymour et al. *(49)* in epileptic humans fed a KD and has been suggested by Rho et al. *(50)* as a possible link to seizure resistance in rodents fed a KD. Exhaled acetone has also recently been shown to provide a good estimate of ketonemia *(51,52)*.

3.4. Role of Calorie Restriction

Calorie restriction appears to be a critical part of the success of KDs in acute models, as it is in clinical practice. However, few experimental studies have administered KDs on a calorie-restricted basis. The role of calorie restriction is not addressed here (*see* Chapter 19).

4. EFFICACY OF THE KD AGAINST ACUTE SEIZURE MODELS

4.1. Chemoconvulsants

The fairly recent resurgence of clinical interest in the KD appears to reflect both a long track record of success, particularly at Johns Hopkins, and publicity driven by the Charlie Foundation (Santa Monica, California). Experimental interest in the KD derives from its effectiveness against both epilepsy and acutely induced seizures and from awareness that it resembles fasting and is within the range of mammals' physiological adaptive responses. The KD has been shown to be effective against a wide variety of epileptic types in humans *(53)* and against a variety of proconvulsants in experimental animals.

This list of proconvulsants includes agents that induce their effects through each of the four major classes of ion channels that Rho and Sankar *(54)* have summarized as being the targets of the most clinically significant AEDs. Those targets, and examples of proconvulsants acting at them, are chloride channels associated with the GABA$_A$ receptor (PTZ, BIC, PTX), sodium and calcium channels associated with two types of ionotropic glutamate receptor (*N*-methyl-D-asparate [NMDA] and kainate) and voltage-dependent sodium channels (MET and MES). In addition, Snead *(55,56)* has shown that γ-butyrolactone/γ-hydroxybutyrate (GBL/GHB) activate low-threshold T-type Ca^{2+} channels secondary to activation of GABA$_B$ and specific GHB receptors. Antagonists of the GABA$_B$ receptor are candidate antiabsence drugs *(57)*, and T-type Ca^{2+} channels appear to be the target of ethosuximide *(58)*, an effective antiabsence drug, although there is some controversy in this regard *(59)*. $GABA_B$ receptors and T-type Ca^{2+} channels have also been implicated in absence seizures of lethargic mice *(60)*.

4.1.1. Low-Dose PTZ

PTZ is thought to decrease the mean open time of the $GABA_A$ channel by binding allosterically at the PTX site *(61)*. Administration of the classical (LCT) KD to Sprague-Dawley rats has been shown to increase the resistance to PTZ-induced threshold seizures, as demonstrated in at least two routes of administration. In the first, in comparison to controls, rats maintained on a KD exhibited a greater resistance to PTZ when it was infused into the tail vein *(29,30,36,37,41,62)*, a technique developed by Pollock and Shen *(63)*. In the second, Harney et al. *(43)* showed that rats maintained on an LCT KD were more resistant to repetitive, low doses (10 mg/kg) of PTZ than were controls.

4.1.2. Maximal-Dose PTZ, BIC, and PTX

BIC and PTX have been shown to be $GABA_A$ competitive and allosteric antagonists, respectively *(64)*. It is noteworthy, however, that the relationship between GABA receptors and both BIC and PTX is not a simple one *(64,65)*. When PTZ was injected in a dose that induced generalized seizures in 100% of control animals (50 mg/kg in this study), the cohorts of rats maintained on various KDs exhibited fewer seizures than did control animals *(31)*. Furthermore, the seizure score for the KD group was significantly reduced. By contrast, in another study by the same group of investigators, the MCT KD did not confer protection against threshold PTZ seizures (70 mg/kg) and was actually proconvulsant against maximal PTZ-induced seizures (85 mg/kg) *(26)*. Curiously, findings in mice have been nearly the opposite of those described in rats. Uhlemann and Neims *(38)* found that a version of the LCT KD gave protection against tonic extension induced by BIC injection but did not alter the response to PTZ (85 mg/kg).

4.1.3. γ-Butyrolactone/γ-Hydroxybutyrate

Evidence based on a very small number of observations *(66)* suggests that the LCT KD reduces the latency to, number, and duration of spike-wave discharges (SWD) evoked by injection of GBL (100 mg/kg ip) in a model of absence seizures developed by Snead *(67)*. GBL is metabolized to GHB, which is an agonist for both $GABA_B$ receptors and specific GHB receptors *(68)*.

4.1.4. Strychnine

Strychnine is a glycine receptor antagonist. In the single study that has been reported, the classical KD was found to have no effect against strychnine-induced seizures in rats *(66)*.

4.1.5. Kainate

Acute injection of a single dose of kainic acid sufficient to induce status epilepticus (10 mg/kg, ip and sc) evoked more severe seizures and caused more deaths during the period of status in rats fed a classical KD than in those fed an isocaloric rodent chow diet *(66)*.

Chronically, if kainate-treated animals are maintained after recovery from status epilepticus, spontaneous seizures develop (69). Although latency and severity of post-status epilepticus spontaneous seizures did not differ significantly between animals fed control and KDs, the KD-fed rats had fewer seizures of shorter duration (70). Also, hippocampal neurons in brains from animals fed the KD showed less mossy fiber sprouting than did those of rats fed the control diet following kainate-induced status epilepticus, and there was evidence of reduced hyperexcitability in hippocampal area CA1 (71). It was also found that early introduction of the KD to rats, rendered spontaneously epileptic following induction of status epilepticus by kainate injection, reduced the incidence of recurrent seizures (72). A similar reduction in seizure incidence was not seen in rats switched to the KD 14 d after induction of status epilepticus. Interestingly, however, early introduction of the KD resulted in poorer performance in the water maze test and diminished weight gain comparison to either controls or rats that began the KD at 14 d after status epilepticus. For further discussion of KD vs chronic models of epilepsy, see Chapter 22.

4.1.6. FLUROTHYL

Rho et al. *(73)* showed that the KD increased latency to first clonus induced by flurothyl inhalation in juvenile mice fed the diet for 7 and 12 d but had no effect on the first clonus of adults fed the diet for as much as 15 d. The diet was not anticonvulsant for the later tonic extension in juvenile mice regardless of the duration of ketogenic feeding, but it did delay tonic extension in the adults. The mechanism by which flurothyl induces seizures remains unknown *(74)*, although such seizures can be blocked by drugs acting either at $GABA_A$ receptors *(74)* or at NMDA receptors *(75)*.

4.2. Electroconvulsive Stimuli

4.2.1. Minimum Electroshock Threshold

Electroshock depolarizes neurons directly and generates synchronous discharges that result in seizures. The relationship between seizures generated by electroshock and diet is varied and can depend on the intensity of the shock being administered. Millichap et al. *(76)* showed that a KD (beef fat) protected female mice from the lowered threshold to MES induced by ip injection of water (100 mL/kg) and that the protection was independent of BHB levels. In early experimental investigations of the KD, Appleton and DeVivo *(19,77)* described elevation of minimum electroshock threshold (MET) in adult rats. Nakazawa et al. *(78)* also found elevation of MET in mice by an MCT KD. Otani et al. *(40)*, however, found that their MCT KD lowered MET in mice.

4.2.2. MAXIMAL ELECTROSHOCK

Variable effects of KDs on seizures following MES have also been described. In one of the earliest studies, Davenport and Davenport *(79)* found that a calorie-restricted normal diet failed to protect male rats against MES, making maximal seizures more severe, i.e., increased extension time; the diet also lowered the threshold for MET. As noted earlier, Thavendiranathan et al. *(26)* found that an (MCT) KD afforded no change in MET but was actually proconvulsant for MES seizures. Bough et al. *(62)* also found that MES seizures were more severe in rats fed the classical KD. The increased MES severity was found both in rats that showed elevation of PTZ threshold (tail-vein infusion) and in seizure-naive rats. Likhodii et al. *(31)* also found elevated PTZ threshold but more severe seizures provoked by MES in rats fed a variety of KDs.

4.2.3. ELECTRICAL KINDLING

We know of only one published study of the effects of the KD on (amygdala) kindled seizures. In this study, the KD afforded transient (2 wk) elevation of seizure threshold and after-discharge threshold, without any consequences for either after-discharge or seizure duration, or for any observed behaviors *(80)*.

4.3. Hyperbaric Oxygen

Rats subjected to 24–36 h of fasting and/or dehydration showed increased latency to seizures induced by hyperbaric oxygen (0.5 MPa, approx 5 atm) *(81,82)*. Chavko et al. *(82)* showed that BHB levels were elevated and glucose levels were lowered. Furthermore, despite elevation of ketonemia to twice the level seen during fasting (achieved by infusion of 1,3-butanediol, a metabolic precursor of BHB), seizure latency remained at control values. Restoration of normal levels of blood glucose in the fasted animal *increased* seizure latency.

4.4. Audiogenic Stimuli

Rats made deficient in Mg^{2+} were found to be more prone to audiogenic seizures (decreased latency, increased incidence and severity) when fed a KD *(83)*. Curiously, Mg^{2+}-deficient rats showed no change in latency but had reduced incidence and severity of such seizures when they were fasted, suggesting that consumption of KDs is not equivalent to fasting.

4.5. Caveats

As White et al. *(84)* have cautioned, it is unwise to "speculate about the mechanism of action of a drug based solely on its ability to prevent seizures induced by a chemoconvulsant with a known mechanism of action." The effectiveness of systemic application of convulsant drugs depends on access to the brain across the blood–brain barrier and may be affected by actions on receptors on nonnervous tissue, complicating interpretation of physiological and behavioral responses *(85)*. Once across the blood–brain barrier, a drug may have actions on receptors on neurons in many different parts of the CNS, and the overall effect may be dose dependent and difficult to predict. We might add that it is also unwise to speculate about the mechanism of ictogenesis of proconvulsant drugs even when the mechanism of drug action is well known.

As noted above, it has been shown repeatedly that the KD elevates the threshold to PTZ-induced seizures but makes MES seizures more severe. In addition to the different targets of these proconvulsant treatments, Miller et al. *(86)* have shown that different structures in the brain are involved in seizures induced by either PTZ or MES. As determined by blockade with GVG, PTZ-induced seizures involve extensive structures including the reticular formation, the diencephalon, and descending motor pathways. By contrast, only the substantia nigra appeared to mediate MES-induced seizures. Although these observations indicate that there are differences in the parts of the brain involved in these two types of experimental seizure, it is important to emphasize that the anatomical pattern described is defined by the agent (GVG) used to block seizures of both origins. Injection of GVG into the substantia nigra did not block PTZ-induced seizures. By contrast, Okada et al. *(87)* were able to block PTZ-induced seizures by injecting a GABA agonist (muscimol) into the substantia nigra. Reconciliation of these seemingly inconsistent findings may depend on differences in the rate of action of a direct GABA agonist (muscimol) versus the comparatively long time course of GABA elevation following enzyme inactivation by GVG, as demonstrated by Gale and Iadorola *(17)*. The substantia nigra appears to be a key control point for seizure propagation, and it seems likely that many such control points will be found. Okada et al. *(87)* also showed that in contrast to its action in substantia nigra, muscimol was proconvulsant when focally injected into the pedunculopontine nucleus. The identity and importance of such sites will likely depend on such variables as the type of epilepsy or, for experimental work, the nature of the proconvulsant drug, the nature of specific anticonvulsant strategies, including drugs, diets, metabolic status, physiological stressors, gender, and circadian and other biological rhythms. Clearly, the consequences of altered levels of transmitters (or agonists, or antagonists) for ictogenesis depend on the neural circuits affected, and targeting is nonspecific when neuroactive agents are applied systemically.

The KD and GVG are not the only treatments that distinguish between PTZ- and MES-induced seizures. Nimodipine and PCA 50922, both calcium channel antagonists, each protected mice against seizures induced by sc injection of PTZ (100 mg/kg) but showed no effect on MES-induced seizures *(88)*. Conversely, the histamine antagonist clobenpropit afforded mice no protection against PTZ-induced (85 mg/kg, sc) seizures but did reduce MES severity *(89)*. Seizure protection against both PTZ- and MES-induced seizures was demonstrated in both rats and mice following administration of D-23129 (retigabine) *(90),* an anticonvulsant with demonstrated actions at both M channels *(91)* and $GABA_A$ receptors *(92)*.

Acute models help to define the many variables affecting seizure generation and propagation and hint at the number of genes likely to be involved in human epilepsies. Perhaps a few major themes will emerge, with many specific modifiers.

5. SUMMARY

5.1. What Might the Ability of the KD to Block Seizures Tell Us?

From a very broad perspective, acute studies of the KD show that excitability and synchrony, key features of seizures and epilepsy in the CNS, are markedly dependent on the quantity (*ad libitum;* calorie restricted) and quality (chow, high fat, high carbohydrate) of the substrate that is being used to support metabolism. As Lack *(93)* indicated decades ago, food is one of the major factors limiting mammalian populations. Yet, humans living in developed countries and experimental animals living in regulated animal care facilities have unlimited access to food and balanced diets. Indeed, it is often necessary to justify NOT feeding laboratory animals *ad libitum,* despite recognition of the value of food restriction by National Institutes of Health Guidelines (*see* ref. *94*). Caloric restriction and intermittent dependence on bodily stores of carbohydrates and fats are nearer the norm for animals in the wild and for many populations, and these were most likely the conditions our ancestors endured in the not-so-distant past *(95)*. We tend to view calorie restriction and consumption of KDs as protective against seizures; but we could also view the abundance of unrestricted high-quality foods as permissive, if not causative, of the incidence of seizures seen in human populations in developed countries. Epilepsy is, however, more common in undeveloped countries *(96)* for a variety of reasons *(97–99),* including malnutrition. Indeed, rats consuming "malnutritious" diets are more prone to seizures *(100)*.

The effectiveness of the KD against a wide range of human epilepsies and against a variety of proconvulsants in experimental animals suggests that the diet alters a variety of neuronal substrates. For example, the diet may affect receptors involved in the production of epileptic or experimental seizures; it may alter fundamental neurochemistry, e.g., transmitter synthesis/degradation or release/reuptake; it may change receptor abundance or subtype; or it may affect neuronal/glial energy supply and maintenance of homeostasis. Mechanistic studies of the KD are in their infancy, despite earlier assertions purporting to describe underlying actions of KD *(76,100)*. Rather, most experimental studies of the KD, including our own, e.g., ref. *29,* consist of attempts either to determine the relevancy of animal models to the use of KDs to control human epileptic seizures or to identify important conditions or correlates of success against seizures. Except for the epileptic mutant strains that have been developed or characterized fairly recently (*see* reviews, refs. *102* and *103*), animal studies have involved either normal, nonepileptic animals subjected to acute seizures, i.e., chemoconvulsants/electroshock, or animals subjected to more chronic treatments that have caused them to develop spontaneous seizures, i.e., pilocarpine, kainate, or kindling.

5.2. Seizures and Metabolism

In general, KDs, calorie restriction, and starvation are protective against small doses of proconvulsants in that they elevate seizure threshold, but they are either ineffective or proconvulsant for treatments that provoke maximal seizures (MES, maximal PTZ, doses of kainate that induce status epilepticus). An attractive hypothesis that might account for this pattern of observations is one that invokes potassium channels sensitive to adenosine triphosphate (ATP) and low-threshold calcium channels. These potassium channels bind either adenosine diphosphate (ADP) or ATP. When bound to ATP, the channels are closed; when bound to ADP the channels are opened *(104)*. If metabolism, as indicated by overall ATP production, is depressed, then the ratio of ATP to ADP will decrease and the proportion of K_{ATP} channels bound to ATP will decrease and those bound to ADP will increase. An increase in the number of channels as K_{ADP} would increase the membrane conductance to K^+, causing the membrane to approach the potassium equilibrium potential E_K, meaning that it would hyperpolarize. One consequence of such hyperpolarization could be that threshold is elevated, as a result of the requirement for more depolarizing current to reach threshold.

If the cell membrane included a sizable (difficult-to-specify) number of low-threshold calcium channels, a second consequence of the hyperpolarization would be deinactivation (activation) of these channels. Any stimulus, e.g., MES, that forced depolarization might then activate some critical number of these low-threshold calcium channels, leading to a more severe seizure. Clearly, the explanation for dietary elevation of threshold seizures and exacerbation of maximal seizures offered here is critically dependent on the voltage sensitivity and kinetics of all the voltage-gated channels affecting cell excitability: sodium, potassium, and calcium channels, in the least.

5.3. Energy

A larger difficulty for the hypothesis just advanced is that a key part of it is in conflict with experimental data. Intuitively, it makes sense to anticipate that starvation and calorie restriction, and perhaps KDs, result in reduced availability of energy-containing metabolites. It has been shown repeatedly, however, that brain energetics are either unchanged *(42)* or improved when animals consume KDs and develop ketonemia *(27,78)*. Zeigler et al. *(105)* have shown that a KD results in a general increase in protein phosphorylation in rat brains and that elevation of ketone bodies in the incubation medium promotes phosphate uptake by brain slices. Similarly, Pan et al. *(106)* have shown increased levels of high-energy phosphates, including ATP, in a variety of human epileptic patients maintained on a KD.

Elevated rates of phosphorylation and levels of high-energy phosphates may not, however, be the variables most relevant to the hypothesis. Baukrowitz et al. *(107)* and Shyng and Nichols *(108)* have independently shown that inhibition of K_{ATP} channels by ATP is highly dependent on regulation by phosphatidylinositol (PIP). Elevation of PIP_2 levels can dramatically reduce the ATP-mediated inhibition of K_{ATP} channels. In 2001 Yamada et al. *(109)* showed that ATP-sensitive potassium channels in substantia nigra, where they are most abundant, were protective against generalized seizures induced by hypoxia. This class of potassium channel is widely distributed and has been shown to modulate smooth muscle contraction, thereby regulating cerebral circulation *(110)*. It is also important in control of membrane potential and catecholamine release by adrenal chromaffin cells *(111)*. As Szot describes in Chapter 20, catecholamines are important mediators of seizure protection by KDs.

Carbon budgets vary with diet, and the possible relevance of such variation to seizure control is poorly understood. Kekwick and Pawan *(112)* found that isocaloric high-carbohydrate and high-fat diets were utilized differently by mice. The greater non-CO_2 carbon loss of the high-fat diet was shown to reflect the loss of body fat and the inefficient use of fat-based carbon on such diets. Hawkins et al. *(113)* reported that the brains of rats starved for 2 d showed little change from glucose to ketone body utilization, unlike the large reduction (>25%) of brain glucose metabolism described in humans by Hasselbalch et al. *(114)*. Brain infusion of BHB has been shown to reduce body weight without a reduction in food consumption, as happened when glucose was infused *(115)*, but intracerebroventricular (ICV) infusion of BHB resulted in increased adiposity despite the decrease in weight *(116)*, a phenomenon we have noted in rats fed a calorie-restricted KD (Bough and Eagles, unpublished data).

5.4. Comparisons With Drugs

There are few comparisons between the KD and AEDs. We showed that the KD is about as effective as 300 mg/kg valproate in elevating the threshold of PTZ-induced seizures *(30)*. Furthermore, we observed that valproate and the KD have additive effects, suggesting the KD and VPA may act synergistically against PTZ-induced seizures. Curiously, of the classical anticonvulsants, VPA is among the most widely effective but, like the KD, is also among the least understood. It has been shown to reduce low-threshold calcium currents *(117)* and to have phenytoin-like effects against repetitive discharge in neurons *(118);* yet both effects are weak, and the mechanism by which valproate affords protection against absence epilepsy and a wide variety of convulsive seizure types remains uncertain *(20)*. Some medications that reduce convulsions by acting on GABA receptors or channels worsen absence seizures *(68)*. Perhaps the nearly unique ability of VPA (and the KD) to block absence seizures as well as convulsive and myoclonic seizure types *(119)* reflects these two different cellular actions.

5.5. Neurotoxicity and Memory Deficits

Chronic administration of a calorie-restricted KD did not affect neurobehavioral function *(41)*. By comparison, acute administration of high doses of VPA and phenytoin, singly, resulted in decreased neurobehavioral function as assessed in a standard battery of tests *(30)*. Additionally, the performance of animals maintained on a KD was similar to that of controls in the Morris water maze and open-field test *(80)*. From these data it was concluded that spatial memory and exploratory behavior are not altered as a result of diet treatment, further suggesting that chronic consumption of a KD does not markedly alter neurobehavioral function in rats.

6. CONCLUSION

In terms of the breadth of its anti-ictal (and antiepileptic) efficacy the KD seems to stand alone. Its effectiveness against acute threshold convulsive and nonconvulsive seizures, but not against maximal seizures, its effectiveness in alleviating the symptoms of glucose transporter deficiency *(120)*, the action of ICV BHB *(115,116)* and of the KD *(41)* in elevating metabolism, its elevation of phosphorylation in the brain, e.g., ref. *105,* and its alteration of transmitter synthesis (121–123) *(see* also Chapter 15) all argue for a role in altering fundamental metabolic processes as a key to the mechanism(s) by which the KD, calorie restriction, and starvation alter seizures and epilepsy. Perhaps our newfound ability to sequence and insert genes and to study their products, combined with more conventional approaches, will enable us to discover the basis of the epilepsies and how they can be alleviated.

REFERENCES

1. Prasad AN, Stafstrom CE, Holmes GL. Alternative epilepsy strategies: the ketogenic diet, immunoglobulins, and steroids. Epilepsia 1996;37 (Suppl 1):S81–S95.
2. Merritt HH, Putnam TJ. Sodium diphenylhydantoinate in the treatment of convulsive disorders. J Am Med Assoc 1938;111:1068–1073.
3. Richards RK, Everett GM. Analgesic and anticonvulsive properties of 3,5,5-trimethyloxazoliidine-2,4-dione (Tridione). Fed Proc 1944;3:39.
4. Krall RL, Penry JK, White BG, Kupferberg HJ, Swinyard EA. Antiepileptic drug development: II. Anticonvulsant drug screening. Epilepsia 1978;19:409–428.
5. Schachter SC. Current evidence indicates that antiepileptic drugs are anti-ictal, not antiepileptic. Epilepsy Res 2002;50:67–70.
6. Jacobs MP, Fischbach, GD, Davis, MR, Dichter MA, Dingledine R, Lowenstein DH, Morrell MJ, Noebels JL, Rogawski MA, Spencer SS, Theodore WH. Future directions for epilepsy research. Neurology 2001;57:1536–1542.
7. Meldrum B. Do preclinical seizure models preselect certain adverse effects of antiepileptic drugs? Epilepsy Res 2002;50:33–40.
8. Sankar R, Weaver DF. Basic principles of medicinal chemistry. In: Engel J Jr, Pedley TA (eds.). Epilepsy: A Comprehensive Textbook, Vol. 2. Philadelphia, Lippincott-Raven, 1997, pp. 1394–1403.
9. MacLean MJ, Macdonald RL. Multiple actions of phenytoin on mouse spinal cord neurons in cell culture. J Pharmacol Exp Ther 1983;227:779–789.
10. Schwarz J, Grigat G. Phenytoin and carbamazepine: potential- and frequency-dependent block of Na$^+$ currents in mammalian myelinated nerve fibers. Epilepsia 1989;30:286–294.
11. Jung MJ, Lippert B, Metcalf BW, Bohlen P, Schechter PJ. Gamma-vinyl GABA (4-amino-hex-5-enoic acid), a new selective irreversible inhibitor of GABA-T; effects on brain GABA metabolism in mice. J Neurochem 1977;29:797–802.
12. Browne TR, Mattson RH, Penry JK, Smith DB, Treiman DM, Wilder BJ, Ben-Menachem E, Napoliello MJ, Sherry KM, Szabo GK. Vigabatrin for refractory complex partial seizures. Multicenter single-blind study and long-term follow-up. Neurology 1987;37:184–189.
13. Sayin Ü, Cengiz S, Altug T. Vigabatrin as an anticonvulsant against pentylenetetrazol seizures. Pharmacol Res 1993;28:325–331.

14. Hosford DA, Wang Y. Utility of the lethargic (LH/LH) mouse model of absence seizures in predicting the effects of lamotrigine, vigabatrin, tiagabine, gabapentin, and topiramate against human absence seizures. Epilepsia 1997;38:408–414.

15. Schechter PJ, Trainier Y, Jung MJ, Sjoerdsma A. Antiseizure activity of γ-acetylenic γ-aminobutyric acid: a catalytic irreversible inhibitor of γ-aminobutyric acid transaminase. J Pharmacol Exp Ther 1977;201:606–612.

16. Schechter PJ, Trainier Y. Effect of elevated brain GABA concentration on the actions of bicuculline and picrotoxin in mice. Psychopharmacology 1977;54:145–148.

17. Gale K, Iadorola MJ. Seizure protection and increased nerve terminal GABA: delayed effects of GABA transaminase inhibition. Science 1980;208:288–291.

18. Gale K. Role of the substantia nigra in GABA-mediated anticonvulsant actions. In: Delgado-Escueta, Ward AA, Woodbury DM, Porter RJ (eds.). Basic Mechanisms of the Epilepsies: Molecular and Cellular Approaches. Raven, New York, Advances in Neurology, Vol. 44, 1986, pp. 343–364.

19. Appleton DB, DeVivo DC. An animal model for the ketogenic diet. Epilepsia 1974;15:211–227.

20. Macdonald RL. Cellular effects of antiepileptic drugs. In: Engel J Jr and Pedley TA (eds.). Epilepsy: A Comprehensive Textbook, Vol. 2. Philadelphia, Lippincott-Raven, 1997, pp. 1383–1391.

21. Llinás R, Yarom Y. Properties and distribution of ionic conductances generating electroresponsiveness of mammalian inferior olivary neurones in vitro. J Physiol 1981;315:569–584.

22. Swinyard EA. Laboratory evaluation of antiepileptic drugs. Epilepsia 1969;10:107–119.

23. Wilder RM. The effects of ketonemia on the course of epilepsy. Mayo Clin Bull 1921;2:307–308.

24. Freeman JM, Kelly MT, Freeman JB. The Epilepsy Diet Treatment: An Introduction to the Ketogenic Diet. Demos, New York, 1994.

25. Huttenlocher PR, Wilbourn AJ, Signore JM. Medium-chain triglycerides as a therapy for intractable childhood epilepsy. Neurology 1971;21:1097–1103.

26. Thavendirinathan P, Mendonca A, Dell C, Likhodii SS, Musa K, Iracleous C, Cunnane SC, Burnham WM. The MCT ketogenic diet: effects on animal seizure models. Exp Neurol 2000;161:696–703.

27. DeVivo DC, Leckie MP, Ferrendelli JS, McDougal DB Jr. Chronic ketosis and cerebral metabolism. Ann Neurol 1978;3:331–337.

28. Al-Mudallal AS, LaManna JC, Lust WD, Harik SI. Diet-induced ketosis does not cause cerebral acidosis. Epilepsia 1996;37:258–261.

29. Bough KJ, Eagles DA. A ketogenic diet increases the resistance to pentylenetetrazole-induced seizures in the rat. Epilepsia 1999;40:138–143.

30. Bough KJ, Eagles DA. Comparison of the anticonvulsant efficacies and neurotoxic effects of valproic acid, phenytoin, and the ketogenic diet. Epilepsia 2001;42:1345–1353.

31. Likhodii SS, Musa K, Mendonca A, Dell C, Burnham WM, Cunnane SC. Dietary fat, ketosis, and seizure resistance in rats on the ketogenic diet. Epilepsia 2000;41:1400–1410.

32. DeVivo DC, Fujimoto K, Leckie MP, Agrawal HC. Subcellular distribution of ketone body metabolizing enzymes in the rat brain. J Neurochem 1976;26:635–637.

33. DeVivo DC. The effects of ketone bodies on glucose utilization. In: Passoneau JV, Hawkins RA, Lust WD, Welsh FA (eds.). Cerebral Metabolism and Neural Function. Williams & Wilkins, Baltimore, 1980, pp. 243–254.

34. Yeh Y-Y, Sheehan PM. Preferential utilization of ketone bodies in the brain and lung of newborn rats. Fed Proc 1985;44:2352–2358.

35. Adam PAJ, Räihä N, Rahiala E-L, Kekomäki. Oxidation of glucose and D-β-OH-butyrate by the early human fetal brain. Acta Paediatr Scand 1975;64:17–24.

36. Bough KJ, Valiyil R, Han FT, Eagles DA. Seizure resistance is dependent upon age and calorie restriction in rats fed a ketogenic diet. Epilepsy Res 1999;35:21–28.

37. Bough KJ, Chen RS, Eagles DA. Path analysis shows that increasing ketogenic ratio, but not β-hydroxybutyrate, elevates seizure threshold in the rat. Dev Neurosci 1999;21:400–406.

38. Uhlemann ER, Neims AH. Anticonvulsant properties of the ketogenic diet in mice. J Pharmacol Exp Ther 1972;180:231–238.

39. Huttenlocher PR. Ketonemia and seizures: metabolic and anticonvulsant effects of two ketogenic diets in childhood epilepsy. Pediatr Res 1976;10:536–540.

40. Otani K, Yamatodani A, Wada H, Mimaki T, Yabuuchi T. Effect of ketogenic diet on convulsive threshold and brain monoamine levels in young mice. No To Hattatsu 1984;16:196–204.

41. Bough KJ, Yao SG, Eagles DA. Higher ketogenic diet ratios confer protection from seizures without neurotoxicity. Epilepsy Res 2000;38:15–25.

42. Harik SI, Al-Mudallal AS, LaManna JC, Lust WD, Levin BE. Ketogenic diet and the brain. Ann N Y Acad Sci 1997;835:218–224.

43. Harney JP, Madara J, Madara J, I'Anson H. Effects of acute inhibition of fatty acid oxidation on latency to seizure and concentrations of β-hydroxybutyrate in plasma of rats maintained on calorie restriction and/or the ketogenic diet. Epilepsy Res 2002;49:239–246.

44. Thio LL, Wong M, Yamada KA. Ketone bodies do not directly alter excitatory or inhibitory hippocampal synaptic transmission. Neurology 2000;54:325–331.

45. Cullingford TE, Eagles DA, Sato H. The ketogenic diet upregulates expression of the gene encoding the key ketogenic enzyme mitochondrial 3-hydroxy-3-methylglutaryl-CoA synthase in rat brain. Epilepsy Res 2002;49:99–107.

46. Cullingford TE, Dolphin CT, Bhakoo KK, Peuchen S, Canevari L, Clark JB. Molecular cloning of rat mitochondrial 3-hydroxy-3-methylglutaryl-CoA lyase and detection of the corresponding mRNA and of those encoding the remaining enzymes comprising the ketogenic 3-hydroxy-3-methylglutaryl-CoA cycle in central nervous system of suckling rat. Biochem J 1998;329:373–381.

47. Daniel PM, Love ER, Moorehouse SR, Pratt OE, Wilson P. Factors influencing utilisation of ketone-bodies by brain in normal rats and rats with ketoacidosis. Lancet 1971;2:637–638.

48. Sokoloff L. Metabolism of ketone bodies by the brain. Ann Rev Med 1973;24:271–280.

49. Seymour KJ, Bluml S, Sutherling J, Sutherling W, Ross B. Identification of cerebral acetone by ^{1}H-MRS in patients with epilepsy controlled by ketogenic diet. MAGMA 1999;8:33–42.

50. Rho JM, Anderson GD, Donevan SD, White HS. Acetoacetate, acetone, and dibenzylamine (a contaminant in 1-(+)-beta-hydroxybutyrate) exhibit direct anticonvulsant actions in vivo. Epilepsia 2002;43:358–361.

51. Likhodii SS, Musa K, Cunnane SC. Breath acetone as a measure of systemic ketosis assessed in a rat model of the ketogenic diet. Clin Chem 2002;48:115–120.

52. Musa-Veloso K, Likhodii SS, Cunnane SC. Breath acetone is a reliable indicator of ketosis in adults consuming ketogenic meals. Am J Clin Nutr 2002;76:65–70.

53. Freeman JM, Vining EPG, Pillas DJ, Pyzik PL, Casey JC, Kelly MT. The efficacy of the ketogenic diet-1998: A prospective evaluation of intervention in 150 children. Pediatrics 1998;102:1358–1363.

54. Rho JM, Sankar R. The pharmacologic basis of antiepileptic drug action. Epilepsia 1999;40:1471–1483.

55. Snead OC III. Basic mechanisms of generalized absence seizures. Ann Neurol 1995;37:146–157.

56. Snead OC III. Antiabsence seizure activity of specific GABA$_B$ and γ-hydroxybutyric acid receptor antagonists. Pharmacol Biochem Behav 1996;53:73–79.

57. Marescaux C, Vergnes M, Bernasconi R. GABA$_B$ receptor antagonists: potential new antiabsence drugs. J Neural Transm 1992;35:179–188.

58. Coulter DA, Huguenard JR, Prince DA. Characterization of ethosuximide reduction of low-threshold calcium current in thalamic neurons. Ann Neurol 1989;25:582–593.

59. Leresche N, Parri HR, Erdemli G, Guyon A, Turner JP, Williams SR, Asprodini E, Crunelli V. On the action of the anti-absence drug ethosuximide in the rat and cat thalamus. J Neurosci 1998;18:4842–4853.

60. Hosford DA, Clark S, Cao Z, Wilson WA Jr, Lin F-H, Morrisett RA, Huin A. The role of GABA$_B$ receptor activation in absence seizures of lethargic (LH/LH) mice. Science 1992;257:398–401.

61. Huang R-Q, Bell-Horner CL, Dibas MI, Covey DF, Drewe JA, Dillon GH. Pentylenetetrazole-induced inhibition of recombinant γ-aminobutyric acid type A (GABA$_A$) receptors: mechanism and site of action. J Pharmacol Exp Ther 2001;298:986–995.

62. Bough KJ, Matthews PJ, Eagles DA. A ketogenic diet has different effects upon seizures induced by maximal electroshock and by pentylenetetrazole infusion. Epilepsy Res 2000;38:105–114.

63. Pollock GM, Shen DD. A timed intravenous pentylenetetrazol infusion seizure model for quantitating the anticonvulsant effect of valproic acid in the rat. J Pharmacol Methods 1985;13:135–146.

64. Olsen RW, Wong EHF, Stauber GB, King RG. Biochemical pharmacology of the γ-aminobutyric acid receptor/ionophore protein. Fed Proc 1984;43:2773–2778.

65. Seutin V, Johnson SW. Recent advances in the pharmacology of quaternary salts of bicuculline. Trends Pharmacol Sci 1999;20:268–270.

66. Bough KJ, Gudi K, Han FT, Rathod AH, Eagles DA. An anticonvulsant profile of the ketogenic diet in the rat. Epilepsy Res 2002;50:313–325.
67. Snead OC III. γ-Hydroxybutyrate model of generalized absence seizures: further characterization and comparison with other absence models. Epilepsia 1988;29:361–368.
68. Snead OC III. The ontogeny of [^{3}H]γ-hydroxybutyrate and [^{3}H]GABA$_B$ binding sites: relation to the development of experimental absence seizures. Brain Res 1994;659;147–156.
69. Stafstrom CE, Thompson JL, Holmes GL. Kainic acid seizures in the developing brain: status epilepticus and spontaneous recurrent seizures. Dev Brain Res 1992;65:227–236.
70. Muller-Schwarze AB, Tandon P, Liu Z, Yang Y, Holmes GL, Stafstrom CE. Ketogenic diet reduces spontaneous seizures and mossy fiber sprouting in the kainic acid model. NeuroReport 1999;10:1517–1522.
71. Stafstrom CE, Wang C, Jensen FE. Electrophysiological observations in hippocampal slices from rats treated with the ketogenic diet. Dev Neurosci 1999;21:393–399.
72. Su SW, Cilio MR, Sogawa Y, Silveira D, Holmes GL, Stafstrom CE. Timing of ketogenic diet initiation in an experimental epilepsy model. Dev Brain Res 2000;125:131–138.
73. Rho JM, Kim DW, Robbins CA, Anderson GD, Schwartzkroin PA. Age-dependent differences in flurothyl seizure sensitivity in mice treated with a ketogenic diet. Epilepsy Res 1999;37:233–240.
74. Liptáková S, Velísek L, Velísková J, Moshé SL. Effect of ganaxolone on flurothyl seizures in developing rats. Epilepsia 2000;41:788–793.
75. Velísek L, Velísková J, Ptachewich Y, Shinnar S, Moshé SL. Effects of MK-801 and phenytoin on flurothyl-induced seizures during development. Epilepsia 1995;36:179–185.
76. Millichap JG, Jones JD, Rudis BP. Mechanisms of anticonvulsant action of ketogenic diet. Am J Dis Child 1964;107:593–604.
77. Appleton DB, DeVivo DC. An experimental animal model for the effect of ketogenic diet on epilepsy. Proc Aust Assoc Neurol 1973;10:75–80.
78. Nakazawa M, Kodama S, Matsuo T. Effects of ketogenic diet on electroconvulsive threshold and brain contents of adenosine nucleotides. Brain Dev 1983;5:375–380.
79. Davenport VD, Davenport HW. The relation between starvation, metabolic acidosis and convulsive seizures in rats. J Nutr 1948;36:139–151.
80. Hori A, Tandon P, Holmes GL, Stafstrom CE. Ketogenic diet: effects on expression of kindled seizures and behavior in adult rats. Epilepsia 1997;38:750–758.
81. Bitterman N, Skapa E, Gutterman A. Starvation and dehydration attenuate CNS oxygen toxicity in rats. Brain Res 1997;761:146–150.
82. Chavko M, Braisted JC, Harabin AL. Attenuation of brain hyperbaric oxygen toxicity by fasting is not related to ketosis. Undersea Hyperbaric Med 1999;26:99–103.
83. Mahoney AW, Hendricks DG, Bernard N, Sisson DV. Fasting and ketogenic diet effects on audiogenic seizure susceptibility of magnesium deficient rats. Pharmacol Biochem Behav 1983;18:683–687.
84. White HS, Wolf HH, Woodhead JH, Kupferberg HJ. The National Institutes of Health anticonvulsant drug development program: Screening for efficacy. In: French J, Leppik I, Dichter MA (eds.). Advances in Neurology, Antiepileptic Drug Development, Vol. 76. Lippincott-Raven, Philadelphia, 1998, pp. 29–47.
85. Gale K. Chemoconvulsant seizures: advantages of focally-evoked seizure models. Ital J Neurol Sci 1995;16:17–25.
86. Miller JW, McKeon AC, Ferrendelli JA. Functional anatomy of pentylenetetrazol and electroshock seizures in the rat brainstem. Ann Neurol 1987;22:615–621.
87. Okada R, Negishi N, Nagaya H. The role of the nigrotegmental GABAergic pathway in the propagation of pentylenetetrazole-induced seizures. Brain Res 1989;480:383–387.
88. Zapater P, Javaloy J, Román JF, Vidal MT, Horga JF. Anticonvulsant effects of nimodipine and two novel dihydropyridines (PCA 50922 and PCA 50941) against seizures elicited by pentylenetetrazole and electroconvulsive shock in mice. Brain Res 1998;796:311–314.
89. Fischer W, van der Groot H. Effect of clobenpropit, a centrally acting histamine H$_3$-receptor antagonist, on electroshock- and pentylenetetrazole-induced seizures in mice. J Neural Transm 1998;105:587–599.
90. Rostock A, Tober C, Rundfelt C, Bartsch R, Engel J, Polymeropoulos EE, Kutscher B, Löscher W, Honack D, White HS, Wolf HH. D-23129: a new anti-convulsant with a broad spectrum of activity in animal models of epileptic seizures. Epilepsy Res 1996;23:211–223.

 91. Cooper EC. Potassium channels: how genetic studies of epileptic syndromes open paths to new thera-
     peutic targets and drugs. Epilepsia 2001;42 (Suppl 5):S49–S54.
 92. Otto JF, Kimball MM, Wilcox KS. Effects of the anticonvulsant retigabine on cultured cortical neu-
     rons: changes in electroresponsive properties and synaptic transmission. Mol Pharmacol
     2002;61:921–927.
 93. Lack D. The factors limiting mammals. In: Lack D (ed.). The Natural Regulation of Animal Num-
     bers. Clarendon, Oxford, UK, 1954, Chapter 16.
 94. Institute of Laboratory Animal Resources, Commission on Life Sciences, National Research Council.
     Guide for the Care and Use of Laboratory Animals. National Academy Press, Washington, DC, 1996.
 95. Friedman JM. A war on obesity, not the obese. Science 2003;299:856–858.
 96. Bolis CL. Epilepsy in developing countries. In: Penry JK (ed.). Epilepsy. The Eighth International
     Symposium. Raven, New York, 1977, pp. 355–357.
 97. Moshé SL, Albala BJ, Ackermann RF, Engel J Jr. Increased seizure susceptibility of the immature
     brain. Dev Brain Res 1983;7:81–85.
 98. Medina MT, Rosas E, Rubio-Donnadieu F, Sotelo J. Neurocysticercosis as the main cause of late-
     onset epilepsy in Mexico. Arch Intern Med 1990;150:325–327.
 99. Shorvon SD, Bharucha NE. Epilepsy in developing countries: epidemiology, aetiology and health
     care. In: Laidlaw J, Richens A, Chadwickle D (eds.). A Textbook of Epilepsy, 4th ed. Churchill Liv-
     ingston, Edinburgh, 1993, pp. 613–630.
100. Palencia G, Calvillo M, Sotelo J. Chronic malnutrition caused by a corn-based diet lowers the thresh-
     old for pentylenetetrazole-induced seizures in rats. Epilepsia 1996;37:583–586.
101. Withrow CD. The ketogenic diet: mechanisms of anticonvulsant action. In: Glaser GH, Penry JK,
     Woodbury DM (eds.). Antiepileptic Drugs: Mechanisms of Action. Raven, New York, 1980, pp.
     635–642.
102. Noebels JL, Rees M, Gardiner RM. Molecular genetics and epilepsy genes. In: Engel J Jr, Pedley TA
     (eds.). Epilepsy: A Comprehensive Textbook, Vol. 1. Lippincott-Raven, Philadelphia, 1997, pp.
     211–216.
103. Seyfried TN, Todorova MT, Poderycki MJ. Experimental models of multifactorial epilepsies: the EL
     mouse and mice susceptible to audiogenic seizures. Adv Neurol 1999;79:279–290.
104. Dzeja PP, Terzic A. Phosphotransfer reactions in the regulation of ATP-sensitive K+ channels. FASEB
     J 1998;12:523–529.
105. Ziegler DR, Araújo E, Rotta LN, Perry ML, Gonçalves C-A. A ketogenic diet increases protein phos-
     phorylation in brain slices of rats. J Nutr 2002;132:483–487.
106. Pan JW, Bebin EM, Chu WJ, Hetherington HP. Ketosis and epilepsy: ^{31}P spectroscopic imaging at 4.1
     T. Epilepsia 1999;40:703–707.
107. Baukrowitz T, Schulte U, Oliver D, Herlitze S, Krauter T, Tucker SJ, Ruppersberg JP, Fakler B. PIP$_2$
     and PIP as determinants for ATP inhibition of K$_{ATP}$ channels. Science 1998;282:1141–1144.
108. Shyng S-L, Nichols CG. Membrane phospholipid control of nucleotide sensitivity of K$_{ATP}$ channels.
     Science 1998;282:1138–1141.
109. Yamada K, Ji JJ, Yuan H, Miki T, Sato S, Horimoto N, Shimizu T, Seino S, Inagaki N. Protective role
     of ATP-sensitive potassium channels in hypoxia-induced generalized seizure. Science
     2001;292:1543–1546.
110. Faraci FM, Heistad DD. Regulation of the cerebral circulation: role of endothelium and potassium
     channels. Physiol Rev 1998;78:53–97.
111. Thompson RJ, Nurse CA. Anoxia differentially modulates multiple K+ currents and depolarizes
     neonatal rat adrenal chromaffin cells. J Physiol 1998;512.2:421–434.
112. Kekwick A, Pawan GLS. The effect of high fat and high carbohydrate diets on rates of weight loss in
     mice. Metabolism 1964;13:87–97.
113. Hawkins RA, Mans AM, Davis DW. Regional ketone body utilization by rat brain in starvation and
     diabetes. Am J Physiol 1986;250:E169–E178.
114. Hasselbalch SG, Knudsen GM, Jakobsen J, Hageman LP, Holm S, Paulson OB. Brain metabolism
     during short-term starvation in humans. J Cereb Blood Flow Metab 1994;14:125–131.
115. Davis JW, Wirtshafter D, Asin KE, Brief D. Sustained intracerebroventricular infusion of brain fuels
     reduces body weight and food intake in rats. Science 1981;212:81–83.

116. Sun M, Martin RJ, Edwards GL. ICV β-hydroxybutyrate: effects on food intake, body composition, and body weight in rats. Physiol Behav 1997;61:433–436.
117. Kelly KM, Gross RA, Macdonald RL. Valproic acid selectively reduces the low-threshold (T) calcium current in rat nodose neurons. Neurosci Lett 1990;116:233–238.
118. MacLean MJ, Macdonald RL. Sodium valproate, but not ethosuximide, produces use- and voltage-dependent limitation of high frequency repetitive firing of action potentials of mouse central neurons in cell culture. J Pharmacol Exp Ther 1986;237:1001–1011.
119. Stefan H, Snead OC III. Absence seizures. In: Engel J Jr, Pedley TA (eds.). Epilepsy: A Comprehensive Textbook, Vol. 2. Lippincott-Raven, Philadelphia, 1997, pp. 579–590.
120. DeVivo DC, Trifiletti RR, Jacobson RI, Ronen GM, Behmand RA, Harik SI. Defective glucose transport across the blood–brain barrier as a cause of persistent hypoglycorrhachia, seizures, and developmental delay. N Engl J Med 1991;325:703–709.
121. Erecinska M, Nelson D, Daikhin Y, Yudkoff M. Regulation of GABA level in rat brain synaptosomes: fluxes through enzymes of the GABA shunt and effects of glutamate, calcium, and ketone bodies. J Neurochem 1996;67:2325–2334.
122. Yudkoff M, Diakhin Y, Nissim I, Lazarow A, Nissim I. Brain amino acid metabolism and ketosis. J Neurosci Res 2001;66:272–281.
123. Yudkoff M, Diakhin Y, Nissim I, Lazarow A, Nissim I. Ketogenic diet, amino acid metabolism, and seizure control. J Neurosci Res 2001;66:931–940.

19 Caloric Restriction and Epilepsy
Historical Perspectives, Relationship to the Ketogenic Diet, and Analysis in Epileptic EL Mice

Thomas N. Seyfried, Amanda E. Greene, and Mariana T. Todorova

1. EPILEPSY

Epilepsy is a prevalent neurological disease estimated to afflict approx 1% of the US population *(1)*. Epileptic seizures are the clinical manifestation of epilepsy and result from excessive, synchronous, abnormal electrical firing patterns of neurons *(2)*. Many persons with epilepsy manifest idiopathic epilepsy involving partial or generalized seizures without signs of a structural brain disorder *(2–4)*. This contrasts with symptomatic or acquired epilepsy, in which seizures arise from brain injury or disease associated with obvious neurostructural changes. Although some idiopathic epilepsies are inherited as simple Mendelian traits, most idiopathic epilepsies are multifactorial and involve complex gene–environment interactions *(5,6)*.

Despite intensive efforts in the realm of antiepileptic drug research and development, seizures cannot be fully controlled in many patients with epilepsy *(7)*. Moreover, many antiepileptic drugs may produce adverse effects that include somnolence, nervousness, ataxia, diplopia, constipation, confusion, memory difficulties, weight loss, and skeletal defects *(7–10)*. Clearly, new antiepileptic therapies are needed that can manage seizures without reducing quality of life.

2. DIETARY THERAPIES AND EPILEPSY

Dietary therapies for epilepsy are as old as the disease itself and have evolved over the ages to accommodate changes in the ideas about the etiology of epilepsy *(11)*. Antiepileptic diets used during the Greek, Roman, and Renaissance periods were designed to rid the brain of toxic agents thought to underlie the epileptic seizures *(12)*. A strict dietary regimen was recognized as a key for managing or curing the disease. These early antiepileptic diets, however, often comprised vile concoctions of raw animal organs and extracts that induced nausea or vomiting and were frequently administered with purgatives and enemas *(12)*. Restricted food intake over days or weeks would often occur as an unintended consequence of such dietary therapies. This restriction

From: *Epilepsy and the Ketogenic Diet*
Edited by: C. E. Stafstrom and J. M. Rho © Humana Press Inc., Totowa, NJ

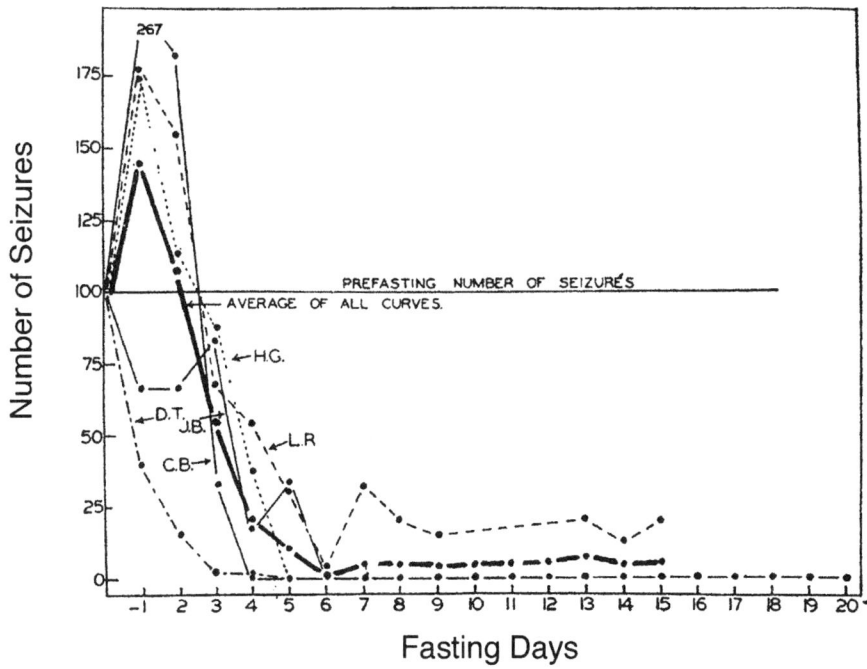

Fig. 1. Influence of fasting on human epileptic seizures as shown by the daily number of seizures during the fasting of five patients who had five or more seizures daily in the prefasting period. The ordinate represents the percentage of seizures taking the prefasting number as 100%. The abscissa represents days of fasting. The heavy solid line is the average of the five curves. From ref. *19,* with permission.

would produce the physiological conditions of fasting in which circulating glucose levels are reduced and ketone levels are elevated *(13–15).* Hence, altered brain energy homeostasis would be expected following antiepileptic dietary therapies that affected circulating levels of glucose and ketone bodies *(11).*

3. FASTING AND THE KETOGENIC DIET

Fasting has been long recognized as an effective antiepileptic therapy for a broad range of epilepsies *(16,17).* Although reference is occasionally made to biblical accounts of fasting as a cure for epileptic seizures (Mark 9:14–29), it is not clear from these passages whether it is the afflicted or the healer who is required to fast. Indeed, biblical scholars interpret these passages to mean that the afflicted could not be cured unless the healer engaged in prayer and fasting *(18).* Despite the ambiguity of biblical interpretations, modern clinical findings indicate that fasting can significantly influence a patient's seizure susceptibility.

Using the water-only diet of Conklin, Lennox and coworkers demonstrated an impressive management of epilepsy in patients having as many as five seizures per day *(16,19).* Seizure incidence actually increased over the first few days of the fast but decreased dramatically after 3 d (Fig. 1). This result is interesting because generally cerebral energy metabolism does not shift from glucose to ketone utilization before approx 3–4 d *(20).* Seizure control through fasting was also associated with reduced blood glucose and increased blood ketone levels. When the fast was broken through food or glucose intake, however, seizure protection was lost. Seizure return was associated with rising blood glucose levels and falling blood ketone levels *(16)*.

Although clinically effective, fasting is impractical for the long-term management of seizures. Consequently, the high-fat, low-carbohydrate ketogenic diet (KD) was developed to mimic the physiological effects of fasting, i.e., resulting in ketosis, without severe food restriction or starvation *(16,21–23)*. The KD is effective in managing intractable seizures in children and may also be effective in managing seizures in adults *(17,24–26)*. The KD is also effective in reducing epileptogenesis and seizures in animal models of epilepsy *(27,28)*. The mechanisms by which the KD inhibits seizure susceptibility remain speculative; however, alterations in brain energy metabolism are likely involved *(11,29,30)*.

The roles of ketone bodies (β-hydroxybutyrate [β-OHB] and acetoacetate) and glucose in the seizure-protective effects of fasting or the KD remain unclear. Plasma ketone levels were associated with seizure protection in some studies but not in others *(27,31–36)*. Because brain ketone utilization can depend on the plasma levels of ketones, glucose, and other metabolites *(37)*, associations between seizure protection and plasma ketone levels may be obscured. Likewise, glucose levels were constant during KD treatment in some studies but reduced during the treatment in others *(27,29,38–40)*. Few studies have investigated the relationship among ketones, glucose, and seizure susceptibility under long-term antiepileptic diet therapies.

4. CALORIC RESTRICTION

In 2001 we showed that in addition to the KD, caloric restriction (CR) alone could reduce seizure susceptibility in epileptic EL mice *(41)*. CR is a natural dietary therapy that improves health, extends longevity, and reduces the effects of neuroinflammatory diseases in humans and rodents *(42–47)*. CR involves a reduction of total dietary energy intake while maintaining adequate levels of vitamins and minerals *(48,49)*. In contrast to prolonged fasting or starvation, which produce clinical hypoglycemia and ketoacidosis, CR lowers glucose levels and raises ketone levels within normal physiological ranges. The shift from glucose to ketone energy produces enhanced vitality and metabolic efficiency *(11,50,51)*.

5. THE EPILEPTIC EL MOUSE

The epileptic EL mouse is a natural model of human idiopathic epilepsy and partial complex seizures with secondary generalization *(6,52)*. Seizures in EL mice originate in or near the parietal lobe and quickly spread to the hippocampus and other brain regions. The seizures commence with the onset of sexual maturity (50–60 d of age) *(6,51–55)*. The seizures are accompanied by electroencephalographic (EEG) abnormalities, vocalization, incontinence, loss of postural equilibrium, excessive salivation, and head, limb, and chewing automatisms (Figure 2) *(52,54,56–59)*. The epilepsy in EL mice also models Gowers' dictum whereby each seizure increases the likelihood of recurrent seizures *(6)*. Adult EL male mice also experience a sexual dysfunction similar to that described in men with temporal lobe epilepsy *(11)*. EL mice express abnormalities of excitatory and inhibitory neurotransmission and develop a hippocampal gliosis

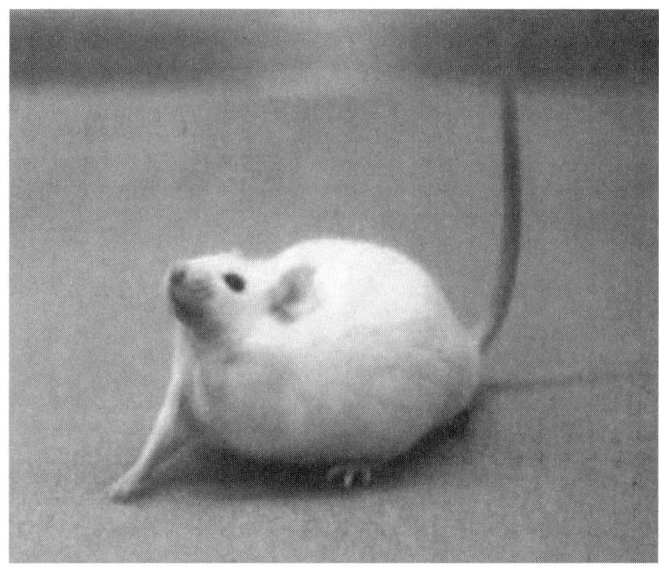

Fig. 2. Epileptic EL mouse. The EL mouse models multifactorial idiopathic epilepsy, exhibiting excessive salivation, and head, limb, swallowing, and chewing automatisms. The arching Straub tail is indicative of seizure spread to spinal cord.

with seizure progression *(60–67)*. The gliosis in EL mice, however, is not associated with obvious hippocampal neuronal loss or synaptic rearrangements to include mossy fiber sprouting *(67,68)*. Gene–environment interactions play a significant role in the determination of seizure frequency and onset in EL mice as with multifactorial human idiopathic epilepsies *(6,69)*. Hence, the EL mouse is a good model for evaluating the effects of dietary therapies on idiopathic epilepsy.

6. INFLUENCE OF CALORIC RESTRICTION ON EL MICE

6.1. Study Design

We used EL mice to evaluate the effects of mild (15%) and moderate (30%) CR on body weight, epileptogenesis, and serum levels of glucose and ketone bodies at both juvenile (30 d) and adult (70 d) ages *(41)*. In addition, we compared the antiepileptic effects of CR with those of the KD in juvenile mice.

All mice were matched for age and body weight before initiation of CR, and all received a regular chow diet that contained a balance of mouse nutritional ingredients and delivered 4.4 kcal per gram of gross energy. We implemented CR in individually housed mice using a total dietary restriction. This involved restricting the amount of food a mouse normally consumed per day under *ad libitum* (AL) conditions. The average daily food intake (grams) was measured under AL conditions in individual male and female mice at both juvenile and adult ages throughout the study *(41)*. Each AL-fed mouse received a known amount of food (approx 50 g), and the difference in chow weight was recorded every 2 d at approximately the same time (11 AM–1 PM). The amount of food given to the CR-fed juvenile mice was 85% (15% CR) of that given to the AL mice daily. At adult ages, the CR-fed mice received 85 and 70% (30% CR) of

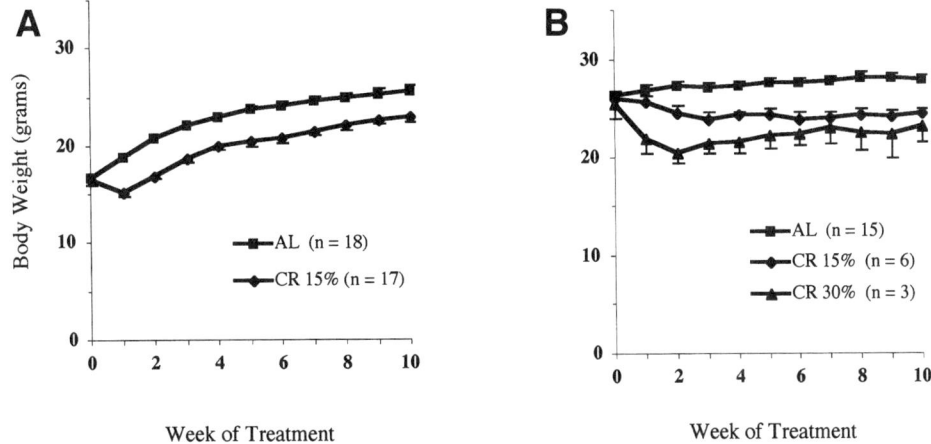

Fig. 3. Influence of CR on body weight in (**A**) juvenile and (**B**) adult EL mice. The mean body weight was significantly lower in the juvenile 15% CR mice than in the AL mice over wk 1–10 ($p <$ 0.01). The reduction in body weight was greater in the 30% CR mice than in the 15% CR mice at the adult ages. Despite the initial weight loss, body weights in both adult CR groups remained stable over wk 3–10. Values are expressed as the mean ± SEM. From ref. *41,* with permission.

the AL amount. The average daily food intake (grams) for the AL-fed mice was determined every other day, and the CR-fed mice were given either 85 or 70% of the daily ration of the AL-fed group.

No adverse side effects were seen in the mice receiving either the 15% CR diet (at juvenile ages) or the 30% CR diet (at adult ages). The CR-fed mice were healthy and more active than the AL-fed mice as assessed by ambulatory and grooming behavior. No signs of vitamin or mineral deficiency were observed in the CR-fed mice. The juvenile EL mice receiving mild CR lost approx 8% of their body weight during the first week of treatment, and their weights remained significantly lower than those of the AL group throughout the study (Figure 3A). Despite this initial body weight loss, the rates of body weight gain beyond wk 2 were similar in the AL-fed and CR-fed mice. These findings, together with the overall healthy appearance of the mice, indicate that mild CR has no adverse effect on global body growth or development. It is important to mention, however, that the young mice were unable to tolerate a moderate CR of 30%. This emphasizes the need for careful health monitoring of young mice following dietary modifications.

The adult AL-fed and CR-fed EL mice were also matched for age and body weight prior to treatment (Figure 3B). The total energy intake of the AL-fed mice was about 30 kcal/d and remained relatively constant over the 10-wk treatment period. The total energy intake of the CR-fed mice was adjusted to 85 (15% CR) or 70% (30% CR) of the AL energy intake. As at juvenile ages, body weights were pooled for males and females because the effects of CR were similar in both sexes. In contrast to the juvenile AL-fed mice, the body weights of the adult AL-fed mice remained relatively constant over the 10-wk testing period. The body weights in the 15 CR and 30% CR groups were about 12 and 15% lower, respectively, than the weights of the AL-fed group and remained stable over the testing period (Figure 3B). The CR-induced reductions in body weights were correlated with the degree of CR.

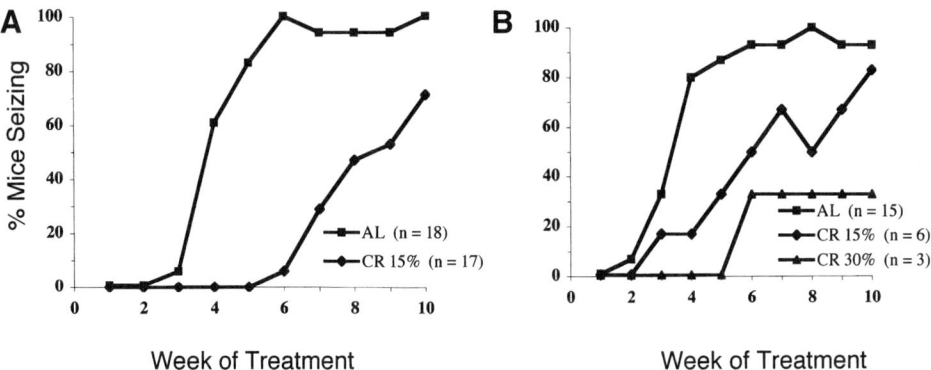

Fig. 4. Influence of CR on seizure susceptibility in (**A**) juvenile and (**B**) adult EL mice. The number of mice seizing was significantly lower in the CR groups than in the control groups. From ref. *41,* with permission.

It is important to emphasize the distinction between CR, malnutrition, and starvation. In contrast to the juvenile mice, which could not tolerate a 30% CR diet, the adult mice showed no adverse effects from the 30% CR diet. Indeed, we find that adult EL mice can easily tolerate a 50% CR diet. In general, adult mice have more body fat and a more stable metabolic rate than juvenile mice. These findings emphasize the importance of age and initial body weight in studies involving CR. CR is designed only to restrict calories, not to restrict essential vitamins or minerals that could produce malnutrition. The therapeutic health benefits of CR are lost if the degree of restriction is too extreme. Excessive calorie restriction produces starvation involving malnutrition, failure to thrive, or kwashiorkor at young ages. The levels of CR that we used, and our findings in EL mice, are consistent with the well-recognized health benefits of mild to moderate diet restriction in rodents *(70).*

6.2. CR Reduces Seizure Susceptibility in Juvenile and Adult EL Mice

We found that mild CR significantly reduced the incidence and delayed the onset (weeks after diet initiation) of seizures in the juvenile EL mice (Fig. 4A). The seizure-protective effects of CR in adult mice were correlated with the degree of CR, where the delay in seizure onset and the reduction in seizure susceptibility was greater in the 30% CR group than in the 15% CR group (Fig. 4B). These findings indicate that CR delays epileptogenesis in EL mice at both juvenile and adult ages and that the antiepileptogenic effect of CR at adult ages is proportional to the degree of CR.

6.3. CR Reduces Plasma Glucose and Elevates β-OHB Levels

CR caused plasma glucose levels to drop significantly after one week in the 15% CR-fed juvenile mice (Fig. 5A). These levels remained significantly lower than those in the AL-fed mice throughout the study but increased gradually in the CR-fed mice after wk 5. In contrast to glucose levels, 15% CR caused plasma β-OHB levels to increase significantly in the juvenile mice (Fig. 5B). These levels were inversely related to those of glucose. In the adult EL mice, the decrease in plasma glucose levels was proportional to the degree of CR (Fig. 5C). As observed in the juvenile mice, the changes in plasma

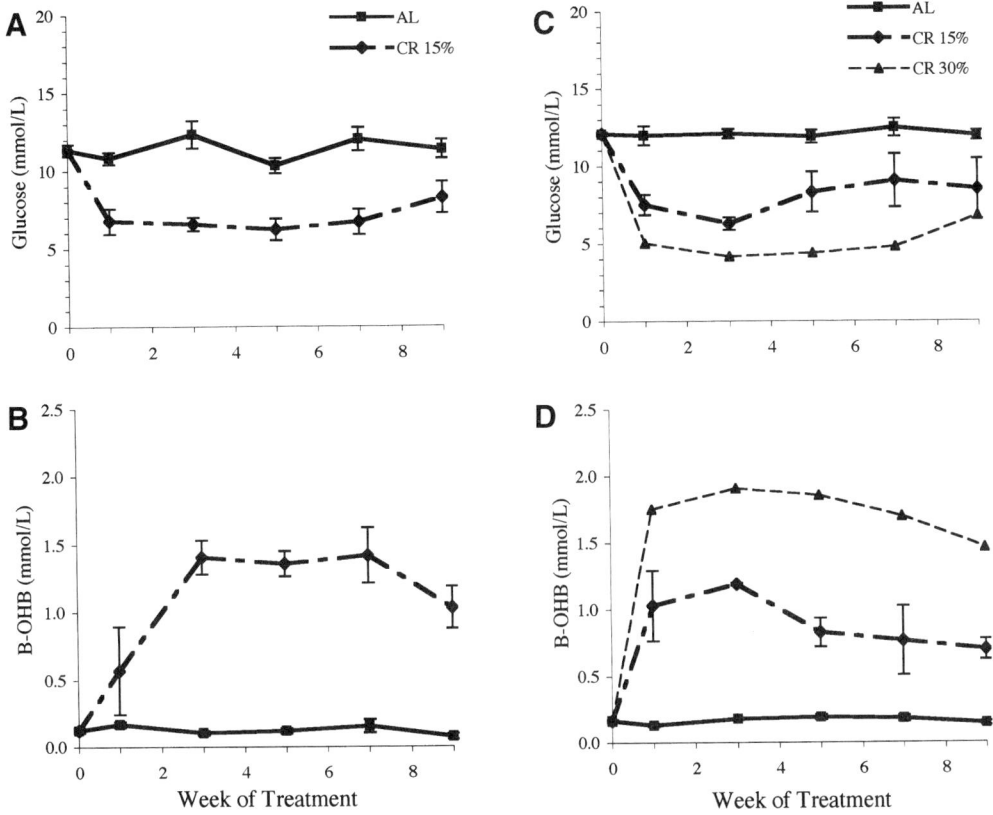

Fig. 5. Influence of CR on plasma glucose and β-OHB levels in juvenile (**A, B**) and in adult (**C, D**) EL mice. At least three animals were analyzed in each group except the adult 30% CR group, in which two animals were analyzed. Values are expressed as the mean ± SEM, or only as the mean for the adult 30% CR group. From ref. *41,* with permission.

glucose levels in the adults were inversely related to the changes in plasma β-OHB levels (Fig. 5D). These findings indicate that reductions in caloric intake cause inverse changes in plasma glucose and β-OHB levels in EL mice.

6.4. Blood Glucose Predicts Blood β-OHB Levels and Seizure Susceptibility in EL Mice

We next analyzed our data by using both simple linear regression and multiple logistic regression to determine if blood glucose levels were predictive of blood β-OHB levels and seizure susceptibility. These statistical analyses included mice considered to be outliers, i.e., mice that experienced CR but showed no changes in body weight, plasma glucose, or β-OHB levels *(41)*. One outlier was found in the juvenile CR group and three outliers were found in the adult CR groups (two in the 15% CR group and one in the 30% CR group). The outliers were considered to be nonrestricted for caloric intake and similar to the mice in the AL-fed groups. These findings also emphasize that differences exist among inbred mice for food intake and energy metabolism *(71)*. Hence, the efficacy of CR as an anticonvulsant therapy must be associated with reductions of blood glucose and body weight.

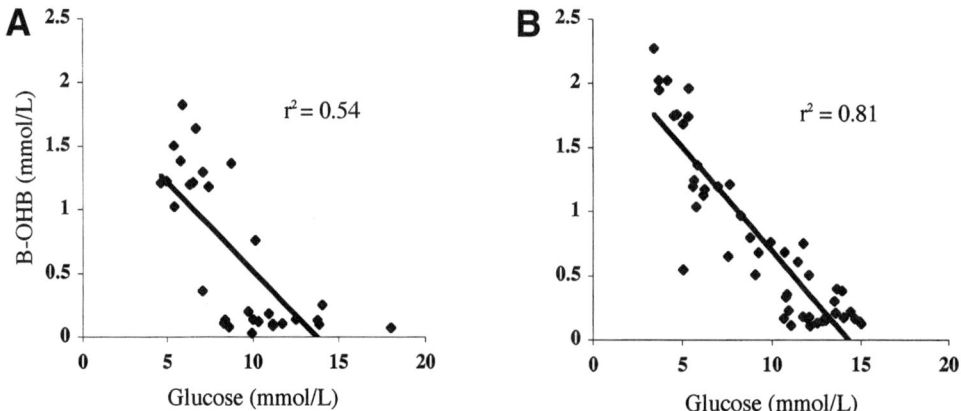

Fig. 6. Linear regression analysis of plasma glucose and β-OHB levels in (**A**) juvenile (*n* = 30) and (**B**) adult (*n* = 50) EL mice. This analysis included the values for plasma glucose and β-OHB levels of individual mice from both the AL and CR groups measured at wk 1,3, 5, 7, and 9. The linear regressions (*r*, correlation coefficient) were highly significant at *p* < 0.001. From ref. *41,* with permission.

We used simple linear regression analysis to examine the relationship between plasma glucose levels (the independent or explanatory *X* variable) and β-OHB levels (the dependent or response *Y* variable) in both the juvenile (Fig. 6A) and adult mice (Fig. 6B). These variables were identified based on physiological and neurochemical studies indicating that plasma glucose levels determine plasma β-OHB levels during periods of fasting *(13)*. This information is important because it addresses the issue of causality: i.e., circulating β-OHB levels are dependent on circulating glucose levels.

The slopes of the regression lines were highly significant, indicating that the plasma β-OHB levels increased as glucose levels decreased in both the juvenile mice and in the adult mice *(41)*. These findings support neurochemical and neurophysiological findings that plasma β-OHB levels are dependent on plasma glucose levels and that glucose levels are predictive of β-OHB levels in all mouse groups.

Based on these observations, we used multiple logistic regression to quantify the risk of seizure associated with changes in plasma glucose levels in the juvenile and the adult mice. Because the simple linear regression indicated that β-OHB levels depend on glucose levels, the β-OHB levels could not be included in the logistic regression analysis *(72)*. In the juvenile and adult mice, prior seizure testing and glucose were significant in predicting seizures. We found that for every decrease in 1 mmol per liter of glucose, the odds of having a seizure decreased by 2.6 and 1.9 in the juvenile and adult mice, respectively *(41)*. Our findings indicate that plasma glucose levels are predictive of seizure susceptibility in EL mice at both juvenile and adult ages. These findings also support recent studies with flurothyl-induced seizures in rats, in which circulating glucose levels were positively correlated with seizure susceptibility *(73)*.

6.5. Comparison of CR and the KD on Epileptogenesis in EL Mice

We next compared the effects of CR with those of the KD on seizure susceptibility in juvenile EL mice, using our data and the previously published data of Todorova et al. *(27)* for the AL feeding of the KD. All the mice were matched for age, sex (male), and

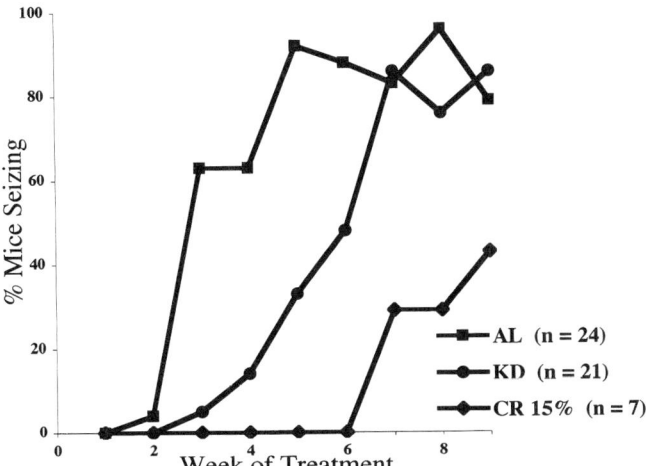

Fig. 7. Influence of CR and the KD on seizure susceptibility in juvenile EL mice. The number of mice seizing was significantly lower in the CR and KD groups than in the AL group. From ref. *41*, with permission.

body weight prior to the analysis *(41)*. We found that the mild 15% CR diet was more effective than the KD in delaying seizure onset and in reducing seizure susceptibility (Figure 7). Our comparative analysis of CR and the KD was restricted to juvenile mice because the AL-fed KD does not inhibit seizure susceptibility in adult EL mice *(74)*. In contrast to CR, which lowers blood glucose levels (Figure 5A), the AL-fed KD does not lower blood glucose levels in the juvenile EL mice *(27)*.

The KD may inhibit epileptogenesis in the juvenile EL mice by prolonging the preweaning period, thereby causing the brain to metabolize ketones for energy *(75,76)*. CR may enhance this effect by also lowering glucose levels. The AL-fed KD is ineffective in reducing seizure susceptibility in adult EL mice, in which glucose levels and body weights are not reduced *(74)*. These findings suggest that the KD may be most effective in reducing seizure susceptibility when blood glucose levels or total calories are also restricted.

7. THE RELATIONSHIP OF THE KD AND CALORIC RESTRICTION IN SEIZURE MANAGEMENT

The KD is most effective in reducing seizure susceptibility in children when administered with fasting or under restricted caloric intake *(17,77)*. Livingston also reported that KD efficacy was associated with body weight reductions of approx 10% and reduced blood glucose levels *(78)*. Our findings in EL mice on the CR diet are consistent with these findings in humans. It is interesting that the anticonvulsant effects of the KD are usually lost in patients who experience a rise in blood glucose levels, i.e., in those who gain weight on the diet or consume carbohydrates *(16,17,21)*. Based on our studies with EL mice, we suggest that the seizure-protective effects of the KD are largely dependent on the maintenance of reduced blood glucose and body weight. We suggest that the KD suppresses seizure susceptibility largely through CR.

8. EVIDENCE THAT THE KD SUPPRESSES SEIZURE SUSCEPTIBILITY THROUGH CALORIC RESTRICTION

In contrast to the KD, CR elevates blood ketone levels naturally through a gradual reduction in blood glucose levels. Although both the KD and CR elevate blood ketone levels, circulating ketone levels alone could not explain the anticonvulsant effects of these diets in either humans or animal models. Indeed, the brain does not generally metabolize ketones for energy unless blood glucose levels are reduced *(11,13)*. We suggest that it is the reduction of blood glucose levels together with an elevation of blood ketone levels that predicts the anticonvulsant efficacy of both the KD and CR. This conclusion comes from our findings that blood glucose predicts both blood ketone levels and seizure susceptibility in EL mice *(41)*. Blood glucose also positively correlates with flurothyl-induced seizures in rats and high glucose may exacerbate human epilepsies *(73)*.

The association between blood glucose levels and seizure susceptibility is less clear in epileptic humans than in animal models of epilepsy, perhaps because of the capricious nature of glucose measurements in humans and from the broad range of glucose levels in "normal" individuals (60–120 mg/dL) *(78,79)*. A normal glucose level for one person could be hypoglycemic or hyperglycemic in another person. Indeed, some children can function normally with blood sugar levels as low as 20 mg/dL *(78)*. The reduction of body weight and restriction of calories in children on the KD implies reduced glucose levels relative to the levels prior to the initiation of the diet. To determine the relationship between glucose and seizure protection under the KD, it would be necessary to monitor glucose levels in children prior to the initiation of the KD. In other words, glucose levels should be monitored both before and during the KD with each child serving as his or her own control. According to Livingston, however, body weight may be a more accurate predictor of diet efficacy than blood glucose levels in children *(78)*. Hence, further studies with animal models of epilepsy are needed to assess the relations among blood glucose levels, body weight changes, and seizure protection with antiepileptic diets.

9. PERSPECTIVES ON THE ANTIEPILEPTIC MECHANISM OF CALORIC RESTRICTION

We propose that CR inhibits seizure susceptibility by shifting brain energy metabolism from glucose to ketone bodies. A CR-induced reduction in glucose utilization and increase in ketone utilization will, on the one hand, reduce the glycolytic energy reserves related to seizure activity and, simultaneously, decrease neuronal excitability through ketone metabolism. This involves multiple metabolic changes that would ultimately shift the neural environment from excitation to inhibition. An outline of these changes (Fig. 8) was recently presented in relation to metabolic control theory for the management of epilepsy *(11)*.

The brain derives almost all its energy from the aerobic oxidation of glucose under normal physiological conditions. Glucose transporters, e.g., GLUT 1, are enriched in the brain capillary endothelial cells and mediate the diffusion of glucose through the blood–brain barrier (Fig. 8). Most of the glucose is metabolized to pyruvate, which enters the mitochondria of neurons and glia and is converted to acetyl-coenzyme A (CoA) before entering the tricarboxylic acid (TCA) cycle. Only a small amount of the pyruvate is converted to lactate under normal conditions *(13)*.

During an epileptic seizure, glucose uptake and metabolism increase more than during any other brain activity *(80,81)*. Glycolytic energy is crucial for maintaining synap-

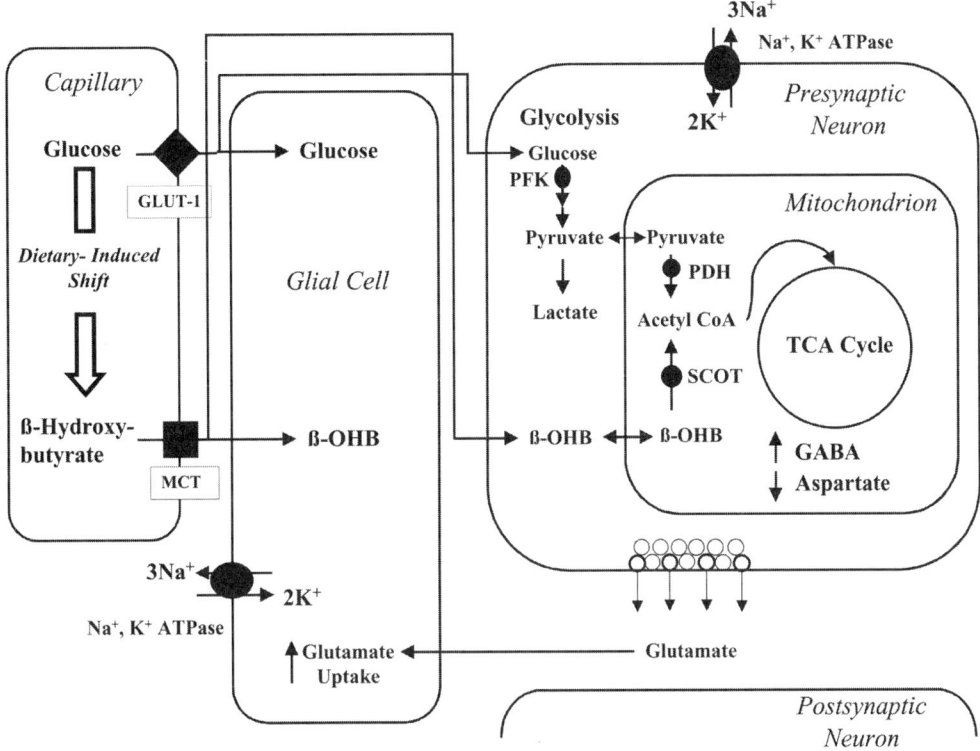

Fig. 8. Perspectives on the metabolic management of epilepsy through a dietary reduction of glucose and elevation of ketone bodies. A dietary reduction in blood glucose levels will increase ketone utilization. This is expected to shift the neural environment from excitation to inhibition (*see* text). Abbreviations: GLUT-1 (glucose transporter), MCT (monocarboxylate transporter), PFK (phosphofructokinase), PDH (pyruvate dehydrogenase), SCOT (succinyl-CoA-acetoacetate-CoA transferase), β-OHB (β-hydroxybutyrate), GABA (γ-aminobutyric acid).

tic activity, and seizures are associated with enhanced glycolysis *(82–86)*. Brain lactate levels also increase significantly during seizure activity *(87,88)*. The seizure-associated lactate increase reflects the rapid increase in glycolytic rate over the cerebral metabolic rate of oxygen, and the maximally activated pyruvate dehydrogenase is the rate-limiting step *(81)*. The pyruvate dehydrogenase fails to metabolize pyruvate to acetyl-CoA at the same rate that pyruvate is produced. Hence, lactate dehydrogenase converts pyruvate to lactate during periods of oxygen deprivation and rapid glucose metabolism, as would occur during epileptic seizures.

Studies indicate that CR downregulates glycolytic enzyme and gene expression in mouse tissues *(89,90)*. Although CR will increase the total energy available to the brain through ketone body metabolism, it will reduce the energy available from glycolysis *(50,91)*. Reduced glycolytic energy could deplete the reserves of immediately available energy necessary for seizure initiation and spread. It is not yet clear, however, to what extent enhanced glycolysis is related to the cause or effects of seizure activity *(11)*.

Although glucose is the preferred metabolic fuel, the mammalian brain will metabolize ketone bodies for energy when blood glucose levels decrease, as during fasting or CR *(13)*. The transport of ketones into the brain occurs through the blood–brain barrier monocarboxylic transporter (MCT-1), whose expression is regulated in part by circulating ketone and glucose levels *(92–94)*. Ketone bodies, being metabolized directly to acetyl-CoA in the mitochondria, bypass cytoplasmic glycolysis and provide brain energy directly through the Krebs cycle *(37,50,95)* (Fig. 8). Reduced blood glucose and increased blood ketone levels may be needed to induce the activity of succinyl-CoA-acetoacetate-CoA transferase (SCOT), a key enzyme required for ketone body metabolism *(20,96)*. In addition to reducing glycolytic energy, ketone body metabolism causes significant increases in the TCA cycle metabolites (from citrate to α-ketoglutarate) and improves metabolic efficiency through an increase in the energy of adenosine triphosphate (ATP) hydrolysis *(50,51,97)*. Thus, a shift in energy metabolism from glucose utilization to ketone utilization could contribute in part to a mechanism by which CR inhibits seizure susceptibility in EL mice.

The metabolism of ketones for energy would also produce multiple changes in the content and distribution of brain neurotransmitters. Ketones stimulate glutamic acid decarboxylase activity that can potentially elevate γ-aminobutyric acid (GABA) content in synaptosomes *(98–100)*. Ketone-induced alterations in TCA cycle metabolites will favor the formation of glutamate over aspartate, thereby reducing brain aspartate, an excitatory neurotransmitter implicated in EL epilepsy *(50,63,64,100)*.

Ketone body metabolism could also increase the activity of the sodium pump in both neurons and glia *(50,101)* (Figure 8). Increased pump activity in neurons could increase the membrane potential, thereby decreasing neuronal excitability *(30,50,80,102)*. Increased pump activity in astroglia, on the other hand, could facilitate glutamate uptake following synaptic release, thereby reducing the duration or spread of seizure activity *(81,103,104)*.

Another effect of prolonged fasting or CR would be a reduction in the cerebral metabolic rate of glucose *(105)*. Generally cerebral energy metabolism shifts from glucose to ketone utilization in humans in approx 3–4 d *(20)*. This period closely parallels that required for seizure control through fasting (Figure 1). CR also elevates circulating glucocorticoids that would further reduce cerebral glucose utilization *(49,106)*. The brain will metabolize ketones for energy more effectively under reduced glucose than under high glucose conditions because reduced glucose stimulates ketone body metabolism and utilization (as a substitute for glucose) *(13,14,20,107)*.

A gradual reduction in blood glucose will force the brain to use ketone bodies as an alternative energy fuel *(107)*. The shift from glucose to ketone metabolism will increase brain ATP and citrate levels, which will inhibit phosphofructokinase and further reduce glycolytic energy *(91,105)*. Slight to moderate shifts in energy metabolism from glucose to ketones would produce global changes in brain excitability that could potentially suppress seizure activity *(11)*.

10. ANTIEPILEPTIC DRUGS, VAGUS NERVE STIMULATION, AND BRAIN ENERGY METABOLISM

Reduced cerebral glucose metabolism occurs not only with CR but also with the use of several common antiepileptic drugs, e.g., phenobarbital, primidone, phenytoin, carbamazepine, vigabatrin, and valproate *(108–112)*. The combination of carbamazepine and valproate causes a reduction in the cerebral metabolic rate of glucose even greater than when that recorded either drug is used alone *(109)*. Decreased nutrient intake and body weight loss are associated with the antiepileptic action of zonisamide and topiramate *(113–115)*, suggesting a mechanism that involves alterations in brain energy metabolism. The inclusion of active body weight controls in clinical trials with these drugs could test this hypothesis. Furosemide and similar diuretics that have anticonvulsant potential inhibit glucose uptake and glycolysis and thus may also alter energy homeostasis *(116,117)*. Vagus nerve stimulation (VNS) is a novel therapy that reduces seizure frequency in patients with refractory seizures *(9)*. The vagus nerve is also known to affect eating behavior, and VNS has been used to treat morbid obesity *(118)*. Because a major biological role of the vagus nerve is systemic energy regulation *(119)*, it is possible that VNS may manage epilepsy in part through effects on brain energy metabolism. Taken together, these findings suggest that changes in cerebral energy metabolism may be common to several epilepsy medications, diets, and therapies.

11. CONCLUSION

We suggest that CR may underlie the anticonvulsant mechanism of the KD and that CR alone may be an effective antiepileptic diet therapy. Moreover, the anticonvulsant action of CR may operate through the combined effects of reducing blood glucose and elevating blood ketones, thereby modulating cerebral energy metabolism. Our preclinical findings in EL mice suggest that CR may be an effective dietary therapy for some human epilepsies because CR is easy to administer and is devoid of the adverse side effects associated with other antiepileptic therapies.

ACKNOWLEDGMENTS

We thank Christine Denny and Julie Kasperzyk for administrative support. The work was supported from the Boston College Research Fund and grants from the National Tay–Sachs and Allied Diseases Association (NTSAD) and National Institutes of Health grant HD39722.

REFERENCES

1. Hauser WA. Incidence and prevalence. In: Engel JJ, Pedley TA (eds.). Epilepsy: A Comprehensive Textbook, Vol. 1. Lippincott-Raven, New York, 1997, pp. 47–57.
2. Engel JJ, Pedley TA. Introduction: what is epilepsy? In: Engel JJ, Pedley TA (eds.). Epilepsy: A Comprehensive Textbook, Vol. 1. Lipponcott-Raven, New York, 1997, pp. 1–10.
3. Baumann RJ. Classification and population studies of epilepsy. In: Anderson VE, Hauser WA, Penry JK, Sing CF (eds.). Genetic Basis of the Epilepsies. Raven, New York, 1982, pp. 11–20.
4. Wolf P. Historical aspects: the concept of idiopathy. In: Malafosse A, Genton P, Hirsch E, Marescaux C, Broglin D, Bernasconi R (eds.). Idiopathic Generalized Epilepsies: Clinical, Experimental, and Genetic Aspects. John Libbey, London, 1994, pp. 3–6.
5. Berkovic SF, Scheffer IE. Epilepsies with single gene inheritance. Brain Dev 1997;19:13–18.
6. Todorova MT, Burwell TJ, Seyfried TN. Environmental risk factors for multifactorial epilepsy in EL mice. Epilepsia 1999;40:1697–1707.
7. Browne TR, Holmes GL. Epilepsy. N Engl J Med 2001;344:1145–1151.
8. Porter RJ, Meldrum BS, Macdonald RL, et al. Antiepileptic drugs. In: Engel JJ, Pedley TA (eds.). Epilepsy: A Comprehensive Textbook, Vol. 2. Lippincott-Raven, New York, 1997, pp. 1379–1670.
9. Wheless JW, Baumgartner J, Ghanbari C. Vagus nerve stimulation and the ketogenic diet. Neurol Clin 2001;19:371–407.
10. Mattson RH. Monotherapy trials: endpoints. Epilepsy Res 2001;45:109–117; discussion, 119, 121–122.

11. Greene AE, Todorova MM, Seyfried TN. Perspectives on the metabolic management of epilepsy through dietary reduction of glucose and elevation of ketone bodies. J Neurochem 2003;86:529–537.

12. Eadie MJ, Bladin PF. A Disease Once Sacred: A History of the Medical Understanding of Epilepsy. John Libby, Eastleigh, UK, 2001, p. 248.

13. Clarke DD, Sokoloff L. Circulation and energy metabolism of the brain. In: Siegel GJ, Agranoff BW, Albers RW, Fisher SK, Uhler MD (eds.). Basic Neurochemistry: Molecular, Cellular and Medical Aspects. Lippincott-Raven, New York, 1999, pp. 637–669.

14. Owen OE, Morgan AP, Kemp HG, Sullivan JM, Herrera MG, Cahill GF, Jr. Brain metabolism during fasting. J Clin Invest 1967;46:1589–1595.

15. Cahill GF, Herrera MG, Morgan AP, et al. Hormone–fuel interrelationships during fasting. J Clin Invest 1966;45:1751–1769.

16. Lennox WG. Epilepsy and Related Disorders, Vol. 1. Little, Brown, Boston, 1960, p. 1168.

17. Freeman JM, Freeman JB, Kelly MT. The Ketogenic Diet: A Treatment for Epilepsy, 3rd ed. Demos, New York, 2000, p. 236.

18. Perkins P. The Gospel of Mark. In: Keck (ed.). The Interpreter's Bible, Vol. VIII: General Articles on the New Testament; The Gospel of Matthew; The Gospel of Mark. Abingdon, Nashville, TN, 1994, pp. 509–773.

19. Lennox WG, Cobb S. Studies in epilepsy: VIII. The clinical effect of fasting. Arch Neurol Psychiat 1928;20:771–779.

20. Bhagavan NV. Medical Biochemistry. Harcourt, New York, 2002, p. 1016.

21. Peterman MG. The ketogenic diet. J Am Med Assoc 1928;90:1427–1429.

22. Peterman MG. The ketogenic diet in epilepsy. J Am Med Assoc 1925;84:1979–1983.

23. Wilder R. The effects of ketonemia on the course of epilepsy. Mayo Clin Proc 1921;2:307–308.

24. Nordli DR Jr, De Vivo DC. The ketogenic diet revisited: back to the future. Epilepsia 1997;38:743–749.

25. Sirven J, Whedon B, Caplan D, et al. The ketogenic diet for intractable epilepsy in adults: preliminary results. Epilepsia 1999;40:1721–1726.

26. Vining EPG. Ketogenic diet. In: Engel JJ, Pedley TA (eds.). Epilepsy: A Comprehensive Textbook, Vol. 2. Lippincott-Raven, New York, 1997, pp. 1339–1344.

27. Todorova M, Tandon P, Madore RA, Stafstrom CE, Seyfried TN. Ketogenic diet inhibits epileptogenesis in EL mice: a genetic model for idiopathic epilepsy. Epilepsia 2000;41:933–940.

28. Bough KJ, Matthews PJ, Eagles DA. A ketogenic diet has different effects upon seizures induced by maximal electroshock and by pentylenetetrazole infusion. Epilepsy Res 2000;38:105–114.

29. DeVivo DC, Leckie MP, Ferrendelli JS, McDougal DB Jr. Chronic ketosis and cerebral metabolism. Ann Neurol 1978;3:331–337.

30. Schwartzkroin PA. Mechanisms underlying the anti-epileptic efficacy of the ketogenic diet. Epilepsy Res 1999;37:171–180.

31. Harney JP, Madara J, I'Anson H. Effects of acute inhibition of fatty acid oxidation on latency to seizure and concentrations of beta hydroxybutyrate in plasma of rats maintained on calorie restriction and/or the ketogenic diet. Epilepsy Res 2002;49:239–246.

32. Rho JM, Anderson GD, Donevan SD, White HS. Acetoacetate, acetone, and dibenzylamine (a contaminant in 1-(+)-beta-hydroxybutyrate) exhibit direct anticonvulsant actions in vivo. Epilepsia 2002;43:358–361.

33. Appleton DB, DeVivo DC. An animal model for the ketogenic diet. Epilepsia 1974;15:211–227.

34. Nakazawa M, Kodama S, Matsuo T. Effects of ketogenic diet on electroconvulsive threshold and brain contents of adenosine nucleotides. Brain Dev 1983;5:375–380.

35. Bough KJ, Valiyil R, Han FT, Eagles DA. Seizure resistance is dependent upon age and calorie restriction in rats fed a ketogenic diet. Epilepsy Res 1999;35:21–28.

36. Rho JM, Kim DW, Robbins CA, Anderson GD, Schwartzkroin PA. Age-dependent differences in flurothyl seizure sensitivity in mice treated with a ketogenic diet. Epilepsy Res 1999;37:233–240.

37. Nehlig A, Pereira de Vasconcelos A. Glucose and ketone body utilization by the brain of neonatal rats. Prog Neurobiol 1993;40:163–221.

38. Al-Mudallal AS, Levin BE, Lust WD, Harik SI. Effects of unbalanced diets on cerebral glucose metabolism in the adult rat. Neurology 1995;45:2261–2265.

39. DeVivo DC, Pagliara AS, Prensky AL. Ketotic hypoglycemia and the ketogenic diet. Neurology 1973;23:640–649.

40. Likhodii SS, Musa K, Mendonca A, Dell C, Burnham WM, Cunnane SC. Dietary fat, ketosis, and seizure resistance in rats on the ketogenic diet. Epilepsia 2000;41:1400–1410.

41. Greene AE, Todorova MT, McGowan R, Seyfried TN. Caloric restriction inhibits seizure susceptibility in epileptic EL mice by reducing blood glucose. Epilepsia 2001;42:1371–1378.

42. Mattson MP, Duan W, Lee J, Guo Z. Suppression of brain aging and neurodegenerative disorders by dietary restriction and environmental enrichment: molecular mechanisms. Mech Ageing Dev 2001;122:757–778.

43. Weindruch R, Walford RL. The Retardation of Aging and Disease by Dietary Restriction. Charles C Thomas, Springfield, IL, 1988, p. 436.

44. Mukherjee P, El-Abbadi MM, Kasperzyk JL, Ranes MK, Seyfried TN. Dietary restriction reduces angiogenesis and growth in an orthotopic mouse brain tumour model. Br J Cancer 2002;86:1615–1621.

45. Mattson MP, Chan SL, Duan W. Modification of brain aging and neurodegenerative disorders by genes, diet, and behavior. Physiol Rev 2002;82:637–672.

46. Eckles-Smith K, Clayton D, Bickford P, Browning MD. Caloric restriction prevents age-related deficits in LTP and in NMDA receptor expression. Mol Brain Res 2000;78:154–162.

47. Duffy PH, Leakey JEA, Pipkin JL, Turturro A, Hart RW. The physiologic, neurologic, and behavioral effects of caloric restriction related to aging, disease, and environmental factors. Environ Res 1997;73:242–248.

48. Mukherjee P, Sotnikov AV, Mangian HJ, Zhou JR, Visek WJ, Clinton SK. Energy intake and prostate tumor growth, angiogenesis, and vascular endothelial growth factor expression. J Natl Cancer Inst 1999;91:512–523.

49. Birt DF, Yaktine A, Duysen E. Glucocorticoid mediation of dietary energy restriction inhibition of mouse skin carcinogenesis. J Nutr 1999;129:571S–574S.

50. Veech RL, Chance B, Kashiwaya Y, Lardy HA, Cahill GF, Jr. Ketone bodies, potential therapeutic uses. IUBMB Life 2001;51:241–247.

51. Sato K, Kashiwaya Y, Keon CA, et al. Insulin, ketone bodies, and mitochondrial energy transduction. FASEB J 1995;9:651–658.

52. Seyfried TN, Poderycki MJ, Todorova MT. Genetics of the EL mouse: a multifactorial epilepsy model. In: Genton P, Berkovic S, Hirsch E, Marescaux C (eds.). Genetics of Focal Epilepsies. John Libbey, London, 1999, pp. 229–238.

53. Uchibori M, Saito K, Yokoyama S, et al. Foci identification of spike discharges in the EEGs of sleeping EL mice based on the electric field model and wavelet decomposition of multimonopolar derivations. J Neurosci Methods 2002;117:51–63.

54. Ishida N, Kasamo K, Nakamoto Y, Suzuki J. Epileptic seizure of EL mouse initiates at the parietal cortex: depth EEG observation in freely moving condition using buffer amplifier. Brain Res 1993;608:52–57.

55. Suzuki J, Kasamo K, Ishida N, Murashima YL. Initiation, propagation and generalization of paroxysmal discharges in an epileptic mutant animal. Jpn J Psychol Neurol 1991;45:271–274.

56. Suzuki J, Nakamoto Y. Seizure patterns and electroencephalograms of EL mouse. Electroencephalogr Clin Neurophysiol 1977;43:299–311.

57. Suzuki J. Paroxysmal discharges in the electroencephalogram of the EL mouse. Experientia 1976;32:336–338.

58. Sato H. The development of EEG background activities in EL mouse. Folia Psychiatr Neurol Jpn 1985;39:581–587.

59. Nakano H, Saito K, Suzuki K. Chronic implantation technique for monopolar EEG monitoring of epileptic seizures in mice. Brain Res Bull 1994;35:261–268.

60. Lambert JD, Fueta Y, Roepstorff A, Andreasen M. Analysis of the kinetics of synaptic inhibition points to a reduction in GABA release in area CA1 of the genetically epileptic mouse, EL. Epilepsy Res 1996;26:15–23.

61. Fueta Y, Kawano H, Ono T, Mita T, Fukata K, Ohno K. Regional differences in hippocampal excitability manifested by paired-pulse stimulation of genetically epileptic EL mice. Brain Res 1998;779:324–328.

62. Ingram EM, Wiseman JW, Tessler S, Emson PC. Reduction of glial glutamate transporters in the parietal cortex and hippocampus of the EL mouse. J Neurochem 2001;79:564–575.

63. Flavin HJ, Seyfried TN. Enhanced aspartate release related to epilepsy in (EL) mice. J Neurochem 1994;63:592–595.

64. Flavin HJ, Wieraszko A, Seyfried TN. Enhanced aspartate release from hippocampal slices of epileptic (EL) mice. J Neurochem 1991;56:1007–1011.

65. Murashima YL, Kasamo K, Suzuki J. Developmental abnormalities of GABAergic system are involved in the formation of epileptogenesis in the EL. Neurosciences 1992;18 (Suppl 2):63–73.

66. Hiramatsu M, Edamatsu R, Suzuki S, Shimada M, Mori A. Regional excitatory and inhibitory amino acid levels in epileptic EL mouse brain. Neurochem Res 1990;15:821–825.

67. Brigande JV, Wieraszko A, Albert MD, Balkema GW, Seyfried TN. Biochemical correlates of epilepsy in the EL mouse: analysis of glial fibrillary acidic protein and gangliosides. J Neurochem 1992;58:752–760.

68. Drage MG, Holmes GL, Seyfried TN. Hippocampal neurons and glia in epileptic EL mice. J Neurocytol 2003; in press.

69. Poderycki MJ, Simoes JM, Todorova M, Neumann PE, Seyfried TN. Environmental influences on epilepsy gene mapping in EL mice. J Neurogenet 1998;12:67–86.

70. Keenan KP, Ballam GC, Soper KA, Laroque P, Coleman JB, Dixit R. Diet, caloric restriction, and the rodent bioassay. Toxicol Sci 1999;52:24–34.

71. Pugh TD, Klopp RG, Weindruch R. Controlling caloric consumption: protocols for rodents and rhesus monkeys. Neurobiol Aging 1999;20:157–165.

72. Lang TA, Secic M. How to Report Statistics in Medicine. American College Physicians, Philadelphia, 1997.

73. Schwechter EM, Veliskova J, Velisek L. Correlation between extracellular glucose and seizure susceptibility in adult rats. Ann Neurol 2003;53:91–101.

74. Mantis JG, Centeno N, Todorova MT, McGowan R, Seyfried TN. Metabolic control of epilepsy in adult EL mice with the ketogenic diet and caloric restriction. Epilepsia 2003; abstract, in press.

75. Nehlig A. Age-dependent pathways of brain energy metabolism: the suckling rat, a natural model of the ketogenic diet. Epilepsy Res 1999;37:211–221.

76. Krebs HA, Williamson DH, Bates MW, Page MA, Hawkins RA. The role of ketone bodies in caloric homeostasis. Adv Enzyme Reg 1971;9:387–409.

77. Freeman JM, Vining EP. Seizures decrease rapidly after fasting: preliminary studies of the ketogenic diet. Arch Pediatr Adolesc Med 1999;153:946–949.

78. Livingston S. Dietary treatment of epilepsy. In: Livingston S (ed.). Comprehensive management of epilepsy in infancy, childhood and adolescence. Charles C Thomas, Springfield, IL, 1972, pp. 378–405.

79. Sacks DB. Carbohydrates. In: Burtis CA, Ashwood ER (eds.). Tietz Fundamentals of Clinical Chemistry. Saunders, New York, 2001, pp. 427–461.

80. McIlwain H. Cerebral energy metabolism and membrane phenomena. In: Jasper HH, Ward AAJ, Pope A (eds.). Basic Mechanisms of the Epilepsies. Little, Brown, Boston, 1969, pp. 83–103.

81. Meldrum B, Chapman A. Epileptic seizures and epilepsy. In: Siegel GJ, Agranoff BW, Albers RW, Fisher SK, Uhler MD (eds.). Basic Neurochemistry: Molecular, Cellular and Medical Aspects. Lippincott-Raven, New York, 1999, pp. 755–768.

82. Li X, Yokono K, Okada Y. Phosphofructokinase, a glycolytic regulatory enzyme has a crucial role for maintenance of synaptic activity in guinea pig hippocampal slices. Neurosci Lett 2000;294:81–84.

83. Meric P, Barrere B, Peres M, et al. Effects of kainate-induced seizures on cerebral metabolism: a combined ^{1}H and ^{31}P NMR study in rat. Brain Res 1994;638:53–60.

84. Ting YL, Degani H. Energetics and glucose metabolism in hippocampal slices during depolarization: ^{31}P and ^{13}C NMR studies. Brain Res 1993;610:16–23.

85. Folbergrova J. Cerebral energy state of neonatal rats during seizures induced by homocysteine. Physiol Res 1993;42:155–160.

86. Ackermann RF, Lear JL. Glycolysis-induced discordance between glucose metabolic rates measured with radiolabeled fluorodeoxyglucose and glucose. J Cereb Blood Flow Metab 1989;9:774–785.

87. During MJ, Fried I, Leone P, Katz A, Spencer DD. Direct measurement of extracellular lactate in the human hippocampus during spontaneous seizures. J Neurochem 1994;62:2356–2361.

88. Cornford EM, Shamsa K, Zeitzer JM, et al. Regional analyses of CNS microdialysate glucose and lactate in seizure patients. Epilepsia 2002;43:1360–1371.

89. Dhahbi JM, Mote PL, Wingo J, et al. Caloric restriction alters the feeding response of key metabolic enzyme genes. Mech Ageing Dev 2001;122:1033–1048.

90. Lee CK, Weindruch R, Prolla TA. Gene-expression profile of the ageing brain in mice. Nat Genet 2000;25:294–297.

91. Kashiwaya Y, Takeshima T, Mori N, Nakashima K, Clarke K, Veech RL. D-beta-Hydroxybutyrate protects neurons in models of Alzheimer's and Parkinson's disease. Proc Natl Acad Sci U S A 2000;97:5440–5444.

92. Pellerin L, Pellegri G, Martin JL, Magistretti PJ. Expression of monocarboxylate transporter mRNAs in mouse brain: support for a distinct role of lactate as an energy substrate for the neonatal vs adult brain. Proc Natl Acad Sci USA 1998;95:3990–3995.

93. Koehler-Stec EM, Simpson IA, Vannucci SJ, Landschulz KT, Landschulz WH. Monocarboxylate transporter expression in mouse brain. Am J Physiol 1998;275:E516–E524.

94. Leino RL, Gerhart DZ, Duelli R, Enerson BE, Drewes LR. Diet-induced ketosis increases monocarboxylate transporter (MCT1) levels in rat brain. Neurochem Int 2001;38:519–527.

95. McIlwain H, Bachelard H. Biochemistry and the Central Nervous System. Churchill Livingstone, New York, 1985, p. 660.

96. Fredericks M, Ramsey RB. 3-Oxo acid coenzyme A transferase activity in brain and tumors of the nervous system. J Neurochem 1978;31:1529–1531.

97. Kashiwaya Y, Sato K, Tsuchiya N, et al. Control of glucose utilization in working perfused rat heart. J Biol Chem 1994;269:25502–25514.

98. Erecinska M, Nelson D, Daikhin Y, Yudkoff M. Regulation of GABA level in rat brain synaptosomes: fluxes through enzymes of the GABA shunt and effects of glutamate, calcium, and ketone bodies. J Neurochem 1996;67:2325–2334.

99. Daikhin Y, Yudkoff M. Ketone bodies and brain glutamate and GABA metabolism. Dev Neurosci 1998;20:358–364.

100. Yudkoff M, Daikhin Y, Nissim I, Lazarow A, Nissim I. Ketogenic diet, amino acid metabolism, and seizure control. J Neurosci Res 2001;66:931–940.

101. Kaur G, Kaur K. Effect of acute starvation on monoamine oxidase and Na+,K+-ATPase activity in rat brain. Mol Chem Neuropathol 1990;13:175–183.

102. Silver IA, Erecinska M. Energetic demands of the Na+/K+ ATPase in mammalian astrocytes. Glia 1997;21:35–45.

103. Pellerin L, Magistretti PJ. Glutamate uptake into astrocytes stimulates aerobic glycolysis: a mechanism coupling neuronal activity to glucose utilization. Proc Natl Acad Sci U S A 1994;91:10625–10629.

104. Petroff OA, Errante LD, Rothman DL, Kim JH, Spencer DD. Glutamate–glutamine cycling in the epileptic human hippocampus. Epilepsia 2002;43:703–710.

105. Redies C, Hoffer LJ, Beil C, et al. Generalized decrease in brain glucose metabolism during fasting in humans studied by PET. Am J Physiol 1989;256:E805–E810.

106. Kadekaro M, Ito M, Gross PM. Local cerebral glucose utilization is increased in acutely adrenalectomized rats. Neuroendocrinology 1988;47:329–334.

107. Haymond MW, Howard C, Ben-Galim E, DeVivo DC. Effects of ketosis on glucose flux in children and adults. Am J Physiol 1983;245:E373–E378.

108. Spanaki MV, Siegel H, Kopylev L, et al. The effect of vigabatrin (gamma-vinyl GABA) on cerebral blood flow and metabolism. Neurology 1999;53:1518–1522.

109. Leiderman DB, Balish M, Bromfield EB, Theodore WH. Effect of valproate on human cerebral glucose metabolism. Epilepsia 1991;32:417–422.

110. Theodore WH, Bairamian D, Newmark ME, et al. Effect of phenytoin on human cerebral glucose metabolism. J Cereb Blood Flow Metab 1986;6:315–320.

111. Theodore WH, DiChiro G, Margolin R, Fishbein D, Porter RJ, Brooks RA. Barbiturates reduce human cerebral glucose metabolism. Neurology 1986;36:60–64.

112. Theodore WH, Bromfield E, Onorati L. The effect of carbamazepine on cerebral glucose metabolism. Ann Neurol 1989;25:516–520.

113. Gadde KM, Francisky DM, Wagner HR, 2nd, Krishnan KR. Zonisamide for weight loss in obese adults: a randomized controlled trial. JAMA 2003;289:1820–1825.

114. Brown RO, Orr CD, Hanna DL, Williams JE, Dickerson RN. Topiramate and weight loss in patients with neurodevelopmental disabilities. Pharmacotherapy 2002;22:831–835.

115. Ormrod D, McClellan K. Topiramate: a review of its use in childhood epilepsy. Paediatr Drugs 2001;3:293–319.
116. Hesdorffer DC, Stables JP, Hauser WA, Annegers JF, Cascino G. Are certain diuretics also anticonvulsants? Ann Neurol 2001;50:458–462.
117. Dimitriadis G, Tegos C, Golfinopoulou L, Roboti C, Raptis S. Furosemide-induced hyperglycaemia: the implication of glycolytic kinases. Horm Metab Res 1993;25:557–559.
118. Roslin M, Kurian M. The use of electrical stimulation of the vagus nerve to treat morbid obesity. Epilepsy Behav 2001;2:S11–S16.
119. Szekely M. The vagus nerve in thermoregulation and energy metabolism. Auton Neurosci 2000;85:26–38.

20 The Role of Norepinephrine in the Anticonvulsant Mechanism of Action of the Ketogenic Diet

Patricia Szot

1. INTRODUCTION

1.1. What We Know About the Anticonvulsant Mechanism of the Ketogenic Diet

From other chapters in this volume, it is apparent that our understanding of the mechanism of action of the ketogenic diet (KD) is limited. Nevertheless, we do know that the KD is an excellent antiepileptic treatment for many children who are refractory to conventional antiepileptic medications. The KD has been shown to be therapeutically effective for a large variety of epilepsies including myoclonic seizures, infantile spasms, and partial and generalized seizures *(1,2)*.

Because the KD suppresses seizure activity when conventional anticonvulsants do not, the anticonvulsant mechanism behind the KD may be different from conventional agents. A change in the source of energy from glucose to ketones such as β-hydroxybutyrate (BHB) has been hypothesized to be a key factor in producing the anticonvulsant effect of the KD, although it is unclear how this change in energy source produces an anticonvulsant effect. The KD may produce myriad changes in the central nervous system (CNS), all of which may act synergistically to produce an anticonvulsant effect. The anticonvulsant effect of the KD is not simply related to changes in electrolytes, acid–base balance, or lipid fluctuations in the brain *(3–6)*. In addition, ketones *per se* do not appear to alter directly the electrophysiology of hippocampal neurons *(7)*. Therefore, the mechanism of the anticonvulsant action of the KD is unknown at the present time.

1.2. GABA and Glutamate

γ-Aminobutyric acid (GABA) and glutamate are the major inhibitory and excitatory neurotransmitters, respectively, in the CNS. However, the ability of GABA or glutamate to alter neuronal activity can be modulated by other neurotransmitter pathways. Other chapters discussed changes in GABA and glutamate associated with the KD; *see,* e.g., Chapter 15 by Yudkoff et al. This chapter deals with one of the modulatory neurotransmitter systems, the noradrenergic nervous system.

From: *Epilepsy and the Ketogenic Diet*
Edited by: C. E. Stafstrom and J. M. Rho © Humana Press Inc., Totowa, NJ

Norepinephrine (NE) is the major neurotransmitter released from noradrenergic neurons; however, it is not released alone. Neuropeptide Y (NPY), galanin, and adenine triphosphate (ATP) are coreleased with NE. This chapter discusses the ability of NE to modulate seizure activity. Chapter 21, by Weinshenker, discusses the anticonvulsant properties of NPY and galanin and their relationship to the KD.

1.3. Noradrenergic Pathways in the CNS

There are two major clusters of noradrenergic neurons in the CNS: the locus coeruleus (LC) and the lateral tegmental neurons. The LC contains the vast majority of noradrenergic cell bodies in the CNS. These neurons send projections to forebrain regions via three different tracts: the central tegmental tract, the central gray dorsal longitudinal fasciculus tract, and the ventral tegmental–medial forebrain bundle. A fourth tract innervates the cerebellum, and a fifth tract innervates the spinal cord. The three forebrain noradrenergic tracts send projections to regions of the brain such as the cerebral cortex, hippocampus, and amygdala, which are known to be involved in seizure activity *(8)*. The general effect of NE in these regions is to inhibit spontaneous discharge *(8)*. Therefore, enhanced noradrenergic activity in these regions could suppress seizure-induced excitability there. The lateral tegmental neurons lie outside the LC and are diffusely scattered throughout the lateral tegmental region. These neurons have limited projections to the forebrain. Lateral tegmental neurons tend to project to the amygdala and septum of the forebrain *(8)*.

2. NOREPINEPHRINE

The innervation pattern of the noradrenergic nervous system and its inhibitory tone in forebrain regions indicate the ability of this nervous system to suppress neuronal activity. However, more evidence is required to establish a modulatory effect of NE in epilepsy. The following criteria would demonstrate the ability of NE to suppress seizure activity physiologically: (1) noradrenergic neurons are activated during a seizure; (2) NE is released; (3) pharmacological agents that bind to noradrenergic receptors reduce seizure activity; and (4) antiepileptic agents alter noradrenergic function in a manner that would confer an anticonvulsant response. This ability of the noradrenergic system to modulate neuronal activity indicates that the KD and the changes induced in NE levels could contribute to the anticonvulsant action of the KD.

2.1. LC Neurons Are Activated During a Seizure and NE Is Released

To determine whether a seizure stimulates a particular region of the brain, studies have employed the immediate early genes (IEGs) as an indirect marker of neuronal activity. The IEG called c-fos (Fos protein) is a transcription factor implicated in a multitude of cellular processes such as differentiation, growth, and apoptosis *(9)*. Significant increases in c-fos mRNA and Fos protein expression in the LC have been observed with a large variety of convulsant agents, including sound, pentylenetetrazol (PTZ), maximal electroshock, kainic acid (KA), amygdala kindling, picrotoxin, and flurothyl *(10–17)*. The elevation of c-fos mRNA expression in the LC following a seizure corresponds very closely to the intensity (severity) of the seizure *(12,17)*. Further evidence for the involvement of the LC is seen with the increase in the utilization of glucose. Active neurons (as observed with a seizure) will utilize more glucose than nonactive neurons. Studies measuring the uptake of [^{14}C] 2-deoxyglucose (2-DG) have shown that the LC region undergoes an increase in 2-DG utilization *(12,18)*.

The increased LC neuronal activity induced by a seizure subsequently results in increased release of NE from noradrenergic terminals in forebrain regions, as measured by in vivo microdialysis *(19,20;* Szot, unpublished observation). Following a seizure, there are changes in gene expression in noradrenergic neurons for the regulation of NE synthesis, perhaps a consequence of increased NE release. Expression of both tyrosine hydroxylase (TH), the rate-limiting enzyme in the synthesis of NE, and the NE plasma membrane transporter protein (NET) mRNA are elevated in the LC following PTZ- and KA-induced seizures *(11,21)*. The amount of NE released with chronic seizures (kindling) *(22,23)* or with status epilepticus induced by bicuculline *(24)*, KA *(25)*, soman *(26)*, or pilocarpine *(27,28)* can be so extensive that the content of NE in many terminal forebrain regions is significantly reduced up to a week after the seizure. This reduction in NE tissue content is not owing to the administration of a convulsant agent because NE tissue content is not reduced unless a seizure is induced *(26)*. These data demonstrate that noradrenergic neurons are stimulated when a seizure occurs and that NE is released from terminals. The release of NE during a seizure may be a physiological response of the brain to suppress the seizure.

2.2. Loss of Endogenous NE Increases Seizure Susceptibility

If noradrenergic neurons modulate seizure activity, then altering (increasing or decreasing) endogenous NE levels should affect seizure activity. The most convincing data for the modulatory role of the noradrenergic nervous system in epilepsy are observed when endogenous NE levels are reduced. Noradrenergic innervation to the forebrain can be destroyed with noradrenergic neurotoxins such as 6-hydroxydopamine (6-OHDA) or *N*-(2-chloroethyl)-*N*-2-bromobenzylamine (DSP-4). When noradrenergic neurons are lesioned with these neurotoxins, animals exhibit increased susceptibility to a wide variety of convulsant stimuli *(29–33)*.

However, when noradrenergic neurons are lesioned, NE is not the only neurotransmitter lost. As stated earlier, noradrenergic neurons coexpress other cotransmitters such as NPY, galanin, and adenosine, i.e., ATP, and each of these cotransmitters is capable of modulating seizures (discussed in Chapter 21). This creates a problem in interpreting lesion studies because the enhanced seizure susceptibility observed with these neurotoxins cannot be attributed specifically to the loss of NE. Genetically engineered mice that lack NE can be used to circumvent this problem.

The dopamine β-hydroxylase knockout mouse (*Dbh–/–*) selectively lacks the enzyme that is responsible for the conversion of dopamine to NE; therefore, *Dbh–/–* mice lack NE and epinephrine *(34)*. Noradrenergic neurons in *Dbh–/–* mice still synthesize galanin and NPY, indicating the selective loss of NE in noradrenergic LC neurons *(35;* Szot, unpublished observation). *Dbh–/–* mice are significantly more sensitive to seizures induced by flurothyl, PTZ, KA, and sound than are their heterozygous littermates (*Dbh+/–*) *(36)*. The increased sensitivity of *Dbh–/–* mice to convulsant stimuli is also observed as an increase in the expression of *c-fos* mRNA, the IEG that is used as a marker of increased neuronal activity *(36)*. The increased seizure susceptibility and *c-fos* mRNA expression can be normalized in *Dbh–/–* mice when endogenous NE levels are normalized with the administration of L-*threo*-3, 4-dihydroxyphenylserine (DOPS) *(36)*.

The use of genetically engineered mice confirms unambiguously the potent inhibitory effect of endogenous NE on seizure activity. Because reduced NE enhances seizure activity, then hypothetically, subjects with epilepsy should have reduced CNS levels of NE. Animal models of epilepsy that exhibit spontaneous seizures can be used to test this hypothesis. The genetically epilepsy-prone rat (GEPR) is the most studied of these animal models. The increased sensitivity of the GEPR to audiogenic seizures has been closely correlated to the loss of NE. GEPRs have reduced CNS NE tissue content, NE turnover, TH levels, DBH levels, and NE uptake *(37–41)*. Administration of NE, adrenergic agonists, or NE uptake inhibitors inhibit audiogenic seizures in the GEPR *(42–44)*.

Importantly, the GEPR is not the only animal model of epilepsy that exhibits reduced central noradrenergic transmission. The *El* (epileptic) mouse, the *quaking* mouse, and the seizure-sensitive Mongolian gerbil have reduced central NE levels, and their enhanced seizure sensitivity can be ameliorated by the administration of adrenergic receptor agonists *(45–49)*. Central NE levels are also reduced prior to the onset of spontaneous seizures induced by the administration of either cobalt, quinolonic acid, or pilocarpine *(27,28,50,51)*.

These animal models suggest an important role of NE in epilepsy, but other neurotransmitter systems are also involved in spontaneous seizures. In addition, a decrease in central NE is not always observed in animal models of epilepsy. The spontaneous seizures of the *tottering* mouse are closely correlated to a hyperinnervation of the noradrenergic nervous system to forebrain regions, and lesioning the LC in the *tottering* mouse will prevent seizures from occurring *(52)*. This paradox of the *tottering* mouse could be explained if one considers the effect of NE as a modulator. If NE modulates seizure activity by altering either an excitatory or an inhibitory pathway, then depending on which pathway NE is affecting, a proconvulsant or anticonvulsant response is observed. This hypothesis cannot be answered for the *tottering* mouse because the innervation pattern of noradrenergic neurons is unknown.

2.3. Increase in Synaptic NE Levels Is Associated With Anticonvulsant Effect

Stimulation of LC neurons and the consequential release of NE at terminals result in an anticonvulsant effect *(53–55)*. The exception to this rule is the elevation in synaptic NE levels associated with NE uptake inhibitors. Tricyclic antidepressants are pharmacological agents that bind to the NE reuptake transporter protein (NET) and block the uptake of NE from the synapse into the presynaptic noradrenergic terminal. Reuptake is the major mechanism for the removal of NE from the synapse, so when NET is blocked, the synaptic levels of NE increase tremendously. Following administration of NET inhibitors, synaptic NE levels can increase up to sevenfold; *see,* e.g., ref. *56*. The newer serotonin selective reuptake inhibitors (SSRIs) also increase synaptic NE levels to a similar degree as the NET inhibitors; *see,* e.g., ref. *56*. However, the ability of antidepressant agents to modulate seizures, clinically, is variable *(57,58)*. This variability of antidepressants on seizure activity is also mirrored in animal models of epilepsy, where antidepressants may exert an anticonvulsant effect, no effect or even a proconvulsant effect *(45,59–64;* Szot, unpublished observation).

Antidepressants may not exert an anticonvulsant effect because at the doses used to treat depression, the increase in synaptic NE levels is too large—much greater than what is observed when LC neurons are stimulated. This tremendous increase in synaptic NE floods the synapse and surrounding areas, stimulating all the different types of adrenoreceptor (AR). As discussed in the next section, NE can exert an inhibitory and excitatory response depending on the receptor type that is stimulated. Therefore, stimulation of all receptors will negate any specific response. This idea is supported by the recent observation of an anticonvulsant effect against PTZ-, KA-, and cocaine-induced seizures in the NET knockout mouse *(65)*. NET knockout mice have about a twofold increase in synaptic NE *(66)*. This modest increase in synaptic NE (vs acute administration of NET inhibitors) is also observed following stimulation of the vagus nerve *(67,68)* and with the KD (discussed in later sections). The increase in synaptic NE induced by either vagus nerve stimulation (VNS) or KD is also associated with an anticonvulsant effect.

Another possible explanation of why antidepressants may not produce an anticonvulsant effect is that chronic administration of these drugs results in a reduction in noradrenergic neuronal activity and synthesis of NE. These changes in noradrenergic function and receptors may prevent synaptic NE from producing an anticonvulsant effect. The NET knockout mice also have many changes in receptors and neuronal activity *(66)*, yet they maintain the anticonvulsant effect of the elevated NE. It is unclear whether the changes in the noradrenergic nervous system of the NET knockout mouse are similar to the changes in receptors associated with chronic antidepressant treatment.

2.4. Modulation of Seizure Activity With Noradrenergic Receptor Agonists/Antagonists

Iontophoretic application of NE to CNS regions such as the neocortex or hippocampus results in both excitatory and inhibitory responses *(69–73)*. The vast array of ARs is responsible for the variable response of NE. There are four different ARs in the CNS (α_1, α_2, β_1 and β_2), and α_1- and α_2-ARs each have three different subtypes, e.g., α_{1A}-, α_{1B}-, α_{1D}-, α_{2A}-, α_{2B}-, and α_{2C}-AR. Most pharmacological agents distinguish between the four major types of receptor, but not the subtypes. Based on electrophysiological studies, the excitatory response of NE appears to be mediated via the β-receptors and/or α_1-ARs, whereas the inhibitory response is mediated via the α_2-ARs *(74,75)*.

The ability of different AR agonists/antagonists to modulate seizures is quite extensive and complicated. A thorough review of the ability of different AR agonists/antagonists to modify seizure activity has been published *(76)*. In general, these studies indicate that α_2-AR agonists like clonidine are anticonvulsant. However, clonidine has been shown to exert a proconvulsant response *(76; Szot, unpublished observation)*. This dual effect of clonidine on seizure activity may be explained by the complexity of the α_2-AR. In addition to the three different subtypes already discussed for the α_2-AR, the α_{2A}-AR (and to some smaller extent the α_{2C}-AR) are localized both pre- and postsynaptically *(77)*.

The presynaptic α_{2A}-AR acts as an inhibitory autoreceptor to reduce the firing of LC neurons and release of NE; *see*, e.g., refs *78* and *79*. It can be hypothesized that the reduction in NE release owing to the stimulation of the presynaptic α_{2A}-AR would result in a proconvulsant effect. Stimulation of the postsynaptic α_{2A}-AR appears to be responsible for the anticonvulsant effect of α_2-AR agonists *(76; Szot, unpublished observation)*. It is unclear why clonidine exerts an anticonvulsant effect (postsynaptic receptor) against some seizure models and a proconvulsant effect (presynaptic autoreceptor) against others. The other problem with clonidine is that it is nonselective for the three α_2-AR subtypes and binds as well to serotonin and imidazole receptors. The ideal

α_2-AR agonist would be to stimulate just the postsynaptic α_{2A}-AR. Guanfacine is the closest α_2-AR agonist to meet this standard. Guanfacine has been shown to be more selective for the α_{2A}-AR, with little affinity for serotonin and imidazole receptors. At high doses guanfacine has been shown to stimulate the postsynaptic α_{2A}-AR and to enhance spatial working memory, an effect not observed with clonidine *(80,81)*. Recent work with guanfacine in our laboratory has shown an anticonvulsant effect against flurothyl-induced seizures, whereas clonidine produced a proconvulsant effect. Further work needs to be performed to determine whether guanfacine possess an anticonvulsant effect against a variety of different convulsant agents, and its possible future as an anticonvulsant agent. The coadministration of AR agonists with antiepileptics such as valproate has been shown to potentiate the anticonvulsant effect of these antiepileptic therapies *(82,83)*.

2.5. Many Anticonvulsant Agents Alter Noradrenergic Function

If endogenous NE is involved in modulating seizure activity, an intact noradrenergic nervous system should be required for an antiepileptic drug to induce an anticonvulsant effect. Many anticonvulsant agents have been shown to require an intact and functional noradrenergic nervous system to exert an anticonvulsant effect. Lesioning the noradrenergic nervous system or the lack of endogenous NE (dopamine β-hydroxylase knockout mice; *Dbh–/–*mice) attenuates the anticonvulsant effect of phenobarbital, phenytoin, carbamazepine, VNS, and the KD *(82,84–88)*.

It is possible that the loss of noradrenergic function in these models has nothing to do with the lack of anticonvulsant effect; the loss of NE may completely alter the activity of the CNS neuronal network. Another way to determine whether NE is involved in the anticonvulsant action of antiepileptic drugs is to determine whether these medications enhance noradrenergic function. The most compelling data concerning the modulation of the noradrenergic nervous system with antiepileptics come from work with valproate, carbamazepine, and VNS.

Chronic administration of phenytoin, valproate, and carbamazepine increases the tissue content of NE in specific regions of the CNS including the cortex and hippocampus *(89–91)*. Carbamazepine may increase NE levels by reducing the turnover rate of NE or by activating LC noradrenergic neurons; *see,* e.g., refs. *92* and *93,* respectively. The enhancement of NE function does not require chronic treatment. Sands et al. *(94)* showed that valproate significantly increases the expression of TH, the rate-limiting enzyme in the synthesis of NE, with 3 d of treatment, the time required to observe a steady anticonvulsant effect.

Modulation of noradrenergic function is also observed with the newer anticonvulsant therapies. Lamotrigine has been shown to inhibit the uptake of NE in cortical synaptosomal preparations *(95)*. The changes in noradrenergic function induced by these anticonvulsants results in a physiological response; all these anticonvulsants are used therapeutically to treat mood disorders, psychiatric conditions in which the noradrenergic nervous system is a major component in the pathophysiology. What has never been clearly established is whether these anticonvulsants increase extracellular levels of NE—the criterion we hypothesize to be responsible for an anticonvulsant effect.

VNS, like the KD, is an effective nonpharmacological treatment and is used to treat patients who are refractory to conventional antiepileptic drugs. As with the KD and conventional antiepileptic drugs, the mechanism of action of the VNS is unknown. VNS requires the placement of a stimulating electrode on the left vagus nerve trunk. Electrical pulses are delivered, which then lead to stimulation of specific regions of the CNS and suppress seizure activity. Krahl et al. *(87)* showed that the VNS requires an intact noradrenergic nervous system to produce an anticonvulsant response. The LC, the major locus for noradrenergic neurons, is one area in the brain that is activated following stimulation of the vagus nerve; *see,* e.g., refs. *96* and *97.*

More recently, it has been shown that stimulation of the vagus nerve increases synaptic levels of NE about twofold in the hippocampus and amygdala *(67,68).* This change in central NE and the clinical observation that patients with VNS have a change in mood has resulted in the investigation of VNS for the treatment of resistant major depression *(98,99).* An antidepressant response of the VNS is extended to animal models. VNS exhibits an antidepressant effect against the forced swim test (S. Krahl, personnel communication), a response similar to other antidepressant agents that alleviate the symptoms of depression by enhancing synaptic NE levels.

2.6. KD and NE

One approach to determining the mechanism of action of the KD is to determine which neurotransmitter system is required for the KD to exert an anticonvulsant effect. Because so many anticonvulsant agents require an intact noradrenergic nervous system to produce their anticonvulsant effect, we used genetically engineered mice that lack NE (*Dbh–/–* mice) to examine NE's role in the KD. KD did not produce an anticonvulsant effect in the mice that lack NE (*Dbh–/–* mice) but did exert an effect in the control heterozygote littermates *(88).* The *Dbh–/–* mice fed the KD had increased BHB levels similar to their heterozygote littermates fed the KD, indicating that the diet did result in a ketotic state *(88).* The lack of effect of the KD in *Dbh–/–* mice cannot be attributed to elevated plasma glucose levels, which would prevent the shift in energy from glucose to fat because *Dbh–/–* mice have lower plasma levels of glucose than their heterozygote littermates (L. Ste Marie, personnel communication). As discussed earlier with respect to the other anticonvulsant agents, the loss of NE may have monumental effects on CNS neuronal activity. If the KD mediates its anticonvulsant effect through the noradrenergic nervous system, then the KD should increase synaptic NE levels.

To determine whether the KD alters noradrenergic function, NE levels were measured peripherally, i.e., via plasma, in rats fed either the KD or a normal calorie-restricted (NCR) diet. After 3 wk serum NE, epinephrine, and corticosterone levels were measured by radioenzymatic assays *(100,101).* Plasma NE levels in the KD animals were significantly higher than in the NCR animals (Table 1), indicating that 3 wk of the KD results in a significant increase in plasma NE. In contrast, plasma epinephrine and corticosterone levels were not statistically different (Table 1), suggesting that stress did not play a part in producing the increase in plasma NE. In addition, plasma BHB levels at this time were statistically elevated in the KD group, indicating that the KD increases sympathetic tone peripherally. However, the peripheral effects of NE probably are not responsible for an anticonvulsant effect of the KD.

To determine whether the KD alters central noradrenergic tone, in vivo microdialysis was performed on anesthetized animals that were fed either the KD (*n* = 4) or NCR (*n* = 4) as described earlier. A microdialysis probe was placed into the ventral hippocampus of anesthetized rats (urethane 7.5 mg/kg, ip) in a stereotaxic apparatus and artificial cerebrospinal fluid (aCSF) plus 5μ*M* desmethylimipramine (DMI) was infused through

Table 1

Plasma NE, Epinephrine, and Corticosterone Levels

Diet	Norepinephrine	Epinephrine	Corticosterone
NCR ($n = 8$)	6399 ± 871 pg/mL	5280 ± 1186 pg/mL	60.1 ± 13.3 ng/mL
KD ($n = 9$)	11599 ± 1254 pg/mL*	7026 ± 727 pg/mL	70.1 ± 5.6 ng/mL

Note: Starting on postnatal d 37 Sprague-Dawley rats were placed on either the KD or an NCR diet for 3 wk. Rats were fasted overnight prior to the onset of the diet. The Bio-Serve KD AIN-76 diet was used, which contains fat and carbohydrate + protein in a ratio of 6.3:1. The diet was administered to the rats with a 90% calorie intake, which was calculated according to the weight of animals fed a standard rodent chow *ad libitum*. Trunk blood was collected from seizure naïve animals after 3 wk of either the KD or the NCR diet. Plasma samples were stored at –80°C until the radioenzymatic assays were performed. NE and epinephrine were determined by the catechol-*O*-methyltransferase-based radioenzymatic assay *(100,101)*. Plasma corticosterone was measured by an ICI Biomedicals radioenzymatic assay. NCR, Normal Calorie Restricted Diet

* Statistical difference between NCR and KD, $p < 0.05$ with Student's unpaired test.

Table 2

Basal Extracellular NE Levels in the Ventral Hippocampus of KD- or NCR-Fed Rats

Diet	Basal NE level (pg/mL)
NCR ($n = 4$)	104.3 ± 15.8
KD ($n = 4$)	253.5 ± 15.8*

Note: Starting on postnatal d 37 Sprague-Dawley rats were placed on either the KD or an NCR diet for 3 wk. Rats were fasted overnight prior to the onset of the diet. The Bio-Serve KD AIN-76 diet was used, which contains fat and carbohydrate + protein in a ratio of 6.3:1. The diet was administered to the rats with a 90% calorie intakes, which was calculated according to the weight of animals fed a standard rodent chow *ad libitum*. After 3 wk a microdialysis probe was placed into the ventral hippocampus (unilateral) in anesthetized animals. Basal dialysate was collected after a 45-min precollection period from anesthetized animals fed either the KD or the NCR diet for 3 wk. Dialysate samples were analyzed by the same catechol-*O*-methyltransferase-based radioenzymatic assay *(100,101)* used to measure plasma. NCR, Normal Calorie Restricted Diet

* Statistical difference between NCR and KD, $p < 0.05$ with student's unpaired test.

the microdialysis probe. Basal dialysate of rats fed the KD and an NCR diet was collected after a 45-min precollection period. Basal levels of extracellular NE were collected for one 20-min period and analyzed by means of a radioenzymatic assay *(100,101)*. The animals fed the KD had significantly higher basal synaptic NE levels than the NCR-fed animals (Table 2), indicating that the KD results in increased levels of NE in the extracellular space in the ventral hippocampus under basal conditions. The increase in extracellular NE is from a neuronal source because the extracellular levels of NE are undetectable when 5µM DMI is removed (data not shown).

To determine whether the increase in basal synaptic NE was attributable to more NE in the terminals in the hippocampus, high-performance liquid chromatographic (HPLC) analysis was performed to measure the NE tissue content in half brains of rats that had been placed on either the KD or an NCR diet for 3 wk. After the 3 wk, the animals were sacrificed and half the forebrain was removed and frozen on dry ice. The NE content in half a forebrain from animals fed the KD ($n = 15$; 19.9 ± 1.9 ng/mg protein) was not sta-

Table 3
NE Tissue Content in Rats Treated with KD (n = 11) and NCR (n = 11)

Tissue	NE (ng/mg protein)	
	NCR	KD
Hippocampus	15.4 ± 1.2	14.3 ± 0.8
Cortex	18.3 ± 2.1	18.1 ± 2.3
Striatum	5.1 ± 1.3	4.5 ± 0.5
Locus coeruleus	25.5 ± 2.0	22.5 ± 2.1

Note: Starting on postnatal d 37 Sprague-Dawley rats were placed on either the KD or an NCR for 3 wk. Rats were fasted overnight prior to the onset of the diet. The Bio-Serve KD AIN-76 diet was used, which contains fat and carbohydrate + protein in a ratio of 6.3:1. The diet was administered to the rats with a 90% calorie intake, which was calculated according to the weight of animals fed a standard rodent chow *ad libitum.* After 3 wk, animals were sacrificed, brains removed, and specific regions dissected free, frozen, and stored at −80°C. Tissue NE content was measured by HPLC as described elsewhere *(34).* NCR, Normal Calorie Restricted Diet

tistically different from animals fed an NCR diet (n = 16; 18.5 ± 1.3 ng/mg protein). To determine whether minor changes occurred in the content of NE in specific regions of the brain, a second group of rats was placed on the KD or NCR for 3 wk. At the time of sacrifice, the brains were removed and the hippocampus, cortex (frontal and parietal), striatum, and LC were dissected free and frozen on dry ice. The NE content in the KD group was not statistically different from the NCR group in any of the regions studied, although there tended to be a reduction in the tissue content of NE in the KD animals in comparison to NCR animals (Table 3). This indicates that the effects of the KD on noradrenergic neurons is specific: KD enhances the basal release of NE into the synapse.

The KD may elevate both central and peripheral NE levels because the diet was designed to mimic the effects of starvation on seizure susceptibility *(2).* However, the diet enables a sustained effect of starvation; i.e., mainly the blood ketone levels remain elevated during the time the diet is consumed. The plasma levels of ketones (clinical markers of KD effectiveness) rise very quickly during fasting *(102).* Physiologically, fasting has a tremendous effect on the peripheral and central noradrenergic nervous systems: peripherally an increase in plasma NE and tissue content is observed *(102,103).* Centrally, fasting increases the turnover of NE in specific regions of the brain, including the hippocampus and cortex, two regions involved in regulating seizure activity *(104).* Prolonged fasting in mice has been associated with a decrease in NE degrading enzyme monoamine oxidase A mRNA, and an increase in TH mRNA (rate-limiting enzyme in the synthesis of NE) in the LC *(105).* All these changes in noradrenergic neurons occur in fasting *after* an increase in plasma ketones *(102).* These data indicate that following the production of ketones, there is an increase in the peripheral and central extracellular NE levels. Plasma NE levels are elevated approx 72 h after fasting; it is unclear when central extracellular levels are elevated. Further studies are required to determine whether the change in central NE synaptic levels corresponds to the time at which an anticonvulsant response is observed. However, after 3 wk of the KD, an anticonvulsant response is observed and hippocampal synaptic NE levels are elevated, and this increase in NE in the hippocampus could contribute to the anticonvulsant action of the KD.

3. CONCLUSION

NE is an inhibitory neurotransmitter in the CNS that has demonstrated the ability to modulate seizure activity, although it is unclear why its ability to modulate seizures has received little attention. Very little is known concerning the mechanism of action of the KD. The noradrenergic nervous system is clearly involved in the anticonvulsant action of the KD because the loss of endogenous NE prevents an anticonvulsant effect from being produced *(106)*. In addition, the KD elevates NE levels in both the periphery (plasma) and in the CNS, i.e., hippocampus, an effect that is associated with an anticonvulsant response; *see,* e.g., refs. *53–55,65,67,* and *68.* These data indicate that NE, to some degree, contributes to the anticonvulsant action of the KD. The KD differs among antiepileptic therapies because it is effective in treating epilepsies of many different types, e.g., myoclonic seizures, infantile spasms, partial and generalized seizures *(1,2)*, and it is effective when conventional antiepileptic drugs fail. The KD may produce its anticonvulsant effect through multiple neurotransmitter systems, and NE appears to be one of them. Future work will define further the changes in the noradrenergic nervous system that are involved in the anticonvulsant action of the KD.

ACKNOWLEDGMENTS

Special thanks to Thomas Storey, Starr Rejniak, Carol Robbins, and Dr. Kris Bough for the arduous task of feeding the KD to the animals for 3 wk. David Flatness and Sylvia White were responsible for the enzymatic assay that was used to analysis NE in plasma, dialysate, and tissue. I also thank the Pediatric Epilepsy Research Center, University of Washington, for providing the funds to do this research.

REFERENCES

1. Prasad AN, Stafstrom CE, Holmes GL. Alternative epilepsy therapies: the ketogenic diet, immunoglobulins, and steroids. Epilepsia 1996;37 (Suppl 2): S81–S95.
2. Vining EPG, Freeman JM, Ballaban-Gil K, Camfield CS, Camfield PR, Holmes GL, Shinnar S, Shuman R, Trevathan E, Wheless JW. A multicenter study of the efficacy of the ketogenic diet. Arch Neurol 1998;55:1433–1437.
3. Huttenlocher PR, Wilbourne AJ, Signore JM. Medium-chain triglycerides as a therapy for intractable childhood epilepsy. Neurology 1971;21:1097–1103.
4. Appleton DB, DeVivo DC. An animal model for the ketogenic diet. Epilepsia 1974;15:211–227.
5. Huttenlocher PR. Ketonemia and seizures: metabolic and anticonvulsant effects of two ketogenic diets in childhood epilepsy. Pediatr Res 1976;10:536–540.
6. Harik SI, Al-Mudallal AS, LaManna JC, Lust WD, Levin BE. Ketogenic diet and the brain. Ann N Y Acad Sci 1997;835:218–224.
7. Thio LL, Wong M, Yamada KA. Ketone bodies do not directly alter excitatory or inhibitory hippocampal synaptic transmission. Neurology 2000;54:325–331.
8. Cooper JR, Bloom FE, Roth RH. Norepinephrine and epinephrine. In: The Biochemical Basis of Neuropharmacology. Oxford University Press, New York, 2003, pp. 181–233.
9. Curran T, Morgan JI. Fos: an immediate-early transcription factor in neurons. J Neurobiol 1995;26:403–412.
10. Eells JB, Clough RW, Browning RA, Jobe PC. Fos in locus coeruleus neurons following audiogenic seizure in the genetically epilepsy-prone rat: comparison to electroshock and pentylenetetrazol seizure models. Neurosci Lett 1997;233:21–24.
11. Szot P, White SS, Veith RC. Effect of pentylenetetrazol on the expression of tyrosine hydroxylase mRNA and norepinephrine and dopamine transporter mRNA. Mol Brain Res 1997;44:46–54.
12. Szot P, White SS, McCarthy EB, Turella A, Rejniak SX, Schwartzkroin PA. Behavioral and metabolic features of repetitive seizures in immature and mature rats. Epilepsy Res 2001;46:191–203.

13. Silveira DC, Liu Z, de LaCalle S, Lu J, Klein P Holmes GL, Herzog AG. Activation of the locus coeruleus after amygdala kindling. Epilepsia 1998;39:1261–1264.

14. Silveira DC, Liu Z, Holmes GL, Schomer DL, Schachter SC. Seizures in rats treated with kainic acid induced Fos-like immunoreactivity in locus coeruleus. Neuroreport 1998;9:1353–1357.

15. Silveira DC, Schachter SC, Schomer DL, Holmes GL. Flurothyl-induced seizures in rats activate Fos in brain stem catecholaminergic neurons. Epilepsy Res 2000;39:1–12.

16. Willoughby JO, Mackenzie L. Picrotoxin-, kainic acid- and seizure-induced Fos in brainstem, with special reference to catecholamine cell groups. Neurosci Res 1999;33:163–169.

17. Storey TW, Rho JM, White SS, Sankar R, Szot P. Age-dependent differences in flurothyl-induced c-fos and c-jun mRNA expression in the mouse brain. Dev Neurosci 2002;24:294–299.

18. El Hamdi G, Boutroy MJ, Nehlig A. Effects of pentylenetetrazol-induced seizures on dopamine and norepinephrine levels and on glucose utilization in various brain regions of the developing rat. Int J Dev Neurosci 1992;10:301–311.

19. Kokaia M, Kalen P, Bengzon J, Lindvall O. Noradrenaline and 5-hydroxytryptamine release in the hippocampus during seizures induced by hippocampal kindling stimulation: an in vivo microdialysis study. Neuroscience 1989;32:647–656.

20. Bengzon J, Kokaia M, Brundin P, Lindvall O. Seizure suppression in kindling epilepsy by intrahippocampal locus coeruleus grafts: evidence for an alpha-2-adrenoreceptor mediated mechanism. Exp Brain Res 1990;81:433–437.

21. Bengzon J, Hansson SR, Hoffman BJ, Lindvall O. Regulation of norepinephrine transporter and tyrosine hydroxylase mRNAs after kainic acid-induced seizures. Brain Res 1999;842:239–242.

22. Lewis J, Westerberg V, Corcoran ME. Monoaminergic correlates of kindling. Brain Res 1987;403:205–212.

23. Callaghan DA, Schwark WS. Involvement of catecholoamines in kindled amygdaloid convulsions in the rat. Neuropharmacol 1979;18:541–545.

24. Calderini G, Carlsson A, Nordstrom C-H. Monoamine metabolism during bicuculline-induced epileptic seizures in the rat. Brain Res 1978;157:295–302.

25. Nelson MF, Zaczek R, Coyle JT. Effects of sustained seizures produced by intrahippocampal injection of kainic acid on noradrenergic neurons: evidence for local control of norepinephrine release. J Pharmacol Exp Ther 1980;214:694–702.

26. El-Etri MM, Nickell WT, Ennis M, Skau KA, Shipley MT. Brain norepinephrine reductions in soman-intoxicated rats: association with convulsions and AChE inhibition, time course, and relation to other monoamines. Exp Neurol 1992;118:153–163.

27. El-Etri MM, Ennis M, Jiang M, Shipley MT. Pilocarpine-induced convulsions in rats: evidence for muscarinic receptor-mediated activation of locus coeruleus and norepinephrine release in cholinolytic seizure development. Exp Neurol 1993;121:24–39.

28. Cavalheiro EA, Fernandes MJ, Turski L, Naffah-Mazzacoratti MG. Spontaneous recurrent seizures in rats: amino acid and monoamine determination in the hippocampus. Epilepsia 1994;35:1–11.

29. Arnold PS, Racine RJ, Wise RS. Effects of atropine, reserpine, 6-hydroxydopamine and handling on seizure development in the rat. Exp Neurol 1973;40:457–470.

30. Jerlicz M, Kostowski W, Bidzinski A, Hauptman M, Dymecki J. Audiogenic seizures in rats: relation to noradrenergic neurons of the locus coeruleus. Acta Physiol Polonica 1978;29:409–412.

31. Mason ST, Corcoran ME. Catecholamines and convulsions. Brain Res 1979;170:497–507.

32. Trottier S, Lindvall O, Chauvel P, Bjorklund A. Facilitation of focal colbalt-induced epilepsy after lesions of the noradrenergic locus coeruleus system. Brain Res 1988;454:308–314.

33. Sullivan HC, Osorio I. Aggravation of penicillin-induced epilepsy in rats with locus coeruleus lesion. Epilepsia 1991;32:591–596.

34. Thomas SA, Marck BT, Palmiter RD, Matsumoto AM. Restoration of norepinephrine and reversal of phenotypes in mice lacking dopamine β-hydroxylase. J Neurochem 1998;70:2468–2476.

35. Weinshenker D, Szot P, Miller NS, Rust NC, Hohmann JG, Pyati U, White SS, Palmiter RD. Genetic comparison of seizure control by norepinephrine and neuropeptide Y. J Neurosci 2001;21:7764–7769.

36. Szot P, Weinshenker D, White SS, Robbins CA, Rust NC, Schwartzkroin PA, Palmiter RD. Norepinephrine-deficient mice have increased susceptibility to seizure-inducing stimuli. J Neurosci 1999;19:10985–10992.

37. Jobe PC, Ko KH, Dailey JW. Abnormalities in norepinephrine turnover rate in the central nervous system of the genetically epilepsy-prone rat. Brain Res 1984;290:357–360.

38. Dailey JW, Jobe PC. Indices of noradrenergic function in the central nervous system of genetically epilepsy-prone rats. Epilepsia 1986;27:665–670.

39. Browning RA, Wade DR, Marcinczyk M, Long GL, Jobe PC. Regional brain abnormalities in norepinephrine uptake and dopamine β-hydroxylase activity in the genetically epilepsy-prone rat. J Pharmacol Exp Ther 1989;249:229–235.

40. Lauterborn JC, Ribak CR. Differences in dopamine beta-hydroxylase immunoreactivity between the brains of genetically epilepsy-prone and Sprague-Dawley rats. Epilepsy Res 1989;4:161–176.

41. Dailey JW, Mishra PK, Ko KH, Penny JE, Jobe PC. Noradrenergic abnormalities in the central nervous system of seizure-naïve rats. Epilepsia 1991;32:168–173.

42. Mishra PT, Kahle EH, Bettendorf AF, Dailey JW, Jobe PC. Anticonvulsant effects of intracerebroventricularly administered norepinephrine are potentiated in the presence of monoamine oxidase inhibition in severe seizure genetically epilepsy-prone rats (GEPRs). Life Sci 1993;52:1435–1441.

43. Yan QS, Jobe PC, Dailey JW. Thalamic deficiency in norepinephrine release detected via intracerebral microdialysis: a synaptic determinant of seizure predisposition in the genetically epilepsy-prone rat. Epilepsy Res 1993;14:229–236.

44. Yan QS, Dailey JW, Steenbergen JL Jobe PC. Anticonvulsant effect of enhancement of noradrenergic transmission in the superior colliculus in genetically epilepsy-prone rats (GEPRs): a micro-injection study. Brain Res 1998;780:199–209.

45. Chermat R, Doare L, Lachapelle F, Simon P. Effects of drugs affecting the noradrenergic system on convulsions in the quaking mouse. Naunyn Schmiedebergs Arch Pharmacol 1981;318:94–99.

46. Loscher W. Influence of pharmacological manipulation of inhibitory and excitatory neurotransmitter systems on seizure behavior in the Mongolian gerbil. J Pharmacol Exp Therap 1985;233:204–213.

47. Loscher W, Czuczwar SJ. Comparison of drugs with different selectivity for central alpha 1- and alpha 2-adrenoreceptors in animal models of epilepsy. Epilepsy Res 1987;1:165–172.

48. Tsuda H, Ito M, Oguro K, Mutoh K, Shiraishi H, Shirasaka Y, Mikawa H. Involvement of the noradrenergic system in the seizures of epileptic EL mouse. Eur J Pharmacol 1990;176:321–330.

49. Tsuda H, Ito M, Oguro K, Mutoh K, Shiraishi H, Shirasaka Y, Mikawa H. Age- and seizure-related changes in noradrenaline and dopamine in several brain regions of epileptic EL mouse. Neurochem Res 1993;18:111–117.

50. Trottier S, Berger B, Chauvel P, Dedek J, Gay M. Alterations of the cortical noradrenergic system in chronic cobalt epileptogenic foci in the rat: a histofluorescence and biochemical study. Neuroscience 1981;6:1069–1080.

51. Vezzani A, Schwarcz R. A noradrenergic component of quinolonic acid-induced seizures. Exp Neurol 1985;90:254–258.

52. Noebels JL. A single gene error of noradrenergic axon growth synchronizes central neurons. Nature 1984;310:409–411.

53. Libet B, Gleason CA, Wright EW, Feinstein B. Suppression of an epileptiform type of electrocortical activity in the rat by stimulation of the locus coeruleus. Epilepsia 1977;18:451–462.

54. Turski L, Ikonomidou C, Turski WA, Bortolotto ZA, Cavalheiro ES. Review: cholinergic mechanisms and epileptogenesis. The seizures induced by pilocarpine: a novel experimental model of intractable epilepsy. Synapse 1989;3:154–171.

55. Weiss GK, Lewis J, Corcoran ME. Antikindling effect of LC stimulation: mediation by ascending noradrenergic projections. Exp Neurol 1990;108:136–140.

56. Hajos-Korcsok E, McTavish SFB, Sharp T. Effect of a selective 5-hydroxytryptamine reuptake inhibitor on brain extracellular noradrenaline: microdialysis studies using paraxetine. Eur J Pharmacol 2000;407:101–107.

57. Sakakihara Y, Oka A, Kubota M, Ohashi Y. Reduction of seizure frequency with clomipramine in patients with complex partial seizures. Brain Dev 1995;17:291–293.

58. Dailey JW, Naritoku DK. Antidepressants and seizures: clinical anecdotes overshadow neuroscience. Biochem Pharmacol 1996;52:1323–1329.

59. Krijzer F, Snelder M, Bradford D. Comparison of the (pro)-convulsive properties of fluvoxamine and clovoxamine with eight other antidepressants in an animal model. Neuropsychobiology 1984;12:249–254.

60. Clifford DB, Rutherford JL, Hicks FG, Zorumski CF. Acute effects of antidepressants on hippocampal seizures. Ann Neurol 1985;18:692–697.

61. Peterson SL, Trzeciakowski JP, St Mary JS. Chronic but not acute treatment with antidepressants enhances the electroconvulsive seizure response in rats. Neuropharmacology 1985;24:941–946.
62. Applegate CD, Flashman LA, Burchfiel JL. The effects of chronic desmethylimipramine on entirhinal cortical kindling in rats. Brain Res 1986;398:121–127.
63. Kleinrok Z, Gustaw J, Czuczwar SJ. Influence of antidepressant drugs on seizure susceptibility and the anticonvulsant activity of valproate in mice. J Neural Transm Suppl 1991;34:85–90.
64. Yacobi R, Burnham WM. The effect of tricyclic antidepressants on cortex- and amygdala-kindled seizures in the rat. Can J Neurol Sci 1991;18:132–136.
65. Kaminiski R, Shippenburg TS, Witkin JM, Caron MG, Rocha BA. Norepineprhine transporter-deficient mice are less vulnerable to seizures induced by chemoconvulsants. Soc Neurosci Abstr 2002;28:792.2.
66. Xu F, Gainetdinov RR, Wetsel WC, Jones SR, Bohn LM, Miller GW, Wang Y-M, Caron MG. Mice lacking the norepinephrine transporter are supersensitive to psychostimulants. Nat Neurosci 2000;3:465–471.
67. Hassert DL, Miyaswhita T, Williams CL. Alterations in basolateral amygdala norepinephrine after vagal stimulation at a memory modulating intensity. Soc Neurosci Abstr 2002;28:379.10.
68. Miyashita T, Hassert DL, Williams CL. Does peripheral physiological arousal affect the capacity for norepinephrine to modulate memory in the hippocampus. Soc Neurosci Abstr 2002;28:379.11.
69. Nishi H, Watanabe S, Ueki S. Effect of monoamines injected into the hippocampus on hippocampal seizure discharges in the rabbit. J Pharmacobiodyn 1981;4:7–14.
70. Segal M. The action of norepinephrine in the rat hippocampus: intracellular studies in the slice preparation. Brain Res 1981;206:107–128.
71. Szabadi E. Adrenoceptors on central neurons: microelectrophoretic studies. Neuropharmacology 1979;18:831–843.
72. Waterhouse BD. Electrophysiological assessment of monoamine synaptic function in neuronal circuits of seizure susceptible brains. Life Sci 1986;39:807–818.
73. Stanton, PK. Noradrenergic modulation of epileptiform bursting and synaptic plasticity in the dentate gyrus. Epilepsy Res Suppl 1992;7:135–150.
74. Curet O, deMontigny C. Electrophysiological characterization of adrenoreceptors in the rat dorsal hippocampus: I. Receptors mediating the effect of microiontophoretically applied norepinephrine. Brain Res 1988;475:35–46.
75. Licata F, Li-Volsi G, Maugeri G, Ciranna L, Santangelo F. Effects of noradrenaline on the firing rate of vestibular neurons. Neuroscience 1993;53:149–158.
76. Weinshenker D, Szot P. The role of catecholamines in seizure susceptibility: new results using genetically engineered mice. Pharmacol Ther 2002;94:213–233.
77. Bucheler MM, Hadamek K, Hein L. Two α_2-adrenergic receptor subtypes, α_{2A} and α_{2C}, inhibit transmitter release in the brain of gene-targeted mice. Neuroscience 2002;109:819–826.
78. Van Gaalen M, Kawahara H, Kawahara Y, Westerink BHC. The locus coeruleus noradrenergic system in the rat brain studied by dual-probe microdialysis. Brain Res 1997;763:56–62.
79. Kawahara Y, Kawahara H, Westernik BHC. Tonic regulation of the activity of noradrenergic neurons in the locus coeruleus of the conscious rat studies by dual-probe microdialysis. Brain Res 1999;823:42–48.
80. Avery RA, Franowicz JS, Studholme C, van Dyke CH, Arnsten AFT. The alpha-2A-adrenergic agonist, guanfacine, increases regional cerebral blood flow in dorsolateral prefrontal cortex of monkeys performing a spatial working memory task. Neuropsychopharmacology 2000;23:240–249.
81. Birnbaum SG, Podell DM, Arnsten AFT. Noradrenergic alpha-2 receptor agonists reverse working memory deficits induced by the anxiogenic drug, FG7142, in rats. Pharmacol Biochem Behav 2000;67:397–403.
82. Fischer W, Muller M. Pharmacological modulation of central monoaminergic systems and influence on the anticonvulsive effectiveness of standard antiepileptics in maximal electroshock seizure. Biomed Biochim Acta 1988;47:631–645.
83. De Sarro G, Gareri P, Falconi O, De Sarro A. 7-Nitroindazole potentiates the antiseizure activity of some anticonvulsants in DBA/2 mice. Eur J Pharmacol 2000;394:275–288.
84. Quattrone A, Samanin R. Decreased anticonvulsant activity of carbamazepine in 6-hydroxy-dopamine-treated rats. Eur J Pharmacol 1977;41:333–336.

85. Crunelli V, Cervo L, Samanin R. Evidence for a preferential role of central noradrenergic neurons in electrically induced convulsions and activity of various anticonvulsants in the rat. In: Morselli PL, Lloyd KG, Loscher W, Meldrum B, Reynolds EH (eds.). Neurotransmitters, Seizures, and Epilepsy. Raven, New York, 1981, pp. 195–202.

86. Waller SB, Buterbaugh GG. Convulsive thresholds and severity and the anticonvulsant effect of phenobarbital and phenytoin in adult rats administered 6-hydroxydopamine or 5,7-dihydroxytryptamine during postnatal development. Pharmacol Biochem Behav 1985;23:473–478.

87. Krahl SE, Clark KB, Smith DC, Browning RA. Locus coeruleus lesions suppress the seizure-attenuating effects of vagus nerve stimulation. Epilepsia 1998;39:709–714.

88. Szot P, Weinshenker D, Rho JM, Storey TW, Schwartzkroin PA. Norepinephrine is required for the anticonvulsant effect of the ketogenic diet. Dev Brain Res 2001;129:211–214.

89. Baf MH, Subhash NM, Lakshmane KM, Roa BS. Alterations in monoamine levels in discrete regions of rat brain after chronic administration of carbamazepine. Neurochem Res 1994;19:1139–1143.

90. Baf MH, Subhash NM, Lakshmane KM, Roa BS. Sodium valproate induced alterations in monoamine levels in different regions of the rat brain. Neurochem Int 1994;24:67–72.

91. Meshkibaf MH, Subhash MN, Lakshmana KM, Roa BS. Effect of chronic administration of phenytoin on regional monoamine levels in rat brain. Neurochem Res 1995;20:773–778.

92. Waldmeier PA, Baumann B, Fehr P, De Herdt L, Maitre L. Carbamazepine decreases catecholamine turnover in the rat brain. J Pharmacol Exp Ther 1984;231:166–172.

93. Olpe HR, Jones RS. The action of anticonvulsant drugs on the firing of locus coeruleus neurons: selective activating effect of carbamazepine. Eur J Pharmacol 1983;91:107–110.

94. Sands SA, Guerra V, Morilak J. Changes in tyrosine hydroxylase mRNA expression in the rat locus coeruleus following acute or chronic treatment with valproic acid. Neuropsychopharmacology 2000;22:27–35.

95. Southam E, Kirkby D, Higgins GA, Hagan RM. Lamotrigine inhibits monoamine uptake in vitro and modulates 5-hydroxytryptamine uptake in rats. Eur J Pharmacol 1998;358:19–24.

96. Gieroba ZJ, Blessing WW. Fos-containing neurons in medulla and pons after unilateral stimulation of the afferent abdominal vagus in conscious rabbits. Neurosci 1994;59:851–858.

97. Naritoku DK, Terry WJ, Helfert RH. Regional induction of fos immunoreactivity in the brain by anticonvulsant stimulation of the vagus nerve. Epilepsy Res 1995;22:53–62.

98. Elger G, Hoppe C, Falkai P, Rush AJ, Elger CE. Vagus nerve stimulation is associated with mood improvements in epilepsy patients. Epilepsy Res 2000;42:203–210.

99. Sackeim HA, Rush AJ, George MS, Marangell LB, Husain MM, Nahas Z, Johnson CR, Seidman S, Giller C, Haines S, Simpson RK, Goodman RR. Vagus nerve stimulation (VNS) for treatment-resistant depression: efficacy, side effects, and predictors of outcome. Neuropsychopharmacology 2001;25:713–728.

100. Da Prada M, Zurcher G. Simultaneous radioenzymatic determination of plasma and tissue adrenaline, noradrenaline and dopamine within femtomolar range. Life Sci 1976;19:1161–1174.

101. Saller CF, Zigmond MJ. A radioenzymatic assay for catecholamines and dihydrophenylacetic acid. Life Sci 1978;23:1117–1150.

102. Webber RC, MacDonald IA. The cardiovascular, metabolic and hormonal changes accompanying acute starvation in men and women. Br J Nutr 1994;71:437–447.

103. El Fazza S, Somody L, Gharbi N, Kamoun A, Gharib C, Gauquelin-Koch G. Effects of acute and chronic starvation on central and peripheral noradrenaline turnover, blood pressure and heart rate in the rat. Exp Physiol 1999;84:357–368.

104. Wiggens RC, Fuller GN, Seifert WE, Butler IJ, Gottesfeld Z. Catecholamines in rat brain following postnatal undernutrition and nutritional rehabilitation. J Neurosci Res 1982;8:651–656.

105. Jahng JW, Houpt TA, Joh TH, Son JH. Differential expression of monoamine oxidase A, serotonin transporter, tyrosine hydroxylase and norepinephrine transporter mRNA by anorexia mutation and food deprivation. Dev Brain Res 1998;107:241–246.

106. Weinshenker D, Szot P. The role of catecholamines in seizure susceptibility: new results using genetically engineered mice. Pharmacol Ther 2002;94:213–233.

21 Galanin and Neuropeptide Y

Orexigenic Neuropeptides Link Food Intake, Energy Homeostasis, and Seizure Susceptibility

David Weinshenker

1. INTRODUCTION

A key difficulty in determining the mechanism of the anticonvulsant effect of the ketogenic diet (KD) is that it likely influences neuronal excitability via multiple, intergrated systems. It is difficult to imagine that any one particular molecule is solely responsible for its efficacy in treating medically refractory epilepsy. When one is thinking about neuronal excitability, three obvious candidates come to mind; a direct effect of ketone bodies on ion channels, enhanced excitatory glutamatergic transmission, and reduced inhibitory GABAergic transmission. However, despite the existence of these hypotheses for a number of years, none of them have been confirmed, leaving us to consider other mechanisms. One of these, enhancement of norepinephrine (NE) signaling, has recently gained some support based on experiments using microdialysis and genetically engineered mice; *see* ref. *1* and chapter 20, this volume.

The high-fat, low-protein, and low-carbohydrate KD, developed to mimic the effects of starvation on epilepsy, results in a shift in energy metabolism. Therefore, the ideal candidate for mediating the anticonvulsant effects of the KD must link two disparate aspects of physiology: energy balance and seizure susceptibility. The orexigenic (appetite increasing) and anticonvulsant neuropeptides galanin and neuropeptide Y (NPY) fulfill this criterion and should be considered as serious candidates for mediating the anticonvulsant effect of the KD.

2. STRUCTURE AND EXPRESSION OF NPY AND GALANIN

Galanin, a peptide containing 29 amino acids, is one of the most abundant neuropeptides in the mammalian central nervous system. It is found in many different brain regions, including the hypothalamus, dorsal raphé, locus coeruleus (LC), spinal cord, and basal forebrain, and it functions in a wide variety of physiological processes such as regulation of food intake, pain, development, and reproduction *(2–4)*. There are three known galanin receptor subtypes (GALR1, GALR2, and GALR3), all of which are G-protein-coupled receptors *(4)*.

From: *Epilepsy and the Ketogenic Diet*
Edited by: C. E. Stafstrom and J. M. Rho © Humana Press Inc., Totowa, NJ

Like galanin, the 36 amino acid peptide NPY is one of most abundant neuropeptides in the nervous system. NPY and galanin both appear to regulate food consumption, energy expenditure, pain, and reproduction *(2,5,6)*. NPY is expressed in the hypothalamus, hippocampus, cortex, brainstem catecholaminergic nuclei, spinal cord, and sympathetic nervous system, and it signals through at least six (Y_1-Y_6) G protein-coupled receptors *(7–10)*.

3. REGULATION OF FOOD INTAKE BY NPY AND GALANIN

The most pronounced effect of central NPY administration is the stimulation of food consumption in rodents *(2,6)*. This effect is observed in both food-restricted and satiated animals and is elicited via injection of NPY into the lateral ventricles or directly into the hypothalamus. Centrally administered NPY both reduces the latency to feeding initiation and increases acute and chronic meal size. Endogenous NPY expressed in the hypothalamus also affects food intake. NPY mRNA expression is elevated during food deprivation and in genetic models of obesity, and inhibition of NPY signaling can attenuate food intake. Deficiencies have been detected in the NPY system of anorexic mice. These effects are thought to be mediated primarily by NPY-containing neurons in the arcuate nucleus (ARC) of the hypothalamus, which project to the paraventricular nucleus (PVN) of the hypothalamus, known to be a crucial brain region in controlling consummatory behavior *(2,11,12)*. Mice with a genetic deletion of NPY maintain normal body weight and energy balance, suggesting the existence of compensatory mechanisms that are activated in the chronic absence of NPY *(6,13)*.

Galanin, like NPY, increases food intake in rodents when administered intracerebrally or directly into the hypothalamus *(4,14)*. Galanin also appears to exert its orexigenic effects in the PVN, although other hypothalamic regions may also be involved. Galanin receptor antagonists and genetic manipulations of the galanin gene have thus far failed to consistently alter food intake in rodents. Unlike NPY, galanin expression is not typically induced by starvation; for an exception, *see* ref. *15*. This has led to the hypothesis that galanin is linked to food ingestion rather than food deprivation.

4. CONTROL OF NPY AND GALANIN EXPRESSION
BY NUTRITIONAL STATUS

The circulating hormones leptin and insulin have inhibitory effects on the expression of orexigenic neuropeptides. Leptin is a "satiety" hormone that is secreted by fat cells and serves as a signal of energy stores. When energy stores are abundant, leptin levels are high. Leptin decreases food intake via two mechanisms. Leptin activates prepromelanocortin (POMC) neurons in the ARC, which release α-melanocyte-stimulating hormone (α-MSH). α-MSH stimulates cells expressing melanocortin-4 receptors, leading to a decrease in food intake. Conversely, leptin inhibits NPY-containing neurons and decreases the hypothalamic expression of NPY and galanin. Furthermore, NPY expression is induced when leptin levels are low, e.g., during food deprivation and in leptin-deficient rodents, leading to an increase in food intake *(4,11,16,17)*.

Insulin is the primary glucose regulator in the body. When blood glucose levels are high, insulin levels rise and enhance glucose uptake and storage as glycogen. When blood glucose levels are low, insulin levels diminish, and glucose is released into the bloodstream via the actions of glucagon. Insulin, like leptin, inhibits NPY-ergic neurons and suppresses the expression of NPY and galanin in the hypothalamus *(4,12,18,19)*. Taken together, these data indicate that when leptin and insulin levels are low, the expression of NPY and galanin increases, their neurons become more active and peptide release is enhanced.

5. THE RELATIONSHIP BETWEEN NPY, GALANIN, AND FAT

Because the KD is a high-fat diet, it is important to consider the effects of fat ingestion on neuropeptide expression. The relationship between NPY, galanin, and the ingestion of specific nutrients has been examined. Specifically, there appears to be a high correlation between galanin expression and fat ingestion. In animals maintained on selective macronutrient diets, the stimulatory effects of centrally administered galanin on feeding are relatively specific to fat consumption *(20)*. Furthermore, hypothalamic galanin antagonist administration selectively inhibits fat consumption *(21)*. Endogenous hypothalamic galanin levels, as measured by in vivo microdialysis and mRNA *in situ* hybridization, are positively correlated to the amount of fat ingestion in rats, whereas injection of galanin antisense oligonucleotides decreases fat ingestion *(22)*. Importantly, galanin gene expression, peptide production, and peptide release are elevated in rats fed a high-fat diet *(23)*, suggesting that this peptide would be induced by the KD.

Despite this evidence linking galanin to fat ingestion, it is important to note that some studies did not confirm this relationship *(24–26)*. Although NPY does stimulate fat consumption, its effect on carbohydrate consumption is more pronounced *(27)*. NPY expression is actually reduced by a high-fat diet in some situations *(28,29)*, suggesting that the KD may decrease NPY expression in certain brain regions. However, because NPY expression induced by fasting is reduced by the inhibition of fatty acid oxidation *(30)*, the overall effect of the KD on NPY expression is unclear.

6. PUTATIVE EFFECT OF THE KD ON NPY AND GALANIN SYSTEMS

Taken together, these data indicate that starvation conditions induce the expression of galanin and NPY. It stands to reason that these peptides would also be induced by the KD. A combination of the starvation-like phenotype, i.e., ketosis, and low glucose intake elicited by the KD would lead to decreased leptin and insulin. Low leptin and insulin levels would stimulate the activity of NPY-ergic neurons and increase NPY and galanin expression. Furthermore, because fat ingestion may enhance galanin expression, galanin expression would also be increased by chronic consumption of the high-fat KD.

7. NPY AND GALANIN ARE POTENT ENDOGENOUS ANTICONVULSANTS

Pharmacological, physiological, molecular, and genetic experiments have demonstrated the anticonvulsant activity of NPY *(31,32)*. NPY was first identified as a putative endogenous anticonvulsant because NPY expression in the hippocampus, cortex, and amygdala was induced after seizures. Seizures increase hippocampal NPY expression in both GABA-ergic inhibitory neurons, where it is also expressed under basal conditions, and in excitatory granule cells and mossy fibers, which do not normally contain NPY. Pharmacologically administered NPY or NPY receptor agonists are effective anticonvulsants in numerous seizure models, such as picrotoxin, kainic acid, and pentylenetetrazole (PTZ). In vitro and in vivo studies with NPY agonists suggest that NPY inhibits excitatory transmission in the hippocampus via activation of Y_2 and Y_5 receptors.

NPY knockout mice have occasional mild spontaneous seizures and are more susceptible to seizures induced by PTZ and kainic acid (33–35). Mice lacking Y_5 receptors are also seizure sensitive (36,37). Interestingly, the seizure phenotypes of some of these mice are influenced by genetic background, suggesting that other genes interacting with the NPY system can influence its anticonvulsant effect. Finally, seizures induced by kainic acid and by electrical kindling are attenuated in transgenic rats overexpressing NPY in the hippocampus (37a).

Both exogenous and endogenous galanin have potent anticonvulsant activities, which appear to be related to the ability of galanin to inhibit glutamate release (38). Direct application of galanin or galanin agonists attenuates electrically induced hippocampal seizure activity, whereas galanin antagonists exacerbate it (39). Peripherally administered galnon, a galanin receptor agonist that can cross the blood–brain barrier, has anticonvulsant activity against PTZ and electrical seizures (40).

Mice with genetically altered galanin systems also provide strong support for the anticonvulsant activity of galanin. Galanin knockout mice have increased hippocampal excitability and are more susceptible than controls to seizures induced electrically or pharmacologically (38). Kindling epileptogenesis and hippocampal glutamate release are retarded in transgenic mice that ectopically overexpress galanin in hippocampal and cortical neurons (41). Mice overexpressing galanin specifically in noradrenergic neurons have decreased hippocampal excitability and glutamate release and are resistant to seizure induction by perforant path stimulation, PTZ, and kainic acid (38). The anticonvulsant activity of galanin appears to be primarily mediated by the GALR1 galanin receptor because genetic disruption or antisense knockdown of GALR1 receptors results in seizure sensitivity and abolishes the anticonvulsant effect of galnon (40,42).

8. NPY AND GALANIN LINK THE DIETARY ASPECTS OF THE KD TO ITS ANTICONVULSANT EFFECT: A MODEL

A model in which NPY and galanin might mediate the anticonvulsant effect of the KD is depicted in Figure 1. The low glucose content of the KD decreases circulating leptin and insulin levels, which in turn leads to the increased expression of NPY and galanin, the activation of their respective neurons, and enhanced peptide release. Ingestion of large amounts of fat coordinately increases galanin expression. The inhibition of excessive neuronal excitability by NPY and galanin thus contributes to the anticonvulsant effect of the KD.

Some empirical evidence exists that supports this model. First, the administration of a calorically restricted KD indeed results in starvation-like conditions that reduce body weight and inhibit growth (43) and would be expected to promote NPY (and perhaps galanin) expression. Second, reduced insulin and leptin levels are observed in people maintained on the KD (44–48), which again would likely increase the expression of orexigenic neuropeptides. Interestingly, weight gain is a common effect associated with use of many anticonvulsant drugs (49), suggesting that other epilepsy therapies may also activate the NPY and galanin systems. Third, galanin is induced by fat consump-

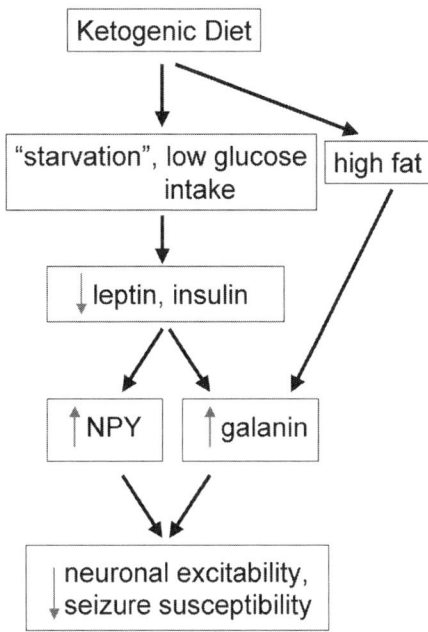

Fig. 1. Model for the mediation of the KD's anticonvulsant effect by NPY and galanin.

tion under some conditions, an effect that would almost certainly occur given the high fat content of the KD. Fourth, inhibition of fatty acid oxidation concurrently reduces ketogenic diet efficacy and NPY/galanin expression *(15,30,50)*.

One appealing aspect of this model is that it leads to a number of predictions that are easily testable.

1. Insulin and leptin levels are decreased by the KD. Although it is clear that insulin levels drop in KD-fed subjects, a rigorous description of the effects of the KD on leptin levels is lacking.
2. Expression of NPY and galanin is increased by the KD in relevant brain regions. The effects of the KD on NPY and galanin levels can be measured by a number of techniques, including mRNA *in situ* hybridization, Northern blotting, the reverse transcriptase polymerase chain reaction, immunocytochemistry, Western blotting, and radioimmunoassay.
3. NPY and galanin are important mediators of the anticonvulsant effect of the KD. The direct contribution of NPY and galanin to the anticonvulsant effects of the KD can be tested by measuring KD efficacy in the presence of NPY or galanin agonists/antagonists, or in genetically engineered mice that either lack or overexpress these neuropeptides.

The primary caveat of this hypothesis is that even though the relationship between nutritional status, NPY, and galanin is firmly established in the hypothalamus, there is no published information on the effects of starvation or fat consumption on the expression of these neuropeptides in regions of the brain implicated in epilepsy. Because most of these studies were focused on food consumption, extrahypothalamic expression of NPY and galanin were not assessed. There are some associations between seizures and hypothalamic activity *(51,52);* it will be critical, however, to directly examine the expression of NPY and galanin in the hippocampus, cortex, and amygdala in animals fed a KD. In support of the model, galanin immunostaining is moderately increased (approx 20%) in the hippocampus of KD-fed rats (J. P. Harney, personal communication).

Another intriguing brain region is the noradrenergic LC, which coexpresses NPY and galanin along with the classical neurotransmitter norepinephrine (NE). Approximately 80% of noradrenergic neurons coexpress galanin, 20% coexpress NPY, and 20% express all three neuromodulators *(53)*. Because NE is already known to be critical for the anticonvulsant effect of the KD, increased NPY and galanin expression in and activation of LC neurons by the KD could enhance the release of at least three known endogenous anticonvulsants; *see* ref. *1* and Chapter 20, this volume.

The specific importance of LC-derived galanin in its anticonvulsant effect has been demonstrated in two ways. First, most of the galanin found in regions of the brain associated with epilepsy such as the hippocampus and cortex comes from LC neurons *(53,54)*. Second, transgenic mice overexpressing galanin specifically in noradrenergic neurons were generated by driving galanin expression with a *Dbh* promoter. These mice have a fivefold increase in galanin mRNA signal levels in the LC and other noradrenergic brainstem nuclei, with very limited ectopic expression *(55)*. *Dbh-galanin* transgenic mice have decreased hippocampal excitability and glutamate release and are resistant to seizure induction by perforant path stimulation, PTZ, and kainic acid *(38)*. Because these mice are similar to animals treated with exogenous galanin and have phenotypes opposite to those produced by galanin antagonists and genetic galanin depletion, it appears that a significant fraction of the anticonvulsant effects of endogenous galanin comes from neurons that coexpress NE. However, galanin that is derived from septal cholinergic neurons that innervate the hippocampus is also likely to contribute to its anticonvulsant effect *(39)*. Although the possibility exists that NPY coreleased with NE is important for seizure susceptibility, it is likely that NPY from other sources plays a primary role. Most of the NPY found in the hippocampus is produced by intrinsic GABA-ergic interneurons. The LC neurons that contain NPY project primarily to the hypothalamus, and despite the existence of noradrenergic projections to the hippocampus and entorhinal cortex, 6-hydroxydopamine lesions of the noradrenergic system do not reduce the NPY content of these epileptic brain regions *(56–58)*. However, NPY produced in noradrenergic neurons could contribute to the anticonvulsant effect of the KD if the KD increased the expression or release of NPY in these neurons.

9. CONCLUSION

The neuropeptides NPY and galanin are intriguing candidates for mediators of the anticonvulsant effect of the KD. These neuropeptides are found in regions of the brain implicated in epilepsy; their expression is modulated by starvation, satiety signals, fat ingestion, and inhibitors of fat metabolism; and they possess robust anticonvulsant activities. The use of molecular, genetic, and pharmacological techniques will reveal whether the mechanism of KD anticonvulsant action involves NPY and galanin. Experiments assessing whether KD efficacy can be enhanced by increasing NPY and galanin signaling will also be of value.

ACKNOWLEDGMENTS

I thank Patricia Szot, Philip Schwartzkroin, Jacob Harney, John Hohman, Ray Dingledine, Richard Palmiter, and Robert Steiner for critical reading of this chapter and helpful suggestions. I also thank Jacob Harney for sharing ideas and unpublished data.

REFERENCES

1. Szot P, Weinshenker D, Rho JM, Storey TW, Schwartzkroin PA. Norepinephrine is required for the anticonvulsant effect of the ketogenic diet. Dev Brain Res 2001;129:211–214.
2. Hökfelt T, Broberger C, Diez M, Xu ZQ, Shi T, Kopp J, Zhang X, Holmberg K, Landry M, Koistinaho J. Galanin and NPY, two peptides with multiple putative roles in the nervous system. Horm Metab Res 1999;31:330–334.
3. Wynick D, Bacon A. Targeted disruption of galanin: new insights from knock-out studies. Neuropeptides 2002;36:132–144.
4. Gundlach AL. Galanin/GALP and galanin receptors: role in central control of feeding, body weight/obesity and reproduction? Eur J Pharmacol 2002;440:255–268.
5. Kalra SP, Horvath TL. Neuroendocrine interactions between galanin, opioids, and neuropeptide Y in the control of reproduction and appetite. Ann N Y Acad Sci 1998;863:236–240.
6. Gehlert DR. Role of hypothalamic neuropeptide Y in feeding and obesity. Neuropeptides 1999;33:329–338.
7. Allen YS, Adrian TE, Allen JM, Tatemoto K, Crow TJ, Bloom SR, Polak JM. Neuropeptide Y distribution in the rat brain. Science 1983;221:877–879.
8. Chronwall BM, DiMaggio DA, Massari VJ, Pickel VM, Ruggiero DA, O'Donohue TL. The anatomy of neuropeptide-Y-containing neurons in rat brain. Neuroscience 1985;15:1159–1181.
9. de Quidt ME, Emson PC. Distribution of neuropeptide Y-like immunoreactivity in the rat central nervous system: II. Immunohistochemical analysis. Neuroscience 1986;18:545–618.
10. Michel MC, Beck-Sickinger A, Cox H, Doods HN, Herzog H, Larhammar D, Quirion R, Schwartz T, Westfall T. XVI International Union of Pharmacology Recommendations for the Nomenclature of Neuropeptide Y, Peptide YY, and Pancreatic Polypeptide Receptors. Pharmacol Rev 1998;50:143–150.
11. Rahmouni K, Haynes WG. Leptin signaling pathways in the central nervous system: interactions between neuropeptide Y and melanocortins. BioEssays 2001;23:1095–1099.
12. Williams G, Bing C, Cai XJ, Harrold JA, King PJ, Liu XH. The hypothalamus and the control of energy homeostasis: different circuits, different purposes. Physiol Behav 2001;74:683–701.
13. Palmiter RD, Erickson JC, Hollopeter G, Baraban SC, Schwartz MW. Life without neuropeptide Y. Recent Prog Horm Res 1998;53:163–199.
14. Crawley JN. The role of galanin in feeding behavior. Neuropeptides 1999;33:369–375.
15. Wang J, Akabayashi A, Yu HJ, Dourmashkin J, Alexander JT, Silva I, Lighter J, Leibowitz SF. Hypothalamic galanin: control by signals of fat metabolism. Brain Res 1998;804:7–20.
16. Jequier E. Leptin signaling, adiposity, and energy balance. Ann N Y Acad Sci 2002;967:379–388.
17. Wilding JP. Neuropeptides and appetite control. Diabetes Med 2002;19:619–627.
18. Schwartz MW, Figlewicz DP, Woods SC, Porte D Jr, Baskin DG. Insulin, neuropeptide Y, and food intake. Ann N Y Acad Sci 1993;692:60–71.
19. Wang J, Leibowitz KL. Central insulin inhibits hypothalamic galanin and neuropeptide Y gene expression and peptide release in intact rats. Brain Res 1997;777:231–236.
20. Tempel DL, Leibowitz KJ, Leibowitz SF. Effects of PVN galanin on macronutrient selection. Peptides 1988;9:309–314.
21. Leibowitz SF, Kim T. Impact of a galanin antagonist on exogenous galanin and natural patterns of fat ingestion. Brain Res 1992;599:148–152.
22. Akabayashi A, Koenig JI, Watanabe Y, Alexander JT, Leibowitz SF. Galanin-containing neurons in the paraventricular nucleus: a neurochemical marker for fat ingestion and body weight gain. Proc Natl Acad Sci U S A 1994;91:10375–10379.
23. Leibowitz SF, Akabayashi A, Wang J. Obesity on a high-fat diet: role of hypothalamic galanin in neurons of the anterior paraventricular nucleus projecting to the median eminence. J Neurosci 1998;18:2709–2719.
24. Corwin RL, Rowe PM, Crawley JN. Galanin and the galanin antagonist M40 do not change fat intake in a fat-chow choice paradigm in rats. Am J Physiol 1995;269:R511–R518.
25. Smith BK, York DA, Bray GA. Effects of dietary preference and galanin administration in the paraventricular or amygdaloid nucleus on diet self-selection. Brain Res Bull 1996;39:149–154.
26. Beck B, Stricker-Krongrad A, Burlet A, Cumin F, Burlet C. Plasma leptin and hypothalamic neuropeptide Y and galanin levels in Long-Evans rats with marked dietary preferences. Nutr Neurosci 2001;4:39–50.

27. Stanley BG, Daniel DR, Chin AS, Leibowitz SF. Paraventricular nucleus injections of peptide YY and neuropeptide Y preferentially enhance carbohydrate ingestion. Peptides 1985;6:1205–1211.

28. Giraudo SQ, Kotz CM, Grace MK, Levine AS, Billington CJ. Rat hypothalamic NPY mRNA and brown fat uncoupling protein mRNA after high-carbohydrate or high-fat diets. Am J Physiol 1998;266:R1578–R1583.

29. Ziotopoulou M, Mantzoros CS, Hileman SM, Flier JS. Differential expression of hypothalamic neuropeptides in the early phase of diet-induced obesity in mice. Am J Physiol Endocrinol Metab 2000;279:E838–E845.

30. Shimokawa T, Kumar MV, Lane MD. Effect of a fatty acid synthase inhibitor on food intake and expression of hypothalamic neuropeptides. Proc Natl Acad Sci U S A 2002; 99:66–71.

31. Vezzani A, Sperk G, Colmers WF. Neuropeptide Y: emerging evidence for a functional role in seizure modulation. Trends Neurosci 1999;22:25–30.

32. Baraban SC. Neuropeptide Y and limbic seizures. Rev Neurosci 1998;9:117–128.

33. Erickson JC, Clegg KE, Palmiter RD. Sensitivity to leptin and susceptibility to seizures of mice lacking neuropeptide Y. Nature 1996;381:415–421.

34. Baraban SC, Hollopeter G, Erickson JC, Schwartzkroin PA, Palmiter RD. Knock out mice reveal a critical antiepileptic role for neuropeptide Y. J Neurosci 1997;17:8927–8936.

35. DePrato Primeaux S, Holmes PV, Martin RJ, Dean RG, Edwards GL. Experimentally induced attenuation of neuropeptide-Y gene expression in transgenic mice increases mortality rate following seizures. Neurosci Lett 2000;287:61–64.

36. Marsh DJ, Baraban SC, Hollopeter G, Palmiter RD. Role of the Y5 neuropeptide Y receptor in limbic seizures. Proc Natl Acad Sci U S A 1999;96:13518–13523.

37a. Vezzani A, Michalkiewicz M, Michalkiewicz T, et al. Seizure susceptibility and epileptogenesis are decreased in transgenic rats overexpressing neuropeptide Y. Neuroscience 2002;110:237–243.

37. Baraban SC. Antiepileptic actions of neuropeptide Y in the mouse hippocampus require Y5 receptors. Epilepsia 2002;43 (Suppl 5):S9–S13.

38. Mazarati AM, Hohmann JG, Bacon A, Liu H, Sankar R, Steiner RA, Wynick D, Wasterlain CG. Modulation of hippocampal excitability and seizures by galanin. J Neurosci 2000;20:6276–6281.

39. Mazarati AM, Liu H, Soomets U, Sankar R, Shin D, Katsumori H, Langel U, Wasterlain CG. Galanin modulation of seizures and seizure modulation of hippocampal galanin in animal models of status epilepticus. J Neurosci 1998;18:10070–10077.

40. Saar K, Mazarati AM, Mahlapuu R, Hallnemo G, Soomets U, Kilk K, Hellberg S, Pooga M, Tolf BR, Shi TS, Hokfelt T, Wasterlain C, Bartfai T, Langel U. Anticonvulsant activity of a nonpeptide galanin receptor agonist. Proc Natl Acad Sci U S A 2002;99:7136–7141.

41. Kokaia M, Holmberg K, Nanobashvili A, Xu ZQ, Kokaia Z, Lendahl U, Hilke S, Theodorsson E, Kahl U, Bartfai T, Lindvall O, Hökfelt T. Suppressed kindling epileptogenesis in mice with ectopic overexpression of galanin. Proc Natl Acad Sci U S A 2001;98:14006–14011.

42. Jacoby AS, Hort YJ, Constantinescu G, Shine J, Iismaa TP. Critical role for GALR1 galanin receptor in galanin regulation of neuroendocrine function and seizure activity. Mol Brain Res 2002;107:195–200.

43. Vining EP, Pyzik P, McGrogan J, Hladky H, Anand A, Kriegler S, Freeman JM. Growth of children on the ketogenic diet. Dev Med Child Neurol 2002;44:796–802.

44. Fery F, Bourdoux P, Christophe J, Balasse EO. Hormonal and metabolic changes induced by an isocaloric isoproteinic ketogenic diet in healthy subjects. Diabetes Metab 1982;8:299–305.

45. Langfort J, Pilis W, Zarzeczny R, Nazar K, Kaciuba-Uscilko H. Effect of low-carbohydrate-ketogenic diet on metabolic and hormonal responses to graded exercise in men. J Physiol Pharmacol 1996;47:361–371.

46. Sankar R, Sotero de Menezes M. Metabolic and endocrine aspects of the ketogenic diet. Epilepsy Res 1999;37:191–201.

47. Fraser DA, Thoen J, Bondhus S, Haugen M, Reseland JE, Djøseland Ø, Forre Ø, Kjeldsen-Kragh J. Reduction in serum leptin and IGF-1 but preserved T-lymphocyte numbers and activation after a ketogenic diet in rheumatoid arthritis patients. Clin Exp Rheumatol 2000;18:209–214.

48. Sharman MJ, Kraemer WJ, Love DM, Avery NG, Gomez AL, Scheett TP, Volek JS. A ketogenic diet favorably affects serum biomarkers for cardiovascular disease in normal-weight men. J Nutr 2002;132:1879–1885.

49. Jallon P, Picard F. Bodyweight gain and anticonvulsants: a comparative review. Drug Safety 2001;24:969–978.

50. Harney JP, Madara J, Madara J, I'Anson H. Effects of acute inhibition of fatty acid oxidation on latency to seizure and concentrations of beta hydroxybutyrate in plasma of rats maintained on calorie restriction and/or the ketogenic diet. Epilepsy Res 2002;49:239–246.

51. Schachter SC. Neuroendocrine aspects of epilepsy. Neurol Clin 1994;12:31–40.

52. Bauer J. Interactions between hormones and epilepsy in female patients. Epilepsia 2001;42 (Suppl 3):S20–S22.

53. Xu ZQ, Shi TJ, Hokfelt T. Galanin/GMAP- and NPY-like immunoreactivities in locus coeruleus and noradrenergic nerve terminals in the hippocampal formation and cortex with notes on the galanin-R1 and -R2 receptors. J Comp Neurol 1998;392:227–251.

54. Hokfelt T, Xu ZQ, Shi TJ, Holmberg K, Zhang X. Galanin in ascending systems. Focus on coexistence with 5-hydroxytryptamine and noradrenaline. Ann N Y Acad Sci 1998;863:252–263.

55. Steiner RA, Hohmann JG, Holmes A, Wrenn CC, Cadd G, Jureus A, Clifton DK, Luo M, Gutshall M, Ma SY, Mufson EJ, Crawley JN. Galanin transgenic mice display cognitive and neurochemical deficits characteristic of Alzheimer's disease. Proc Natl Acad Sci U S A 2001;98:4184–4189.

56. Kohler C, Smialowska M, Eriksson LG, Chanpalay V, Davies S. Origin of the neuropeptide Y innervation of the rat retrohippocampal region. Neurosci Lett 1986;65:287–292.

57. Schon F, Allen JM, Yeats JC, Kent A, Kelly JS, Bloom SR. The effect of 6-hydroxydopamine, reserpine and cold stress on the neuropeptide Y content of the rat central nervous system. Neuroscience 1986;19:1247–1250.

58. Wilcox BJ, Unnerstall JR. Identification of a subpopulation of neuropeptide Y-containing locus coeruleus neurons that project to the entorhinal cortex. Synapse 1990;6:284–291.

22 The Neuroprotective and Antiepileptogenic Effects of the Ketogenic Diet

Jong M. Rho

1. INTRODUCTION

The ketogenic diet (KD) is an effective nonpharmacological treatment for patients with intractable epilepsy and is designed to reproduce the biochemical changes seen upon fasting. The typical KD is composed mostly of fats and results in the production of ketone bodies (β-hydroxybutyrate [BHB], acetoacetate, and acetone) that provide, under certain conditions, the major metabolic substrates for the brain. The diet is highly effective in children, resulting in a greater than 50% improvement in seizure frequency in two-thirds of patients and complete cessation of seizures in 7–10%; it is effective against both partial and generalized seizures (1,2). In approx 20% of patients, anticonvulsant medications can be successfully discontinued without recurrence of seizures.

It is this last observation that forms the basis of the intriguing hypothesis that the KD may possess antiepileptogenic properties, i.e., effects that may ameliorate or even cure the disease process itself, not merely quench repetitive seizure activity. Despite several anecdotal accounts of an enduring effect of the ketogenic diet, however, the most compelling data suggesting a potential antiepileptogenic effect were presented in 2001 by Hemingway et al. (3). These investigators studied the long-term outcome of 150 children with medically refractory epilepsy who were enrolled prospectively in a long-term KD trial. One year after starting the diet, 7% had become seizure free, and 20% had a greater than 90% reduction in seizure frequency; interestingly, 3–6 yr after beginning the KD, a greater percentage of patients (13%) became seizure free.

Intriguing as such observations may be, it is difficult to determine whether patients who remain seizure free after cessation of a KD (following full seizure control for at least 2 yr) have had a spontaneous remission of their epilepsy, have had amelioration owing to lack of damaging repetitive seizure activity, or have experienced a true direct antiepileptogenic effect of the KD. Despite the limitations of clinical speculation, results obtained from the study of animal models have provided some insights, as well as new questions.

From: *Epilepsy and the Ketogenic Diet*
Edited by: C. E. Stafstrom and J. M. Rho © Humana Press Inc., Totowa, NJ

Any discussion of neuroprotection and its implications regarding epileptogenesis must begin with a clear definition of terms *(4)*. The common misconception is that the terms "neuroprotective" and "antiepileptogenic" are synonymous. However, it is clear that epilepsy can develop without overt evidence of neuronal damage (however defined), and neuronal damage does not necessarily lead to epilepsy *(5)*. Thus, there should be some caution in interpreting causality. Much of the discussion in this chapter pertains to neuroprotection; only occasional references are made to the concept of antiepileptogenesis.

2. EXPERIMENTAL STUDIES

2.1. Effects of the KD on Kindling

Numerous animal studies have demonstrated the anticonvulsant effects of the KD. However, the vast majority of these studies have been conducted in normal, nonepileptic animals that experienced acutely provoked seizures following various forms of KD treatment, which have varied widely in terms of dietary composition, duration, age at initiation, species, and modes of seizure induction (for review, *see* ref. *6*). Thus, the relevance of these studies to the human condition—in which a KD is administered to patients *after* a medically refractory epilepsy has been established— is open to debate.

Hori et al. *(7)* were the first to demonstrate the long-term effects of a KD in a chronic epilepsy model. Adult male Sprague-Dawley rats at postnatal d 40–42 (P40–42) were stereotactically implanted with stimulating electrodes positioned in the right basolateral amygdala, after which the animals were subjected to electrical kindling following a standard paradigm. Kindled seizures were graded according to a well-known behavioral scale *(8)*. Ten days after being fully kindled, animals were treated with either a ketogenic diet (with a 4:1 ratio by weight of fats to protein, but no carbohydrate; Purina Laboratories) or standard rodent chow. After-discharge threshold and duration (ADT, ADD) and stage 5 seizure threshold and duration (ST, SD) were assessed weekly for 5 wk. During the third week, the investigators studied the impact of a KD on learning and memory, employing the standard Morris water maze and open-field tests.

Animals treated with the KD maintained steady weight gain, as did the controls, and were found to have significant elevations in blood β-hydroxybutyate during the treatment period. More importantly, KD-fed animals exhibited an elevated ADT and ST relative to controls, but this effect was transient, lasting only 2 wk; this loss of protection occurred despite the maintenance of ketonemia. On the other hand, there were no significant differences between groups with respect to ADD or SD. Furthermore, KD treatment did not affect performance on either the water-maze or open-field tests.

Although kindling as a model of epileptogenesis has been established in at least a dozen animal models (but not in humans, for obvious reasons), and is viewed as highly relevant to the genesis of human partial epilepsy by many investigators, several features of the kindling model do not replicate the human condition. First, kindling is induced in normal (not epileptic) brain, and thus initiation of epileptogenesis differs from the clinical situation in which either genetic or secondary symptomatic etiologies are present. Second, "seizures" or after-discharges occur during the process of epileptogenesis, not after a latent period before the epileptic condition is achieved. Third, kindled animals do not typically experience spontaneous seizures. Finally, compounds tested in the kindling model are administered before the stimulations commence, not afterward *(9)*.

2.2. Effects of a KD in the Kainic Acid Model

Another widely employed animal model of partial epilepsy is the kainic acid model. Kainic acid (a structural analog of glutamate) is an excitatory amino acid that has a high affinity for limbic structures in the brain *(10)*. It induces prolonged seizures, which in adult animals, reliably produce selective hippocampal lesions with a topography similar to that seen with mesial temporal sclerosis in humans *(11–13)*. Adult rats acutely experiencing kainic acid-induced seizures usually develop chronic epilepsy after a clear latent period *(14)*. However, such development of spontaneous seizures is age dependent; immature rats rarely develop spontaneous seizures in response to kainic acid and also resist neuropathological damage, suggesting that they are relatively protected from the long-term deleterious effects of this excitotoxin *(15–17)*.

There are both experimental and clinical data demonstrating that synaptic reorganization, e.g., axonal sprouting, in the hippocampus occurs as a consequence of recurrent seizures and/or neuronal degeneration and could play a role in the development or maintenance of the epileptic state *(18–20)*. Such sprouting is believed to be a response to death of target cells in the hilus and hippocampal CA3 regions. Perhaps the most widely studied anatomic change is "mossy fiber sprouting" seen in dentate granule cells *(18–20)*. Sprouting can be identified with a histological technique, i.e., the Timm stain, which exploits the high zinc concentrations of mossy fibers and their terminals. However, sprouting appears to be an age-dependent phenomenon in that very young animals (up to P15 in rats) do not reorganize in response to kindling or chemoconvulsant-induced status epilepticus *(21)*.

The first evidence that a KD can retard epileptogenesis in an animal model was demonstrated by Muller-Schwarze and colleagues *(22)*. These investigators employed the kainic acid model in adult rats to ask whether a KD could reduce spontaneous seizure activity and synaptic reorganization. Rats underwent kainic acid-induced status epilepticus (12–15 mg/kg), after which they were treated with either a KD (of a formulation similar to that used by Hori et al. in ref. *7*) or a standard diet. As expected, KD-fed animals were significantly ketotic compared with those treated with standard chow. Spontaneous recurrent seizures were recorded by using a closed-circuit video recording system, and routine histology and Timm histochemistry were conducted on hippocampal tissue taken from animals after an 8-wk treatment period.

Spontaneous recurrent seizure frequency and duration were both significantly lower in the KD-treated group ($p < 0.05$ for both measures) in comparison to controls. All rats that experienced kainic acid-induced status epilepticus had evidence of neuronal damage on routine cresyl violet staining, but the KD did not appear to alter the degree of damage seen in both CA1 and CA3 subfields of the hippocampus. In contrast, there was a substantial reduction in the extent of Timm histochemistry (indicative of decreased mossy fiber sprouting) in the KD-fed animals. One potentially confounding factor is whether the observed changes might be attributable to differences in the severity of status epilepticus induced by kainic acid prior to KD treatment. This was not the case, however: Muller-Schwarze et al. *(22)* reported that the clinical parameters of the initial status epilepticus were similar in both dietary groups.

Preliminary reports addressing the effects of a KD in the rat kainic acid model yielded somewhat opposing results. Bough et al. *(23)* treated adult Sprague-Dawley rats with a KD prior to treatment with kainic acid (administered either subcutaneously or intraperitoneally). Rats fed a KD experienced more severe seizures and greater mortality than control animals, and this exacerbation of kainic acid-induced seizures was seen irrespective of route of administration. Similarly, in immature (P20) Sprague-Dawley rats, Ko et al. *(24)* found that a 14-d KD pretreatment exacerbated hippocampal neuronal damage in the CA1 and CA3 subfields 72 h after kainic acid injection, although no significant differences were seen in seizure latencies between the two groups.

The seemingly conflicting results of the aforementioned studies may be explained in part by the timing of ketogenic diet initiation. Muller-Schwarze et al. *(22)* initiated the KD after spontaneous recurrent seizures had manifested, whereas Bough et al. *(23)* administered the KD prior to induction of acute seizures with kainic acid. In the case of KD treatment prior to kainic acid exposure in immature rats *(24)*, there may be developmental differences as well. It could be surmised that the profound metabolic shifts induced by a KD may somehow predispose or precondition the brain to excitotoxic injury, but it is unclear how this might occur. Certainly, vulnerability to neuronal injury depends on both species and strain *(25–27)*.

Although the relationships between kainic acid, seizures, and brain damage have been studied extensively in the rat brain, comparable data do not exist for mice. There is even less information about the effects of kainic acid on developing mice. In a more recent study, Noh et al. *(28)* examined the effects of a KD on kainic acid-induced hippocampal cell death in the ICR strain of mice. Mice were given a single dose of kainic acid (25 mg/kg, ip) after a 1-mo treatment with a KD (4:1 ratio of fats to protein + carbohydrate; Harlan Teklad TD 96355) or standard diet beginning at P21, and histological assessment of injury was made 2 d following kainic acid treatment. Methods used included routine cresyl violet staining, TUNEL staining (*in situ* DNA nick-end labeling, indicative of DNA fragmentation) and proapoptotic caspase-3 immunoreactivity.

KD-fed mice exhibited a significantly ($p < 0.0001$) prolonged seizure latency to kainic acid, but there were no changes in behavioral seizure severity as assessed using a modified Racine scale. Administration of kainic acid resulted in typical cellular loss and pyknosis in the CA1 and CA3 hippocampal subfields of control diet-treated animals. Further, marked TUNEL-positive cells were identified in these regions. Additionally, these investigators used semiquantitative reverse transcriptase polymerase chain reaction to demonstrate a substantial increase in caspase-3 mRNA expression in the hippocampus. Strikingly, KD treatment resulted in a substantial decrease in the number of TUNEL-positive cells and caspase-3 immunoreactivity, suggesting that prior KD treatment affords protection against kainic acid-induced neuronal death.

The contrast between the results of Noh et al. *(28)* and the preliminary study by Bough et al. *(23)*, despite the similar approach of KD treatment prior to kainic acid exposure, may reflect species and/or strain, as well as age differences. Although Muller-Schwarze et al. *(22)* addressed the issue of whether attenuation of the initial kainic acid-induced status epilepticus might account for the long-term effects of a KD on spontaneous recurrent seizure activity and mossy fiber sprouting, the findings of Noh et al. *(28)* are less certain in this regard because seizure latency was significantly impacted by prior KD treatment. Certainly, even though the paradigm used by Noh et al. *(28)* does not replicate the human situation, the results of these investigators suggest that the KD may provide protection against later brain injury.

2.3. Effects of a KD on the EL Mouse

Not all epilepsies arise from remote symptomatic causes, and it is increasingly apparent that many idiopathic epilepsies are the result of mutations in genes that are directly or indirectly involved in regulating neuronal membrane excitability *(29)*. Thus far, there has been only one report examining the effects of a KD on a genetically determined epilepsy model *(30)*. The seizure-susceptible EL mouse is an inbred strain that has been extensively described as a model of multifactorial idiopathic partial epilepsy with secondary generalization *(31–34)*. Generalized seizures generally manifest by P60–70 and persist throughout later life, but it is well known that environmental stimulation such as repetitive handling, e.g., by holding mice by their tails, can induce seizures and facilitate epileptogenesis beginning at P30 *(34)*.

Todorova et al. *(30)* treated male EL mice aged P30 with either a KD (Purina, 4.75:1 ratio of fats to proteins and no carbohydrate) or a normal diet (Agway chow). Over a 10-wk period, mice were tested for seizure activity induced by handling once a week, and plasma β-hydroxybutyrate measurements were made to ensure ketonemia. Although neither control nor KD-treated mice had seizures during the first week of dietary treatment, seizure susceptibility scores in the KD-fed group were significantly lower than in the control mice after 3 wk; however, this difference disappeared by wk 7. Overall, KD treatment delayed seizure onset in young EL mice by one month, but similar to what had been reported by Hori et al. *(7)* in the kindling model, seizure protection was transient. In essence, the epileptogenesis curve, i.e., mean seizure severity score vs time, was shifted to the right.

3. POTENTIAL NEUROPROTECTIVE MECHANISMS

The few studies described in the preceding section represent the scant literature on the effects of a KD on animal models of neuroprotection and epileptogenesis. Collectively, the published data suggest that the KD may exert neuroprotective and antiepileptogenic actions. It is then appropriate to ask the following: "What mechanisms contribute crucially toward such effects?"

There are two general experimental lines of evidence suggesting potential neuroprotective effects of a ketogenic diet. The first relates to the role of polyunsaturated fatty acids (PUFAs) as potent neuroprotective agents via actions on neurotransmitter receptors and ion channels *(35,36)*. The second involves the ketosis that accompanies the KD, or to a lesser extent, caloric restriction *(37)*. Fasting has long been known to enhance seizure control, and indeed the KD was designed to mimic this physiological and biochemical state; but the neuroprotective benefits arising from such a regimen have only recently been elucidated *(38–40)*.

Although there are likely many putative mechanisms that could contribute to neuroprotection, the remainder of this chapter focuses on the role of fatty acids, ketones, and γ-aminobutyric acid (GABA, the major inhibitory neurotransmitter in the mammalian central nervous system). These three substrates converge at the level of the mitochondria, the important cellular organelles that are indisputably the central players in determining cellular injury or death (41,42).

3.1. Fatty Acids and the KD

The standard KD formulation includes a preponderance of fats over protein and carbohydrates. Clinically as well as experimentally, the ketogenic potential is expressed as a ratio of grams of fat to grams of carbohydrate plus protein. A 4:1 or 3:1 ratio is usually used in clinical practice, and sometimes higher ratios are used in experimental models. Maintaining such a high ketogenic potential usually entails a diet composed of fatty foods, creams, and special oils.

Of the fats that constitute various forms of a KD, PUFAs have received by far the most attention. There is now an abundant literature describing the health benefits of PUFAs, particularly for cardiovascular diseases (35,43–45). Specifically, PUFAs have been implicated in the prevention of coronary artery disease and fatal ventricular arrhythmias, and in decreasing the risk of sudden cardiac arrest (35,43–45). The putative mechanisms accounting for such effects involve PUFA inhibition of fast, voltage-dependent sodium channels (46,47) and L-type calcium channels (48).

Given these compelling observations, what is the evidence for PUFA action on epileptic brain? PUFAs may help reduce seizure activity (49–51) and were found to be elevated in patients treated with the KD (52). Recalling their effects against cardiovascular disease, it is believed that PUFAs may exert anticonvulsant actions through modulation of voltage-gated ion channels (53,54). And although the inhibitory effects of PUFAs have been appreciated for some time, there is increasing evidence that they may provide neuroprotective actions as well (36,55). Although the mechanisms of neuroprotection afforded by PUFAs remain to be fully elucidated, it has been hypothesized that opening of pre- and postsynaptic potassium channels may dampen the excitotoxicity induced by transient global ischemia and kainic acid (36).

Another important mechanism by which fatty acids might afford neuroprotection is via mitochondrial uncoupling proteins (UCPs). It is well established that fatty acids can upregulate the activity of UCPs, several of which have been identified in the mammalian brain (56–58). Mitochondrial UCPs possess a number of functions, all related to their primary role in diminishing the proton gradient across the inner mitochondrial membrane. The net effect of this action is to reduce ATP synthesis, reduce calcium influx into the mitochondrial matrix, dissipate heat, and reduce the production of reactive oxygen species (ROSs) (56). The reduction of calcium influx and ROS production are highly relevant to neuroprotection.

Mitochondrial ROS production is intimately linked to the mitochondrial membrane potential ($\Delta\Psi$). A higher $\Delta\Psi$ increases and promotes ROS production through increased electron shunting. UCPs dissipate $\Delta\Psi$ by increasing proton conductance, and this effect subsequently decreases ROS formation. Even a modest reduction of $\Delta\Psi$ can significantly reduce ROS production (59). In support of this concept, it was demonstrated that when fatty acids increased UCP-2 expression and activity ROS production (as well as) in immature hippocampus, dramatic protection against kainate-induced neuronal death resulted (58). Even more germane to the current discussion is the preliminary study by Sullivan et al. (60), who demonstrated that a KD increased mitochondrial uncoupling and decreased ROS production in mouse hippocampus.

The five known uncoupling proteins (UCP-1–UCP-5) differ greatly in terms of tissue distribution and physiological import *(57)*. Although the functional significance of brain UCPs is incompletely understood, there is emerging evidence that UCP-2 plays an important role both in neuromodulation and neuroprotection *(56,58)*. Overexpression of UCP-2 *(61)* or UCP-5 *(62)* decreases ROS production. At this time, the roles of both UCP-4 and UCP-5, almost exclusively localized to the central nervous system, remain unclear *(57)*. However, preliminary data *(63)* suggest that these, too, may exert neuroprotective actions.

3.2. Ketone Bodies and the KD

Despite decades of clinical experience with the KD, the mechanisms underlying its anticonvulsant actions remain poorly understood. Among the numerous mechanistic hypotheses advanced to explain the anticonvulsant activity of the KD *(64)* are the following; (1) changes in brain pH, e.g., acidosis, which would favor neuronal inhibition through proton-sensitive ion channels *(65)*; (2) direct inhibitory actions of fatty acids, i.e., PUFAs *(66)*; (3) changes in energy metabolism, reflected in part by ketone body production and metabolism *(67–69)*; and (4) neurotransmitter alterations *(70–73)*. Because of the striking ketosis associated with the KD and the ease with which BHB can be measured, much of the attention in this field has focused on the role of ketone bodies as mediators. However, direct evidence for a specific mechanism involving ketones has not emerged.

Investigators have observed that ketosis is necessary but not always sufficient for seizure control with the KD, and it is well known that seizure control gradually improves within the first few weeks of KD initiation, as serum ketone levels steadily increase. Interestingly, seizure control can be abruptly lost when ketosis is broken, usually through ingestion of carbohydrates *(74)*. Furthermore, blood BHB levels appear to correlate directly with seizure control in children placed on a KD *(75)*. These observations, nevertheless, have suggested a direct role for ketone bodies in limiting seizure activity.

Data from animal studies largely support these clinical observations, but even with prominent ketosis, i.e., >4mM, protection against acutely induced seizure activity is not universally seen *(76)*. Nevertheless, given the generally strong correlation between elevated blood ketone levels and enhanced seizure control with the KD *(75)*, it is important to resolve whether ketones are directly responsible for blocking neuronal excitability and/or synchrony, either acutely and/or chronically. This is also of practical importance to the future development of ketone analogs that could retain biological activity without the risk of adverse effects ordinarily encountered in clinical practice *(77)*.

Thio et al. *(78)* utilized standard cellular electrophysiological techniques to help answer this question. In their hands, acute application of BHB and acetoacetate did not affect *(1)* excitatory postsynaptic potentials (EPSPs) and population spikes in CA1 pyramidal neurons after Schaffer collateral stimulation, (2) spontaneous epileptiform activity in the hippocampal–entorhinal cortex slice seizure model, and (3) whole-cell currents evoked by glutamate, kainate, and GABA in cultured hippocampal neurons. Our own electrophysiological data in cultured rat and mouse neocortical neurons support these findings (Rho et al., unpublished data); over a wide concentration range (300µM–10mM), BHB and acetoacetate did not affect GABA$_A$ receptors, ionotropic glutamate receptors, or voltage-gated sodium channels (known molecular targets of most anticonvulsant medications). However, there are two major limitations of these studies: (1) ketones were infused acutely, not chronically; and *(2)* both culture and perfusion media contained glucose, which would be expected to prevent a "ketotic" environment.

Although it remains unclear whether ketone bodies can exert direct effects on membrane excitability, there are nevertheless some intriguing data demonstrating neuroprotective actions which may ultimately be relevant for seizure control. For example, both BHB and acetoacetate have been shown to provide direct neuroprotective effects *(38,39)*. In the former study, D-β-hydroxybutyrate (4mM) protected cultured mesencephalic neurons from the toxic effects of MPP$^+$ (the heroin analog 1-methyl-4-phenylpyridinium, which induces death of dopaminergic neurons in the substantia nigra) and hippocampal neurons from the lethal effects of the amyloid protein fragment Aβ$_{1-42}$ *(38)*. Additionally, Garcia and Massieu *(39)* showed that acetoacetate provided partial protection against cerebellar granule cell damage induced by the simultaneous inhibition of glutamate uptake and the mitochondrial electron transport chain in vitro; interestingly, BHB at a concentration of 5mM did not show any protective effects in their model.

3.3. The KD and GABA

Although most studies focusing on brain injury have addressed "excitotoxic," i.e., glutamatergic, mechanisms, there is also evidence that activation of GABA$_A$ receptors can help protect the brain from the consequences of exogenous injury *(79,80)* and perhaps seizures. Many anticonvulsant medications such as phenobarbital are believed to act principally by positively modulating postsynaptic GABA$_A$ receptors *(81)*. These pharmacological agents may also possess neuroprotective properties. There are numerous reports to support this concept. For example, brief treatment with phenobarbital (coadministered with kainic acid) protected against excitotoxic damage in the dentate gyrus of adult rats, eliminated the increased susceptibility to kindling associated with kainic acid, and reduced mossy fiber sprouting, which has been associated with long-term hyperexcitability *(82)*. Phenobarbital, widely prescribed in children with epilepsy, prevented kainic acid-associated brain injury in prepubescent rats *(83)*. Vigabatrin, an irreversible inhibitor of the GABA-transaminase (GABA-T), has been reported to be neuroprotective in both the perforant pathway stimulation model of status epilepticus *(84)* and kainic acid seizure model in mature rats *(85)*, but not in the lithium–pilocarpine model of temporal lobe epilepsy *(86)*.

However, long-term exposure of the brain to ketone bodies (or other substrate[s] associated with the ketotic state) may influence GABA production, release, reuptake, or degradation. In support of this possibility, ketone bodies have been reported to increase the content of GABA produced from radiolabeled precursors in synaptosomes isolated from rat brain *(70)*. Furthermore, elevated concentrations of GABA have been reported in forebrain and cerebellar homogenates of KD-fed mice *(72)*. In contrast, utilizing colorimetric assays, Al-Mudallal et al. *(65)* found no significant elevations in brain GABA levels in rats treated with a KD. Thus, the question of whether the KD enhances GABA-ergic inhibition in the brain remains unclear.

3.4. The KD and Dentate Gyrus Excitability

There are scant data addressing the effects of a KD on functional synaptic transmission, largely because of difficulties in replicating the relevant biochemical milieu in vitro: standard culture bathing medium contains $10 mM$ glucose, which is likely to counter the ketotic environment that may be crucial for an anticonvulsant effect. Bough et al. *(87)* were the first to evaluate the effects of a KD on cellular excitability *in vivo;* extracellular field recordings were made in the dentate gyrus of KD- and control-fed animals and standard electrophysiological parameters of inhibition and excitation were examined. The dentate gyrus was chosen because of its important role in modulating hippocampal excitability and its relevance to the process of epileptogenesis.

Field recordings were conducted in Sprague-Dawley rats fed one of three diets: ketogenic calorie restricted (KCR), normal calorie restricted (NCR), or normal *ad libitum* (NAL) after more than 28 d of treatment. Both KCR and NCR groups exhibited significantly elevated blood BHB levels. Animals fed either KCR or NCR exhibited a rightward shift in input–output curves (indicating reduced excitability) and a greater degree of paired-pulse inhibition (30-ms interpulse interval, paired pulses delivered at 0.1 or 1 Hz) compared with NAL controls. Furthermore, KCR and NCR groups showed less paired-pulse facilitation than did the NAL group (stimulated at 1 Hz), elevated maximum dentate activation threshold, and attenuated spreading depression-like events. However, only KD treatment significantly inhibited the "kindling-like" prolongation of discharge duration after repeated stimulation.

These data indicated that caloric restriction and subsequent ketosis (either with KCR or NCR) are associated with decreased network excitability in the dentate gyrus, a structure critically involved in seizure genesis. Furthermore, the results suggested that the KD, in addition to its anticonvulsant action, may be antiepileptogenic. Finally, at a mechanistic level, because it has been established that enhanced fast-feedback inhibition in the dentate gyrus (as determined with a standard paired-pulse paradigm) is indicative of increased $GABA_A$ receptor activation *(88),* this study also supports the hypothesis that KD and caloric restriction (or caloric restriction alone) can enhance GABA-ergic inhibition in the dentate gyrus network.

4. CONCLUSION

Despite over eight decades of clinical use, little is known of the mechanisms through which the KD induces an anticonvulsant effect. Given that the KD is highly effective in the treatment of medically refractory epilepsy (irrespective of seizure type), exploration of novel mechanisms that could contribute crucially to seizure control, neuroprotection, and perhaps antiepileptogenesis is of paramount importance for the future of epilepsy therapeutics. Admittedly, research addressing the neuroprotective and antiepileptogenic potential of the KD is still in its infancy. Yet, there are already tantalizing and intriguing observations that should spur both clinical and basic investigators to expedite the study of this unusual but effective dietary form of medical therapy, one that juxtaposes the complexities of brain function with the myriad metabolic processes that depend on multiple organs and multiple systems.

REFERENCES

1. Vining EPG, Freeman JM, Ballaban-Gil K, Camfield CS, Camfield PR, Holmes GL, Shinnar S, Shuman R, Trevathan E, Wheless JW. A multicenter study of the efficacy of the ketogenic diet. Arch Neurol 1998;55:1433–1437.
2. Freeman JM, Vining EPG, Pillas DJ, Pyzik PL, Casey JC, Kelly MT. The efficacy of the ketogenic diet—1998: a prospective evaluation of intervention in 150 children. Pediatrics 1998;102:1358–1363.

3. Hemingway C, Freeman JM, Pillas DJ, Pyzik PL. The ketogenic diet: a 3- to 6-year follow-up of 150 children enrolled prospectively. Pediatrics 2001;108:898–905.

4. Cole AJ, Dichter M. Neuroprotection and antiepileptogenesis: overview, definitions, and context. Neurology 2002;59 (9 Suppl 5):S1–S2.

5. Baram TZ, Eghbal-Ahmadi M, Bender RA. Is neuronal death required for seizure-induced epileptogenesis in the immature brain? Prog Brain Res 2002;135:365–375.

6. Stafstrom CE. Animal models of the ketogenic diet: what have we learned, what can we learn? Epilepsy Res 1999:37:241–259.

7. Hori A, Tandon P, Holmes GL, Stafstrom CE. Ketogenic diet: effects on expression of kindled seizures and behavior in adult rats. Epilepsia 1997;38:750–758.

8. Racine RJ. Modification of seizure activity by electrical stimulation: II. Motor seizure. Electroencephalogr Clin Neurophysiol 1972;32:281–294.

9. Pitkanen A. Drug-mediated neuroprotection and antiepileptogenesis: animal data. Neurology 2002;59 (9 Suppl 5):S27–S33.

10. Ben-Ari Y, Riche D, Ghilini G, Naquet R. Electrographic, clinical and pathological alterations following systemic administration of kainic acid, bicuculline or pentylenetetrazol: metabolic mapping using the deoxyglucose method with special reference to the pathology of epilepsy. Neuroscience 1981;6:1361–1391.

11. Falconer MA, Serafetinides EA, Corsellis JAN. Etiology and pathogenesis of temporal lobe epilepsy. Arch Neurol 1964;10:233–248.

12. Scheibel ME, Crandall PH, Scheibel AB. The hippocampal–dentate complex in temporal lobe epilepsy. Epilepsia 1974;15:55–80.

13. Lothman EW, Collins RC. Kainic acid induced limbic seizures: metabolic, behavioral, electroencephalographic and neuropathological correlates. Brain Res 1981;218:299–318.

14. Cavalheiro EA, Riche DA, Le Gal La Salle G. Long-term effects of intrahippocampal kainic acid injection in rats: a method for inducing spontaneous recurrent seizures. Clin Neurophysiol 1982;53:581–589.

15. Albala BJ, Moshé SL, Okada R. Kainic acid-induced seizures: a developmental study. Dev Brain Res 1984;13:139–148.

16. Holmes GL, Thompson JL. Effects of kainic acid on seizure susceptibility in the developing brain. Dev Brain Res 1988;39:51–59.

17. Sperber EF, Haas KZ, Stanton PK, Moshé SL. Resistance of the immature hippocampus to seizure-induced synaptic reorganization. Dev Brain Res 1991;60:88–93.

18. Tauck DL, Nadler JV. Evidence of functional mossy fiber sprouting in hippocampal formation of kainic acid-treated rats. J Neurosci 1985;5:1016–1022.

19. Sutula T, Cascino G, Cavazos J, Parada I, Ramirez L. Mossy fiber synaptic reorganization in the epileptic human temporal lobe. Ann Neurol 1989;26:321–330.

20. Cavazos JE, Golarai G, Sutula TP. Mossy fiber synaptic reorganization induced by kindling: time course of development, progression, and permanence. J Neurosci 1991;11:2795–2803.

21. Sperber EF, Haas KZ, Moshé SL. Developmental aspects of status epilepticus. Int Pediatr 1992;7:213–222.

22. Muller-Schwarze AB, Tandon P, Liu Z, Yang Y, Holmes GL, Stafstrom CE. Ketogenic diet reduces spontaneous seizures and mossy fiber sprouting in the kainic acid model. Neuroreport 1999;10:1517–1522.

23. Bough KJ, Fetner JD, Eagles DA. A ketogenic diet exacerbates kainate-induced seizures in the rat. Soc Neurosci Abstr 1998;24:1208.

24. Ko TS, Soo AC, Kim DW, Kim KJ. Ketogenic diet: Effects on hippocampal c-*fos* expression and neuronal death after kanic acid-induced seizures in immature rats. Epilepsia 1999;40 (Suppl 7):79.

25. Golden GT, Smith GG, Ferraro TN, Reyes PF, Kulp JK, Fariello RG. Strain differences in convulsive response to the excitotoxin kainic acid. Neuroreport 1991;2:141–144.

26. Golden GT, Smith GG, Ferraro TN, Reyes PF. Rat strain and age differences in kainic acid induced seizures. Epilepsy Res 1995;20:151–159.

27. Schauwecker PE, Steward O. Genetic determinants of susceptibility to excitotoxic cell death: implications for gene targeting approaches. Proc Natl Acad Sci U S A 1997;94:4103–4108.

28. Noh HS, Kim YS, Lee HP, Chung KM, Kim DW, Kang SS, Cho GJ, Choi WS. The protective effect of a ketogenic diet on kainic acid-induced hippocampal cell death in the male ICR mice. Epilepsy Res 2003;53:119–128.

29. Noebels JL. Exploring new gene discoveries in idiopathic generalized epilepsy. Epilepsia 2003;44 (Suppl 2):16–21.

30. Todorova MT, Tandon P, Madore RA, Stafstrom CE, Seyfried TN. The ketogenic diet inhibits epileptogenesis in EL mice: a genetic model for idiopathic epilepsy. Epilepsia 2000;41:933–940.

31. Fueta Y, Matsuoka S, Mita T. Crossbreeding analysis of the mouse epilepsy. Sangyo Ika Daigaku Zasshi 1986;20:417–420.

32. Seyfried TN, Brigande JV, Flavin HJ, Frankel WN, Rise ML, Wieraszko A. Genetic and biochemical correlates of epilepsy in the EL mouse. Neuroscience 1992;18 (Suppl 2):9–20.

33. Frankel WN, Valenzuela A, Lutz CM, Johnson EW, Dietrich WF, Coffin JM. New seizure frequency QTL and the complex genetics of epilepsy in EL mice. Mamm Genome 1995;6:830–838.

34. Todorova MT, Burwell TJ, Seyfried TN. Environmental risk factors for multifactorial epilepsy in EL mice. Epilepsia 1999;40:1697–1707.

35. Leaf A, Kang JX, Xiao YF, Billman GE, Voskuyl RA. The antiarrhythmic and anticonvulsant effects of dietary n-3 fatty acids. J Membr Biol 1999;172:1–11.

36. Lauritzen I, Blondeau N, Heurteaux C, Widmann C, Romey G, Lazdunski M. Polyunsaturated fatty acids are potent neuroprotectors. EMBO J 2000;19:1784–1793.

37. Merry BJ. Molecular mechanisms linking calorie restriction and longevity. Int J Biochem Cell Biol 2002;34:1340–1354.

38. Kashiwaya Y, Takeshima T, Mori N, Nakashima K, Clarke K, Veech RL. D-β-Hydroxybutyrate protects neurons in models of Alzheimer's and Parkinson's disease. Proc Natl Acad Sci U S A 2000;97:5440–5444.

39. Garcia O, Massieu L. Strategies for neuroprotection against L-trans-2,4-pyrrolidine dicarboxylate-induced neuronal damage during energy impairment in vitro. J Neurosci Res 2001;64:418–428.

40. Veech RL, Chance B, Kashiwaya Y, Lardy HA, Cahill GFJr. Ketone bodies, potential therapeutic uses. IUBMB Life 2001;51:241–247.

41. Calabrese V, Scapagnini G, Giuffrida Stella AM, Bates TE, Clark JB. Mitochondrial involvement in brain function and dysfunction: relevance to aging, neurodegenerative disorders and longevity. Neurochem Res 2001;26:739–764.

42. Newmeyer DD, Ferguson-Miller S. Mitochondria: releasing power for life and unleashing the machineries of death. Cell 2003;112:481–490.

43. Leaf A, Kang JX. Prevention of cardiac sudden death by n-3 fatty acids: a review of the evidence. J Intern Med 1996;240:5–12.

44. Nordoy A. Dietary fatty acids and coronary artery disease. Lipids 1999;34:S19–S22.

45. Leaf A, Kang JX, Xiao YF, Billman GE. Clinical prevention of sudden cardiac death by n-3 polyunsaturated fatty acids and mechanism of prevention of arrhythmias by n-3 fish oils. Circulation 2003;107:2646–2652.

46. Xiao Y-F, Kang JX, Morgan JP, et al. Blocking effects of polyunsaturated fatty acids on Na^+ channels of neonatal rat ventricular myocytes. Proc Natl Acad Sci U S A 1995;92:11000–110004.

47. Xiao Y-F, Wright SN, Wang GK, et al. n-3 Fatty acids suppress voltage-gated Na^+ currents in HEK293t cells transfected with the α-subunit of the human cardiac Na^+channel. Proc Natl Acad Sci U S A 1998;95:2680–2685.

48. Xiao Y-F, Gomez AM, Morgan JP, et al. Suppression of voltage-gated L-type Ca^{2+} currents by polyunsaturated fatty acids in adult and neonatal rat cardiac myocytes. Proc Natl Acad Sci U S A 1997;94:4182–4187.

49. Yehuda S, Carasso RL, Mostofsky DI. Essential fatty acid preparation (SR-3) raises the seizure threshold in rats. Eur J Pharmacol 1994;254:193–198.

50. Voskuyl RA, Vreugdenhil M, Kang JX, Leaf A. Anticonvulsant effect of polyunsaturated fatty acids in rats, using the cortical stimulation model. Eur J Pharmacol 1998;341:145–152.

51. Schlanger S, Shinitzky M, Yam D. Diet enriched with omega-3 fatty acids alleviates convulsion symptoms in epilepsy patients. Epilepsia 2002;43:103–104.

52. Fraser DD, Whiting S, Andrew RD, Macdonald EA, Musa-Veloso K, Cunnane SC. Elevated polyunsaturated fatty acids in blood serum obtained from children on the ketogenic diet. Neurology 2003;60:1026–1029.

53. Vreugdenhil M, Bruehl C, Voskuyl RA, Kang JX, Leaf A, Wadman WJ. Polyunsaturated fatty acids modulate sodium and calcium currents in CA1 neurons. Proc Natl Acad Sci U S A 1996;93:12559–12563.

54. Xiao Y-F, Li X. Polyunsaturated fatty acids modify mouse hippocampal neuronal excitability during excitotoxic or convulsant stimuli. Brain Res 1999;846:112–121.
55. Blondeau N, Widmann C, Lazdunski M, Heurteaux C. Polyunsaturated fatty acids induce ischemic and epileptic tolerance. Neuroscience 2002;109:231–241.
56. Horvath LT, Diano S, Barnstable C. Mitochondrial uncoupling protein 2 in the central nervous system: neuromodulator and neuroprotector. Biochem Pharmacol 2003;1917–1921.
57. Mattson MP, Liu D. Mitochondrial potassium channels and uncoupling proteins in synaptic plasticity and neuronal cell death. Biochem Biophys Res Commun 2003;304:539–549.
58. Sullivan PG, Dube C, Dorenbos KD, Steward O, Baram TZ. Mitochondrial uncoupling protein-2 protects the immature brain from excitotoxic neuronal death. Ann Neurol 2003;53:711–717.
59. Votyakova TV, Reynolds IJ. $\Delta\psi$m-dependent and -independent production of reactive oxygen species by rat brain mitochondria. J Neurochem 2001;79:266–277.
60. Sullivan PG, Rippy NA, Dorenbos KA, Steward O, Rho JM. A ketogenic diet enhances respiratory uncoupling and decreases reactive oxygen species production in mitochondria isolated from mouse cortex. Epilepsia 2002;43 (Suppl 7):258.
61. Li LX, Skorpen F, Egeberg K, Jorgensen IH, Grill V. Uncoupling protein-2 participates in cellular defense against oxidative stress in clonal beta-cells. Biochem Biophys Res Commun 2001;282:273–277.
62. Kim-Han JS, Reichert SA, Quick KL, Dugan LL. BMCP1: a mitochondrial uncoupling protein in neurons which regulates mitochondrial function and oxidant production. J Neurochem 2001;79:658–668.
63. Sullivan PG, Rippy NA, Rho JM. A ketogenic diet increases the expression of mitochondrial uncoupling proteins UCP2, UCP4 and UCP5/BMCP1 in mouse hippocampus. Epilepsia 2003;44(Suppl 9):283.
64. Schwartzkroin PA. Mechanisms underlying the anti-epileptic efficacy of the ketogenic diet. Epilepsy Res 1999;37:171–180.
65. Al-Mudallal AS, LaManna JC, Lust, WD, Harik SI. Diet-induced ketosis does not cause cerebral acidosis. Epilepsia 1996;37:258–261.
66. Cunnane S, Musa K, Ryan M, Whiting S, Fraser D. Potential role of polyunsaturates in seizure protection achieved with the ketogenic diet. Prostaglandins Leukotienes Essent Fatty Acids 2002;67:131–135.
67. Appleton DB, DeVivo DC. An animal model of the ketogenic diet. Epilepsia 1974;15:211–227.
68. Pan JW, Bebin EM, Chu WJ, Hetherington HP. Ketosis and epilepsy: [31]P spectroscopic imaging at 4.1 T. Epilepsia 1999;40:703–707.
69. Seymour KJ, Bluml S, Sutherling J, Sutherling W, Ross BD. Identification of cerebral acetone by ^{1}H-MRS in patients with epilepsy controlled by ketogenic diet. MAGMA 1999;8:33–42.
70. Erecinska M, Nelson D, Daikhin Y, Yudkoff M. Regulation of GABA level in rat brain synaptosomes: fluxes through enzymes of the GABA shunt and effects of glutamate, calcium, and ketone bodies. J Neurochem 1996;67:2325–2334.
71. Szot P, Weinshenker D, Rho JM, Storey TW, Schwartzkroin PA. Norepinephrine is required for the anticonvulsant effect of the ketogenic diet. Dev Brain Res 2001;129:211–214.
72. Yudkoff M, Daikhin Y, Nissim I, Lazarow A, Nissim I. Brain amino acid metabolism and ketosis. J Neurosci Res 2001;66:272–281.
73. Yudkoff M, Daikhin Y, Nissim I, Lazarow A, Nissim I. Ketogenic diet, amino acid metabolism, and seizure control. J Neurosci Res 2001;66:931–940.
74. Huttenlocher P. Ketonemia and seizures: metabolic and anticonvulsant effects of two ketogenic diets in childhood epilepsy. Pediatr Res 1976;10:536–540.
75. Gilbert DL, Pyzik PL, Freeman JM. The ketogenic diet: seizure control correlates better with serum beta-hydroxybutyrate than with urine ketones. J Child Neurol 2000;15:787–790.
76. Thavendiranathan P, Mendonca A, Dell C, Likhodii SS, Musa K, Iracleous C, Cunnane SC, Burnham WM. The MCT ketogenic diet: effects on animal seizure models. Exp Neurol 2000;161:696–703.
77. Ballaban-Gil K, Callahan C, O'Dell C, Pappo M, Moshé S, Shinnar S. complications of the ketogenic diet. Epilepsia 1998;39:744–748.
78. Thio LL, Wong M, Yamada KA. Ketone bodies do not directly alter excitatory or inhibitory hippocampal synaptic transmission. Neurology 2000;54:325–331.
79. Saji M, Reis D. Delayed transneuronal death of substantia nigra neurons prevented by γ-aminobutyric acid agonist. Science 1987;235:66–69.
80. Lyden PD, Lonzo L. Combination therapy protects ischemic brain in rats. A glutamate antagonist plus a gamma-aminobutyric acid agonist. Stroke 1994;25:189–196.

81. Macdonald RL and Olsen RW. GABA$_A$ receptor channels. Annu Rev Neurosci 1994;17:569–602.
82. Sutula T, Cavazos J, Golarai G. Alteration of long-lasting structural and functional effects of kainic acid in the hippocampus by brief treatment with phenobarbital. J Neuroscience 1992;12:4173–4187.
83. Mikati MA, Holmes GL, Chronopoulos A, Hyde P, Thurber S, Gatt A, Liu Z, Werner S, Stafstrom CE. Phenobarbital modifies seizure-related brain injury in the developing brain. Ann Neurol 1994;36:425–433.
84. Ylinen AM, Miettinen R, Pitkanen A, Gulyas AI, Freund TF, Riekkinen PJ Sr. Enhanced GABAergic inhibition preserves hippocampal structure and function in a model of epilepsy. Proc Natl Acad Sci U S A 1991;88:7650–7653.
85. Halonen T, Miettinen R, Toppinen A, Tuunanen J, Kotti T, Riekkinen PJ Sr. Vigabatrin protects against kainic acid-induced neuronal damage in the rat hippocampus. Neurosci Lett 1995;195:13–16.
86. Andre VV, Ferrandon A, Marescaux C, Nehlig A. Vigabatrin protects against hippocampal damage but is not antiepileptogenic in the lithium–pilocarpine model of temporal lobe epilepsy. Epilepsy Res 2001;47:99–117.
87. Bough KJ, Schwartzkroin PA, Rho JM. Calorie restriction and ketogenic diet diminish neuronal excitability in rat dentate gyrus in vivo. Epilepsia 2003;44:752–760.
88. Kapur J, Stringer JL, Lothman EW. Evidence that repetitive seizures in the hippocampus cause a lasting reduction of GABAergic inhibition. J Neurophysiol 1989;61:417–426.

Afterword

A Parent's Perspective on Childhood Epilepsy: The Things I Wish They Had Told Us

Jim Abrahams

IMPRESSION: It is my impression that Charlie has a mixed seizure disorder, mostly likely a variation of Lennox–Gastaut syndrome. Parents are fully aware of the ramifications of this diagnosis. Although there are many traditional combinations and permutations of drugs that could be used here, I agree with the current approach. It is my understanding that the next drug to be tried is a combination of Felbamate and Tegretol with which I have no problem. I would also consider the combination of Felbamate with Valproate with perhaps a benzodiazepine. In addition, one wonders if the Felbamate could be pushed to an even higher dose than it is now, since we really do not know what the maximum dose of Felbamate is in young children. Another possibility is high-dose Valproate monotherapy. One other alternative therapy which I have mentioned to the family, but only reluctantly because of the high incidence of side-effects is high-dose ACTH. The problem is that while high-dose ACTH may be effective in stopping the seizures, they almost always recur as the dose is tapered. This makes one wonder if the risk–benefit ratio justifies the use of this somewhat dangerous mode of therapy. Finally, I think that if all pharmacological or theraputic modalities fail, I would seriously consider a corpus callosotomy on this child. A corpus callosotomy would not be curative of all the seizure types, but may help the most troublesome part of his seizure complex, i.e. the "drops."

It's not really necessary to mention the name of the doctor who wrote the foregoing excerpt from a medical report we received on our son, Charlie. Suffice it to say he was the fifth pediatric neurologist my wife and I had taken Charlie to see in the year he had been experiencing seizures—four of these physicians ran pediatric neurology departments at esteemed university hospitals around the United States. They all concurred. Yes, there were some variations in drug combinations suggested, and I'm sure that to a certain extent this report dates itself in that there are new drugs available today. But I begin with this "impression" not so much for what it says, but rather for what it omits—what it and all the doctors who examined Charlie never told us.

Today, 9 years later, I think back to those days, and realize how much time was lost, how much unnecessary damage was done to Charlie's life, and as a result, how much needless pain was, and continues to be, experienced by Charlie and all of us who love

From: *Epilepsy and the Ketogenic Diet*
Edited by: C. E. Stafstrom and J. M. Rho © Humana Press Inc., Totowa, NJ

him—all because information was not shared. I know the value of "ifs," but sometimes I can't help myself: if only the first time we walked into a neurologist's office someone had handed us a pamphlet, recommended a book, or taken the time to tell us just some of the following information we have learned since then...

TREATING KIDS WITH DIFFICULT-TO-CONTROL SEIZURES IS 20% SCIENCE AND 80% ART

It was not long after we received the doctor's report just quoted that I was watching a CNN report on childhood epilepsy and there was one of the doctors who had seen Charlie making that statement. (Actually he'd said "10% science and 90% art," but since then I've put the art versus science question to many neurologists and none peg it lower than 75% art, so I've rounded the number down). "Hold on a second," I thought when I heard the CNN broadcast. Those were lab coats Charlie's doctors were wearing, not smocks to protect them from splattering paint! They were scientists! Interior decorating is an art form—not pediatric neurology. In discussing the subject with me, a world-renowned pediatric neurologist likened treating difficult cases to fishing. Just as you return to one fishing hole time and again after you've had luck once, so too a neurologist will return to the same drug combination time and again after one success.

To a parent, this is a big deal. Clearly it puts the onus on the parent of the sick child to ask a key question, "Based on what?" Similarly I believe it puts a duty on the doctor to advise a patient if he is basing a statement on anecdote, experience, or science. An example: Lennox–Gastaut syndrome features the full gamut of seizure types. Charlie suffered most of them—including tonic–clonic seizures. We were instructed at the time by his doctors that a tonic–clonic seizure, if allowed to continue for over 30 minutes, could damage his young brain. Therefore, at 30 minutes, drug intervention with Valium or Ativan would be necessary. We lived 10 minutes from a hospital. So, whenever Charlie would begin one of his many tonic–clonic seizures, the first thing we did was make note of the time. Twenty minutes into the seizure, we'd get into the car and take off for the hospital. Certainly, as we sat there trying to comfort our son during his many tonic–clonic seizures, every parental instinct in us told us that these prolonged misfirings of his brain had to be damaging and we should put a stop to them earlier, if possible. But we were typical, terrified parents and never questioned the source of the magical "30 minutes."

We never asked, "Based on what?" Several years later, after Charlie's seizures had been controlled by the ketogenic diet, and both his physical and mental delays were apparent, I attended an epilepsy conference and learned that the 30-minute rule had been shortened to 5 minutes. Now tonic–clonic seizures could damage the brain in 5 minutes. All those hours of holding Charlie when we could have stopped his seizures had in fact been detrimental. The 30-minute rule was not scientific. There were no blinded studies documenting the long-term effects of tonic–clonic seizures of more or less than 30 minutes. At best, the 30-minute rule was based on anecdote, and at worst it was based on lore. I wish we had asked, "Based on what?" or that someone had told us. I wish we had known the art-versus-science percentage.

"THERE'S NO SCIENCE BEHIND IT"

This was an argument selectively used by several physicians who saw Charlie. Monotherapy, then multiple drugs, and finally surgery failed to slow his seizures. He started to lose abilities he once had and, like most parents, we became more desperate. Holistic approaches, Chinese herbs, neck realignment and a host of non-Western approaches were suggested. The medical argument against them was: no science—"We don't understand the mechanisms, therefore we can't endorse it." I'd have no problem with that notion, were it spread evenly across the playing field. But it's not. From the naive patient's point of view, when that argument is used to overrule "nontraditional" therapies, but omitted from Western recommendations, there is the assumption that Western approaches are backed by science. So, for example, when Dilantin was added to Charlie's daily Felbatol, Tegretol, and benzodiazapine, in the absence of any cautionary thought regarding "no science," I wrongly assumed (and probably never questioned) that modern science was at work.

Nancy and I dutifully coerced Charlie to swallow all that stuff around the clock and watched the terrible side effects. Far from our minds was the notion he might be a guinea pig. If not a "crap shoot," the chance of this drug combo stopping even some of his seizures and leaving him with any acceptable quality of life was beyond remote. What's more, the effects of the simultaneous use of these potent drugs on his one-year-old brain were and are completely without scientific documentation. We assumed naively that if there were no medical books on the interactions and efficacy of that combination of drugs, certainly there were articles. As a matter of fact, I came to learn, there is no hard science regarding efficacy or side effects behind any multiple drug combinations in the treatment of pediatric epilepsy.

Again, my problem is more than trying multiple drug combinations. What I wish they had told us is that the "there's no science behind it" argument is used to dissuade families from some approaches and omitted from others at the doctor's discretion.

SEVENTY PERCENT OF NEW EPILEPSY PATIENTS HAVE THEIR SEIZURES CONTROLLED WITH THE FIRST EPILEPTIC DRUG THEY TRY—ALMOST IRRESPECTIVE OF WHICH DRUG IT IS

After the first drug fails, there is a 10–15% chance the second drug will work and only a 20% chance drugs will ever control a child's seizures. In other words, after a second antiepileptic drug fails, four out of five children will not achieve seizure control with drugs alone.

I've been told by some that this fact, were it known by many parents, would rob them of hope. I disagree. If someone had told us, it would have robbed us of complacency.

A COUPLE OF DRUG FACTS

1. The minimum criterion for the Food and Drug Administration (FDA) to approve a new antiepileptic drug, assuming the drug's side effects are not prohibitive, is that the drug stop 50% of the seizures in at least 50% of the children (who do not drop out of the study because of intolerance, noncompliance, or other reasons). In other words, if 100 kids test a new drug and 25 drop out of the study, 38 must have at least a 50% reduction in seizures. Thus a new drug that does not stop seizures can still be approved by the FDA. For the parent of a child with difficult-to-control seizures, there is always the "buzz," the promise about the next drug—the next "great white hope"—to arrive on the market. Very few of us know this liberal criterion for FDA approval.

2. In 1993 a new drug, Felbatol, met federal requirements and was approved by the FDA for children with difficult-to-control seizures. It was produced by a company named Carter-Wallace. I wrote to Carter-Wallace to get their annual stock-holders' report. From this report, it was clear that in the 2 years prior to the release of Felbatol, the company spent $20 million—not on research and development, but on marketing the drug. In 1993 there were about 1200 pediatric neurologists in the United States to whom the advertising campaign was aimed. I'll let you do the math: $20 million to convince 1200 folks to prescribe a drug! I certainly wish someone had told us that bit of information before we allowed Charlie to spend all those sleepless nights while he was on Felbatol, which did not help to control his seizures.

LEGAL STANDARD OF CARE REGARDING PROVISION OF INFORMATION

The legal standard of care in America today, regarding physicians sharing information with patients, is that physicians are required to tell their patients, in general, the same information colleagues would share with their own patients under similar circumstances. Practically speaking, that means that if, in a court of law, a doctor can get several other doctors to testify that they would have told their patients substantially what the defendant had told his or her patient, the standard of care has been satisfied. This is not to suggest that legalities were ever a consideration regarding Charlie's case; it is only to provide information I wish I had had, the bottom line regarding information sharing by a physician.

Especially for Charlie, whose seizures were difficult to control and the art-versus-science thing was clearly applicable, I as the patient's dad, always assumed that the doctors would lay out a range of treatments and together we would decide on the correct course of action—in essence, a doctor–patient partnership. I assumed an informed joint decision-making process. I was wrong.

Certainly Nancy and I didn't pretend to have the medical expertise. But then of course the doctors didn't live with Charlie and had no real knowledge of his family, its agony, and his living circumstances. And of course none of the doctors we saw had ever held their own child during a seizure. Unfortunately, informed joint decision making turned out to be wishful thinking. Information was always provided on a need-to-know basis and then in a seemingly reluctant manner. In fact, there was almost a physical chill when more than limited probing and suggesting occurred.

THE KETOGENIC DIET

Throughout Charlie's epilepsy, I remember crying hardest with Nancy when we received the copy of the report that begins this afterword. It seemed so hopeless. And yes, we were "fully aware of the ramifications" of Charlie's diagnosis. So, as a way to prepare Charlie and the rest of us for what seemed to be many more years of seizures, drugs, and "progressive retardation," I started doing some research. To my surprise, in epilepsy texts dating back to the 1920s (and in every decade from the 1920s through the present) from Hopkins, the Mayo Clinic, and many other highly regarded institutions, there was consistent anecdotal documentation regarding the ketogenic diet and its efficacy (roughly one-third of the kids who tried it became seizure free, one-third were significantly improved, and for one third it was ineffective). The documentation covered literally thousands of children with epilepsy. In addition, the diet's side effects were minimal compared with many of those Charlie had experienced from drugs. I learned that there was still a dietician at Johns Hopkins who had over 40 years of experience with the diet. So, one month after receiving that gloomy report, we took Charlie to Baltimore. At Johns Hopkins they put him on the diet. His seizures dropped from dozens a day to zero within 48 hours of its initiation, and he was off all medication in another month.

I don't want to minimize the difficulty of the diet, but it was a walk on the beach next to the drugs and continued seizure activity. More importantly, we had our son back! Today Charlie is 11 years old, off the diet, and has been free of seizures and drugs for years.

I asked his doctors why they left it to us to learn about the diet they all had heard of. Their answers: (1) it was too difficult; (2) being high in fat, it might be unhealthy; and (3) there was no science behind the diet. Too difficult? What could be more difficult than watching your child slip into retardation via drugs and seizures? Unhealthy? Compared to what? No science? No need to deal with that subject again.

THE MEDICAL DESTINY OF EACH OF US AND OUR CHILDREN IS LARGELY UP TO US

To think otherwise can be damaging. There is a tendency when we walk into a doctor's office to want to hand over our problem to the doctor and say, "Here it is, please fix it." It's comfortable, it's easy, and more often than not, it works. Just as we take comfort in deferring to them, many doctors are unwilling to confide in us that we may have stepped into one of Western medicine's black holes. There are many black holes, and they are deep, and kids with difficult-to-control seizures are in one of them.

So what does that mean? It means that our medical problems and our children's medical problems are precisely that—OURS. At first, that's a pretty intimidating and perhaps a seemingly foolish concept, both to us and to some physicians. After all, they went through years of education. They've seen countless patients in their practices. And then we walk into their offices with a disease we probably don't even know how to spell. How presumptuous and perhaps foolish of us, the patients, to ask and then pursue the hard questions, learn the side effects, get the second opinions, do the research, and participate in the cure—in short, to become proactive.

Ironically, the "side effect" of participating in our medical destinies may not only lead to getting better sooner. It is empowering. Though I would do almost anything to go back and have Charlie not suffer epilepsy, the experience has been empowering. Regardless of whether responsibility for informing ourselves confirms what we learn from our physicians, it's nevertheless empowering. As fate would have it, I am writing this afterword from a hospital bed where I am fighting leukemia. But the bed I am lying in, the treatment I am undergoing, and the doctor who is helping me are not arbitrary. Though my diagnosis was shocking and treatment was needed immediately, there was time to find information, interview oncologists, and even visit hospitals before setting sail on a course. Mercifully, I found a bright, compassionate doctor who believes in informed joint decision making. We take control of so many lesser issues in our families' lives—meals, bedtimes, TV hours—why not have that same attitude with the most important issue, our families' health? In the worst case, we have learned something new; in the best case, we have improved either our lives or the lives of our children. There is no downside.

Epilogue

The story of the ketogenic diet is a fascinating one, a saga as compelling as any in clinical medicine. From both teleological and evolutionary perspectives, it makes abundant sense that dietary factors should be important in influencing brain physiology. The aphorism *"We are what we eat"* is a popular reminder that our station in life is often correlated with the perceived rarity and value of foodstuffs available for personal consumption. However, "what we eat" has become an even more timely consideration given the recent dramatic increase in obesity seen in both children and adults living in the United States, an ominous development that heralds an impending epidemic of diabetes, cardiovascular disease, and other long-term health consequences. Furthermore, the attainment of significant weight loss and a lean body habitus—a mantra promulgated by the media—has become a psychological holy grail, one that promises bountiful happiness and self-esteem, despite potential negative health effects of nutritional deprivation. The ketogenic diet emerged as a rediscovered therapy for medically refractory epilepsy in the context of this dichotomy of physical extremes, and the obsession with food or the avoidance of it.

Pharmaceutical agents have often been portrayed as the magic bullets to cure "what ails us." Although significant advances have been made in the design and clinical validation of compounds that are devoid of significant side effects and drug interactions, in most areas of medicine, we have not been blessed with truly revolutionary therapies. Our collective efforts as a clinical and research community have been humbled by the ever-increasing realization that disease processes are inherently complex, representing dynamic tapestries woven from the elusive fabric of both genetic and environmental substrates.

There is now a growing literature attesting to the health benefits of caloric restriction, relative ketosis, and the ingestion of polyunsaturated fatty acids. At both clinical and basic science levels, it is increasingly apparent that a multitude of dietary factors can have a profound impact on disease risk and progression. Given the potential of the ketogenic diet to protect neurons from injury or death, whether this is a consequence of diminishing the damaging effects of seizures or direct neuroprotective activity, it might be more accurate to state that "We become what we eat."

The ketogenic diet has a natural appeal to patients and their families who have been frustrated with the limitations of modern-day therapies for epilepsy (consisting of seemingly endless trials of anticonvulsant medications, resective or palliative epilepsy surgery, and more recently, the vagus nerve stimulator). The same frustrations draw clinicians and scientists to novel approaches to the treatment of epilepsy, knowledge that will also undoubtedly add to our understanding of how the normal brain functions.

From: *Epilepsy and the Ketogenic Diet*
Edited by: C. E. Stafstrom and J. M. Rho © Humana Press Inc., Totowa, NJ

This volume has attempted to present a balanced perspective between clinical and basic science topics pertinent to the ketogenic diet. Practical aspects have included such topics as how the ketogenic diet originated, instructions on how to calculate and plan a ketogenic diet tailored to the needs of individual patients, how to monitor ketogenic diet effectiveness, potential pitfalls and complications, and challenges for future clinical applications. From the basic scientific perspective, and despite a heightened research interest over the past 10 yr, how the ketogenic diet works remains essentially a mystery. Much remains to be learned about how the brain synthesizes and regulates ketone bodies and fatty acids, the manner in which these and other relevant substrates modulate neuronal excitability, and what mechanisms modify ketogenic diet effectiveness at the molecular, cellular, and neuronal network levels. The application of modern-day research tools to the achievement of a detailed understanding of this age-old therapy will undoubtedly bring novel and surprising insights into the relationships between diet and brain function. It is our hope that the integration of laboratory and clinical data, as represented by the content of this volume, will provide a unique and timely platform for future investigation.

Carl E. Stafstrom, MD, PhD
Jong M. Rho, MD

Appendix A
The Carbohydrate and Caloric Content of Drugs

George Karvelas, Denis Lebel, and Lionel Carmant

As mentioned in several chapters of this volume, complete or even partial loss of ketosis can lead to acute seizure recurrence and can even impair long-term seizure control *(1)*. Although the exact mechanism of action of the ketogenic diet (KD) remains uncertain, maintenance of ketosis is mandatory for improved seizure control *(2)*. For these reasons, and because the amount of carbohydrates and proteins is strictly limited in the KD, strict compliance to the diet is of foremost importance.

In children, the control of caloric intake can be difficult owing to the availability of carbohydrates and calories from different sources. The optimal management of the ketogenic diet requires the collaboration of siblings, school personnel, classmates, and nursing and hospital staff. During the 2 yr or more of the diet, modifications in the use of chronic medications and acute treatment for intercurrent illnesses must also be taken into account. Syrups are usually contraindicated because of their high carbohydrate content in the form of sucrose, maltose, sorbitol, mannitol, alcohol, or starch. A number of caregivers are however unaware that the "sugar-free" label of drug tablets does not guarantee that ketosis will not be affected. These drugs may contain sorbitol, a carbohydrate that does not affect glycemia but will alter ketosis. The knowledge of the carbohydrate and caloric content of these drugs will help physicians, dieticians, and nurses adjust the diet accordingly. We therefore developed a comprehensive table of all commonly used drugs for which the information was available (Table 1) *(3)*.

For some medications, the data are not readily available. We therefore developed a worst-case scenario that in our experience always overestimates the caloric content of these medications (Table 2). To obtain this estimation, one needs to measure the weight of 10 tablets of a given drug, subtract the amount of active material in these tablets, and then divide the result by the number of tablets weighed. We consider this number to represent the maximal carbohydrate content of the pharmaceutical formulation in grams. Extrapolating the energy content by multiplying the calculated number by 4 kcal as the worst-case scenario assumes that all this weight comprises carbohydrates.

From: *Epilepsy and the Ketogenic Diet*
Edited by: C. E. Stafstrom and J. M. Rho © Humana Press Inc., Totowa, NJ

Table 1

Caloric Content of Drugs, Listed by Generic Names

Drug, concentration, and presentation	Commercial name and company	Caloric content (kcal)	
		Carbohydrate[b]	Total[b]
5-Aminosalicylic acid, 250 mg/Tablet	Pentasa (Hoechst Marion Roussel)	0.00	Nd
5-Aminosalicylic acid, 500 mg/Tablet	Pentasa (Hoechst Marion Roussel)	0.00	Nd
Acebutolol HCl, 100 mg/Tablet	Novo-Acebutol (Novopharm)	0.360	0.375
Acebutolol HCl, 200 mg/Tablet	Novo-Acebutol (Novopharm)	0.720	0.749
Acebutolol HCl, 400 mg/Tablet	Novo-Acebutol (Novopharm)	0.025	0.066
Acetaminophen, 16 mg/mL/Liquid	Tempra (Mead Johnson)	Nd	1.78
Acetaminophen, 16 mg/mL/Liquid	Atasol (Carter Horner)	1.44	2.40
Acetaminophen, 16 mg/mL/Liquid	PMS-acetaminophen (Pharmascience)	1.7	Nd
Acetaminophen, 160 mg/Chewable tablet	Tylenol (McNeil)	Nd	2.5
Acetaminophen, 160 mg/Chewable tablet	Tylenol, sugar free (McNeil)	Nd	2.0
Acetaminophen, 32 mg/mL/Liquid	Tempra (Mead Johnson)	Nd	1.78
Acetaminophen, 32 mg/mL/Liquid	Tylenol elixir (McNeil)	Nd	1.76
Acetaminophen, 32 mg/mL/Liquid	Tylenol suspension liquid (raisin) (McNeil)	Nd	2.22
Acetaminophen, 32 mg/mL/Liquid	Tylenol suspension liquid (bubblegum) (McNeil)	Nd	2.40
Acetaminophen, 32 mg/mL/Liquid	PMS-acetaminophen (Pharmascience)	1.7	Nd
Acetaminophen, 325 mg/Tablet	Tylenol (McNeil)	Nd	0.2
Acetaminophen, 325 mg/Tablet	Novo-Gesic (Novopharm)	0.039	Nd
Acetaminophen, 500 mg/Tablet	Tylenol (McNeil)	Nd	0.3
Acetaminophen, 500 mg/Tablet	Novo-Gesic (Novopharm)	0.062	Nd
Acetaminophen, 80 mg/Chewable tablet	Tylenol (McNeil)	Nd	1.2
Acetaminophen, 80 mg/Chewable tablet	Tylenol, sugar free (McNeil)	Nd	1
Acetaminophen, 80 mg/mL/Liquid	Tempra (Mead Johnson)	Nd	1.40
Acetaminophen, 80 mg/mL/Liquid	Tylenol drops (McNeil)	Nd	0.98
Acetaminophen, 80 mg/mL/Liquid	Tylenol suspensions, drops (McNeil)	Nd	2.10
Acetaminophen, 80 mg/mL/Liquid	PMS-Acetaminophen (Pharmascience)	0.36	Nd

Drug	Product		
Acetaminophen, 80 mg/ml/Liquid	Atasol drops (Carter Horner)	1.79	2.40
Acetaminophen-caffeine-codeine phosphate (C15), 300 mg + 15 mg + 15 mg/Tablet	Novo-Gesic C15 (Novopharm)	0.148	0.188
Acetaminophen-caffeine-codeine phosphate (C30), 300 mg + 15 mg + 30 mg/Tablet	Novo-Gesic C30 (Novopharm)	0.154	0.195
Acetaminophen-caffeine-codeine phosphate (C8), 300 mg + 15 mg + 8 mg/Tablet	Novo-Gesic C8 (Novopharm)	0.145	0.184
Acetazolamide, 250 mg/Tablet	Apo-Acetazolamide (Apotex)	Nd	0.79
Acetazolamide, 250 mg/Tablet	Diamox (Berlex)	Nd	1.0
Acetazolamide, 250 mg/Tablet	Novo-Zolamide (Novopharm)	0.100	0.143
Acetylsalicylic acid, 325 mg/Tablet	Novasen Novasen Sp.C. (Novopharm)	0.239	Nd
Acetylsalicylic acid, 650 mg/Tablet	Novasen Novasen SP.C. (Novopharm)	0.479	Nd
Acyclovir, 40 mg/mL/Liquid	Zovirax (Glaxo Wellcome)	1.26	2.62
Alfacalcidol, 0.2 mg/mL/Liquid	One-Alpha (Leo Pharma)	2.63	Nd
Alfacalcidol, 0.25 mg/Capsule	One-Alpha (Leo Pharma)	1.15	Nd
Alfacalcidol, 1 mg/Capsule	One-Alpha (Leo Pharma)	1.15	Nd
Allopurinol, 100 mg/Tablet	Novo-Purol (Novopharm)	0.458	0.484
Allopurinol, 200 mg/Tablet	Novo-Purol (Novopharm)	0.057	0.084
Allopurinol, 300 mg/Tablet	Novo-Purol (Novopharm)	0.346	0.395
Alprazolam, 0.25 mg/Tablet	Novo-Alprazol (Novopharm)	0.416	0.450
Alprazolam, 0.50 mg/Tablet	Novo-Alprazol (Novopharm)	0.413	0.482
Aluminium + magnesium hydroxide, 45 mg + 40 mg/Liquid	Maalox (Novartis Pharma)	Nd	0.04
Aluminium + magnesium hydroxide, /Liquid	Almagel (Atlas laboratories)	0.20	Nd
Aluminium hydroxide, 64 mg/mL/Liquid	Amphogel (Axcan Pharma)	Nd	0.60
Amantadin, 10 mg/mL/Liquid	Symmetrel (Du Pont Pharma)	2.58	Nd
Amiloride HCl/Hydrochlorothiazide, 5/50 mg/Tablet	Novamilor (Novopharm)	0.401	0.412
Aminocaproic acid, 250 mg/mL/Liquid	Amicar (Wyeth-Ayerst)	Nd	2.40
Amitriptylin, 10 mg/Tablet	Novo-Triptyn (Novopharm)	0.039	0.065
Amitriptylin, 25 mg/Tablet	Novo-Triptyn (Novopharm)	0.046	0.063
Amitriptylin, 2 mg/mL/Liquid	Elavil (Merck Sharp & Dohme)	2.63	Nd

(continues)

Table 1
(Continued)

Drug, concentration, and presentation	Commercial name and company	Caloric content (kcal)	
		Carbohydrate[b]	Total[b]
Amitriptylin, 50 mg/Tablet	Novo-Triptyn (Novopharm)	0.082	0.138
Amoxicillin + clavulanic acid, 50 + 12.5 mg/mL/Liquid	Clavulin (SmithKline Beecham Pharma)	0.18	Nd
Amoxicillin + potassium clavulanate, 25 + 6.25 mg/mL/Liquid	Clavulin (SmithKline Beecham Pharma)	0.18	Nd
Amoxicillin + potassium clavulanate, 250 mg + 12.5 mg/Tablet	Clavulin (SmithKline Beecham Pharma)	1.20	Nd
Amoxicillin + potassium clavulanate,	Clavulin (SmithKline Beecham Pharma)	1.80	Nd0
Amoxicillin, 125 mg/Chewable tablet	Amoxil (Wyeth-Ayerst)	Nd	0.50
Amoxicillin, 25 mg/mL/Liquid	Amoxil (Wyeth-Ayerst)	Nd	0.40
Amoxicillin, 25 mg/mL/Liquid	Apo-Amoxi, hypoglucidic (Apotex)	Nd	0.026
Amoxicillin, 25 mg/mL/Liquid	Novamoxin hypoglucidic (Novopharm)	0.48	Nd
Amoxicillin, 25 mg/mL/Liquid	Nu-Amoxi (Nu-Pharm)	1.78	Nd
Amoxicillin, 25 mg/mL/Liquid	Apo-Amoxi (Apotex)	1.79	Nd
Amoxicillin, 25 mg/mL/Liquid	Novamoxin (Novopharm)	2.27	Nd
Amoxicillin, 250 mg/Capsule	Amoxil (Wyeth-Ayerst)	Nd	0.20
Amoxicillin, 250 mg/Capsule	Apo-Amoxi (Apotex)	Nd	0.21
Amoxicillin, 250 mg/Capsule	Nu-Amoxi (Nu-Pharm)	Nd	0.21
Amoxicillin, 250 mg/Capsule	Novamoxin (Novopharm)	0.082	0.126
Amoxicillin, 250 mg/Chewable tablet	Amoxil (Wyeth-Ayerst)	Nd	1.0
Amoxicillin, 50 mg/mL/Liquid	Amoxil (Wyeth-Ayerst)	Nd	0.32
Amoxicillin, 50 mg/mL/Liquid	Apo-Amoxi, hypoglucidic (Apotex)	Nd	0.026
Amoxicillin, 50 mg/mL/Liquid	Novamoxin, hypoglucidic (Novopharm)	0.41	Nd
Amoxicillin, 50 mg/mL/Liquid	Apo-Amoxi (Apotex)	1.78	Nd
Amoxicillin, 50 mg/mL/Liquid	Nu-Amoxi (Nu-Pharm)	1.78	Nd
Amoxicillin, 50 mg/mL/Liquid	Novamoxin (Novopharm)	2.14	Nd

Drug, dosage form	Brand (manufacturer)		
Amoxicillin, 500 mg/Capsule	Amoxil (Wyeth-Ayerst)	Nd	0.40
Amoxicillin, 500 mg/Capsule	Apo-Amoxi (Apotex)	Nd	0.36
Amoxicillin, 500 mg/Capsule	Nu-Amoxi (Nu-Pharm)	Nd	0.36
Amoxicillin, 500 mg/Capsule	Novamoxin (Novopharm)	0.164	0.245
Ampicillin, 100 mg/mL/Liquid	Novo-Ampicillin (Novopharm)	1.87	1.87
Ampicillin, 25 mg/mL/Liquid	Apo-Ampi (Apotex)	Nd	1.82
Ampicillin, 25 mg/mL/Liquid	Nu-Ampi (Nu-Pharm)	Nd	1.82
Ampicillin, 25 mg/mL/Liquid	Novo-Ampicillin (Novopharm)	2.27	2.27
Ampicillin, 250 mg/Capsule	Apo-Ampi (Apotex)	Nd	0.22
Ampicillin, 250 mg/Capsule	Nu-Ampi (Nu-Pharm)	Nd	0.22
Ampicillin, 250 mg/Capsule	Novo-Ampicillin (Novopharm)	0.104	0.148
Ampicillin, 50 mg/mL/Liquid	Apo-Ampi (Apotex)	Nd	1.70
Ampicillin, 50 mg/mL/Liquid	Nu-Ampi (Nu-Pharm)	Nd	1.70
Ampicillin, 50 mg/mL/Liquid	Novo-Ampicillin (Novopharm)	2.16	2.16
Ampicillin, 500 mg/Capsule	Apo-Ampi (Apotex)	Nd	0.39
Ampicillin, 500 mg/Capsule	Nu-Ampi (Nu-Pharm)	Nd	0.39
Ampicillin, 500 mg/Capsule	Novo-Ampicillin (Novopharm)	0.078	0.155
ASA-caffeine-codeine phosphate, 1 tablet/Tablet	Novo A.C. & C. (Novopharm)	0.067	0.067
Atenolol, 100 mg/Tablet	Novo-Atenol (Novopharm)	0.188	0.222
Atenolol, 50 mg/Tablet	Novo-Atenol (Novopharm)	0.094	0.111
Azithromycin, 1000 mg/Powder	Zithromax (Pfizer)	38.828	Nd
Azithromycin, 20 mg/mL/Liquid	Zithromax (Pfizer)	3.15	Nd
Azithromycin, 250 mg/Capsule	Zithromax (Pfizer)	0.928	Nd
Azithromycin, 40 mg/mL/Liquid	Zithromax (Pfizer)	3.16	Nd
Azithromycin, 600 mg/Tablet	Zithromax (Pfizer)	0.348	Nd
Bacampicillin, chlorhydrate, 400 mg/Tablet	Penglobe (Astra Pharma)	Nd	0.10
Bacampicillin, chlorhydrate, 800 mg/Tablet	Penglobe (Astra Pharma)	Nd	0.20
Baclofen, 20 mg/Tablet	Novo-Baclofen (Novopharm)	0.132	0.156
Benzydamine, 0.15 %/Liquid	Novo-Benzydamine (Novopharm)	0.808	Nd
Bisacodyl, 5 mg/Foaming tablet	Dulcolax (Boehringer Ingelheim)	Nd	0.26

(*continues*)

Table 1
(Continued)

Drug, concentration, and presentation	Commercial name and company	Caloric content (kcal)	
		Carbohydrate[b]	Total[b]
Bisacodyl, 5 mg/Tablet	Apo-Bisacodyl (Apotex)	Nd	0.48
Bisacodyl, 5 mg/Tablet	Soflax EX (Pharmascience)	0.12	Nd
Bismuth subsalicylate, 17.6 mg/mL/Liquid	Pepto-Bismol (Procter & Gamble)	1.00	Nd
Bromazepam, 3 mg/Tablet	Novo-Bromazepam (Novopharm)	0.400	0.417
Bumetanide, 1 mg/Tablet	Burinex (Leo Pharma)	0.61	Nd
Bumetanide, 2 mg/Tablet	Burinex (Leo Pharma)	0.74	Nd
Bumetanide, 5 mg/Tablet	Burinex (Leo Pharma)	1.17	Nd
Buspirone, 10 mg/Tablet	Novo-Buspirone (Novopharm)	0.487	0.499
Calcitriol, 1 mg/mL/Liquid	Rocaltrol (Hoffman-La Roche)	8.60	Nd
Calcium gluconate + glucoheptonate, 20 mg/mL/Liquid	Calcium Stanley (Stanley Pharmaceuticals.)	Nd	0.04
Calcium lactobionate,/Liquid	Calcium-Sandoz (Sandoz)	Nd	1.35
Calcium, 500 mg Ca elemen/Capsule	Calsan (Novartis Sante Familiale)	Nd	5.85
Captopril, 100 mg/Tablet	Novo-Captopril (Novopharm)	0.311	0.329
Captopril, 12.5 mg/Tablet	Novo-Captopril (Novopharm)	0.039	0.041
Captopril, 25 mg/Tablet	Novo-Captopril (Novopharm)	0.078	0.082
Captopril, 50 mg/Tablet	Novo-Captopril (Novopharm)	0.156	0.165
Carbamazepine, 100 mg/Chewable table	Tegretol (Novartis Pharma)	Nd	1.08
Carbamazepine, 20 mg/mL/Liquid	Tegretol (Novartis Pharma)	Nd	1.79
Carbamazepine, 200 mg/Tablet	Apo-Carbamazepine (Apotex)	Nd	0.35
Carbamazepine, 200 mg/Tablet	Nu-Carbamazepine (Nu-Pharm)	Nd	0.35
Carbamazepine, 200 mg/Controlled-release tablet	Tegretol CR (Novartis Pharma)	nd	0
Carbamazepine, 200 mg/Tablet	Tegretol (Novartis Pharma)	0.00	Nd
Carbamazepine, 200 mg/Tablet	Novo-Carbamaz (Novopharm)	0.031	0.048
Carbamazepine, 200 mg/Controlled-release tablet	Tegretol (Novartis Pharma)	Nd	2.12
Carbamazepine, 400 mg/Controlled-release tablet	Tegretol CR (Novartis Pharma)	Nd	0

Product (Manufacturer)	Generic, Dose/Form		
Carnitor (Sigma-Tau Pharmaceuticals)	Carnitine, 100 mg/mL/Liquid	0.20	Nd
Ceclor (Eli Lilly)	Cefaclor, 25 mg/mL/Liquid	Nd	2.52
PMS-Cefaclor (Pharmascience)	Cefaclor, 250 mg/Capsule	0.14	Nd
Apo-Cefaclor (Apotex)	Cefaclor, 250 mg/Capsule	0.28	Nd
Ceclor (Eli Lilly)	Cefaclor, 50 mg/mL/Liquid	Nd	2.42
PMS-Cefaclor (Pharmascience)	Cefaclor, 500 mg/Capsule	0.28	Nd
Apo-Cefaclor (Apotex)	Cefaclor, 500 mg/Capsule	0.317	Nd
Ceclor (Eli Lilly)	Cefaclor, 75 mg/mL/Liquid	Nd	2.24
Suprax (Rhône-Poulenc Rorer)	Cefixime, 20 mg/mL/Liquid	2.22	Nd
Suprax (Rhône-Poulenc Rorer)	Cefixime, 400 mg/Tablet	0.396	Nd
Cefzil (Bristol-Myers Squibb)	Cefprozil, 25 mg/mL/Liquid	Nd	1.50
Cefzil (Bristol-Myers Squibb)	Cefprozil, 250 mg/Tablet	0.064	Nd
Cefzil (Bristol-Myers Squibb)	Cefprozil, 50 mg/mL/Liquid	Nd	1.30
Cefzil (Bristol-Myers Squibb)	Cefprozil, 500 mg/Tablet	0.128	Nd
Ceftin (Glaxo Wellcome)	Cefuroxime axetil, 25 mg/mL/Liquid	2.45	2.59
Ceftin (Glaxo Wellcome)	Cefuroxime axetil, 250 mg/Tablet	0.00	Nd
Ceftin (Glaxo Wellcome)	Cefuroxime axetil, 500 mg/Tablet	0.00	Nd
Keflex (Eli Lilly)	Cephalexin, 25 mg/mL/Liquid	Nd	2.48
Novo-Lexin (Novopharm)	Cephalexin, 25 mg/mL/Liquid	2.32	2.32
Pms-Cephalexin (Pharmascience)	Cephalexin, 25 mg/mL/Liquid	2.48	Nd
Novo-Lexin (Novopharm)	Cephalexin, 250 mg/Capsule	0.044	0.109
Apo-Cephalex (Apotex)	Cephalexin, 250 mg/Tablet	Nd	0.51
Nu-Cephalex (Nu-Pharm)	Cephalexin, 250 mg/Tablet	Nd	0.51
Novo-Lexin (Novopharm)	Cephalexin, 250 mg/Tablet	0.075	0.104
PMS-Cephalexin (Pharmascience)	Cephalexin, 250 mg/Tablet	0.51	Nd
Keflex (Eli Lilly)	Cephalexin, 50 mg/mL/Liquid	Nd	2.42
Novo-Lexin (Novopharm)	Cephalexin, 50 mg/mL/Liquid	2.23	2.23
Pms-Cephalexin (Pharmascience)	Cephalexin, 50 mg/mL/Liquid	2.42	Nd
Novo-Lexin (Novopharm)	Cephalexin, 500 mg/Capsule	0.088	0.211
Apo-Cephalex (Apotex)	Cephalexin, 500 mg/Tablet	Nd	1.02

(continues)

Table 1
(*Continued*)

Drug, concentration, and presentation	Commercial name and company	Caloric content (kcal)	
		Carbohydrate[b]	Total[b]
Cephalexin, 500 mg/Tablet	Nu-Cephalex (Nu-Pharm)	Nd	1.02
Cephalexin, 500 mg/Tablet	Novo-Lexin (Novopharm)	0.150	0.213
Cephalexin, 500 mg/Tablet	Pms-Cephalexin (Pharmascience)	1.02	Nd
Chloral hydrate, 100 mg/mL/Liquid	Pms-Chloralhydrate (Pharmascience)	2.0	Nd
Chloral hydrate, 500 mg/Capsule	Novo-Chlorhydrate (Novopharm)	0.00	0.060
Chloramphenicol, 250 mg/Capsule	Novo-Chlorocap (Novopharm)	0.863	0.932
Chlordiazepoxide, 10 mg/Capsule	Novo-Poxide SP.C. (Novopharm)	0.465	0.476
Chlordiazepoxide, 25 mg/Capsule	Novo-Poxide (Novopharm)	0.416	0.426
Chlordiazepoxide, 5 mg/Capsule	Novo-Poxide (Novopharm)	0.482	0.492
Chloroquine, 250 mg/Tablet	Novo-Chloroquine (Novopharm)	0.824	0.988
Chlorpheniramine, 4 mg/Tablet	Novo-Pheniram (Novopharm)	0.032	0.051
Chlorpromazine, 20 mg/mL/Liquid	Largactil (Rhône-Poulenc Rorer)	2.86	Nd
Chlorpromazine, 5 mg/mL/Liquid	Largactil (Rhône-Poulenc Rorer)	3.04	Nd
Chlorpromazine, 10 mg/Tablet	Novo-Chlorpromazine (Novopharm)	0.064	0.094
Chlorpromazine, 100 mg/Tablet	Novo-Chlorpromazine (Novopharm)	0.216	0.243
Chlorpromazine, 20 mg/mL/Liquid	Chlorpromanyl (Technilab)	Nd	3.40
Chlorpromazine, 200 mg/Tablet	Novo-Chlorpromazine (Novopharm)	0.479	0.568
Chlorpromazine, 25 mg/Tablet	Novo-Chlorpromazine (Novopharm)	0.124	0.139
Chlorpromazine, 40 mg/mL/Liquid	Chlorpromanyl (Technilab)	Nd	3.60
Chlorpromazine, 40 mg/mL/Liquid	Largactil (Rhône-Poulenc Rorer)	Nd	Nd
Chlorpromazine, 50 mg/Tablet	Novo-Chlorpromazine (Novopharm)	0.114	0.132
Chlorpropamide, 250 mg/Tablet	Novo-Propamide (Novopharm)	0.933	0.978
Chlorthalidone, 100 mg/Tablet	Novo-Thalidone (Novopharm)	0.037	0.049
Chlorthalidone, 50 mg/Tablet	Novo-Thalidone (Novopharm)	0.037	0.049
Cholestyramine, 4 g/dose/Powder	Novo-Cholamine Light (Novopharm)	0.00	0.00

Cholestyramine, 4 g/dose/Powder	Novo-Cholamine (Novopharm)	16.09	16.09
Cimetidine, 200 mg/Tablet	Novo-Cimetidine (Novopharm)	0.053	0.075
Cimetidine, 300 mg/Tablet	Novo-Cimetidine (Novopharm)	0.059	0.093
Cimetidine, 400 mg/Tablet	Novo-Cimetidine (Novopharm)	0.106	0.150
Cimetidine, 600 mg/Tablet	Novo-Cimetidine (Novopharm)	0.159	0.226
Cimetidine, 800 mg/Tablet	Novo-Cimetidine (Novopharm)	0.211	0.301
Ciprofloxacin, 250 mg/Tablet	Cipro (Bayer)	0.171	Nd
Ciprofloxacin, 500 mg/Tablet	Cipro (Bayer)	0.333	Nd
Ciprofloxacin, chlorhydrate, 100 mg/mL/Liquid	Cipro (Bayer)	6.40	Nd
Cisapride, 1 mg/mL/Liquid	Prepulsid (Jansen-Ortho)	0.80	Nd
Clarithromycin, 250 mg/Tablet	Biaxin (Abbott)	0.21	Nd
Clarithromycin, 25 mg/mL/Liquid	Biaxin pediatric (Abbott)	2.35	Nd
Clarithromycin, 500 mg/Tablet	Biaxin (Abbott)	0.00	Nd
Clindamycin, palmitate, 15 mg/mL/Liquid	Dalacin C (Pharmacia & Upjohn)	Nd	1.20
Clobazam, 10 mg/Tablet	Frisium (Hoechst Marion Roussel)	0.398	Nd
Clomipramine HCl, 10 mg/Tablet	Novo-Clopamine (Novopharm)	0.209	0.212
Clomipramine HCl, 25 mg/Tablet	Novo-Clopamine (Novopharm)	0.00	0.003
Clomipramine HCl, 50 mg/Tablet	Novo-Clopamine (Novopharm)	0.00	0.009
Clonazepam, 0.25 mg/Tablet	PMS-Clonazepam (Pharmascience)	0.26	Nd
Clonazepam, 0.5 mg/Tablet	Rivotril (Hoffman-La Roche)	Nd	0.6
Clonazepam, 0.5 mg/Tablet	PMS-Clonazepam (Pharmascience)	0.13	Nd
Clonazepam, 0.5 mg/Tablet	Apo-Clonazepam (Apotex)	0.48	Nd
Clonazepam, 0.5 mg/Tablet	Clonapam (ICN)	0.72	Nd
Clonazepam, 0.5 mg/Tablet	Rho-Clonazepam (Rhodiapharm)	0.72	Nd
Clonazepam, 1 mg/Tablet	PMS-Clonazepam (Pharmascience)	0.26	Nd
Clonazepam, 1.0 mg/Tablet	Clonapam (ICN)	0.725	Nd
Clonazepam, 1.0 mg/Tablet	Rho-Clonazepam (Rhodiapharm)	0.725	Nd
Clonazepam, 2 mg/Tablet	Rivotril (Hoffman-La Roche)	Nd	0.6
Clonazepam, 2 mg/Tablet	PMS-Clonazepam (Pharmascience)	0.54	Nd
Clonazepam, 2 mg/Tablet	Rho-Clonazepam (Rhodiapharm)	0.722	Nd

(continues)

Table 1
(Continued)

Drug, concentration, and presentation	Commercial name and company	Caloric content (kcal)	
		Carbohydrate[b]	Total[b]
Clonazepam, 2.0 mg/Tablet	Apo-Clonazepam (Apotex)	0.4	Nd
Clonazepam, 2.0 mg/Tablet	Clonapam (ICN)	0.722	Nd
Clonidin, 0.1 mg/Tablet	Novo-Clonidine (Novopharm)	0.418	0.431
Clonidin, 0.2 mg/Tablet	Novo-Clonidine (Novopharm)	0.796	0.822
Clorazepate, 15 mg/Capsule	Novo-Clopate (Novopharm)	0.601	0.632
Clorazepate, 3.75 mg/Capsule	Novo-Clopate (Novopharm)	0.475	0.499
Clorazepate, 7.5 mg/Capsule	Novo-Clopate (Novopharm)	0.463	0.487
Cloxacillin sodium, 250 mg/Capsule	Apo-Cloxi (Apotex)	Nd	0.20
Cloxacillin sodium, 250 mg/Capsule	Nu-Cloxi (Nu-Pharm)	Nd	0.21
Cloxacillin sodium, 500 mg/Capsule	Apo-Cloxi (Apotex)	Nd	0.33
Cloxacillin sodium, 500 mg/Capsule	Nu-Cloxi (Nu-Pharm)	Nd	0.33
Cloxacillin, 25 mg/mL/Liquid	Apo-Cloxi (Apotex)	Nd	1.79
Cloxacillin, 25 mg/mL/Liquid	Nu-Cloxi (Nu-Pharm)	Nd	1.79
Cloxacillin, 25 mg/mL/Liquid	Orbenine (Wyeth-Ayerst)	Nd	2.00
Cloxacillin, 25 mg/mL/Liquid	Novo-Cloxin (Novopharm)	1.80	1.80
Cloxacillin, 250 mg/Capsule	Orbenine (Wyeth-Ayerst)	Nd	0.44
Cloxacillin, 250 mg/Capsule	Novo-Cloxin (Novopharm)	0.139	0.210
Cloxacillin, 500 mg/Capsule	Orbenine (Wyeth-Ayerst)	Nd	0.30
Cloxacillin, 500 mg/Capsule	Novo-Cloxin (Novopharm)	0.00	0.123
Codeine, 5 mg/mL/Liquid	Codeine phosphate (Rougier)	Nd	3.33
Cyclobenzaprine HCl, 10 mg/Tablet	Novo-Cycloprine (Novopharm)	0.533	0.542
Cyclosporine, 100 mg/mL/Liquid	Neoral (Sandoz)	7.00	Nd
Cyproheptadine, 0.4 mg/mL/Liquid	Periactin (Johnson & Johnson Merck consumer pharmaceuticals)	1.80	Nd
Dapsone, 100 mg/Tablet	Avlosulfon (Wyeth-Ayerst)	Nd	0.12

320

Demeclocycline, chlorhydrate, 150 mg/Tablet	Declomycin (Wyeth-Ayerst)	Nd	1.0
Demeclocycline, chlorhydrate, 300 mg/Tablet	Declomycin (Wyeth-Ayerst)	Nd	1.0
Desipramine HCl, 10 mg/Tablet	Novo-Desipramine (Novopharm)	0.003	0.005
Desipramine HCl, 25 mg/Tablet	Novo-Desipramine (Novopharm)	0.007	0.012
Desipramine HCl, 50 mg/Tablet	Novo-Desipramine (Novopharm)	0.010	0.019
Desipramine HCl, 75 mg/Tablet	Novo-Desipramine (Novopharm)	0.010	0.018
Desogestrel-ethinyl estradiol, 0.5 mg/Tablet	Marvelon (Organon.)	0.281	Nd
Desogestrel-ethinyl estradiol, 1 mg/Capsule	Marvelon (Organon.)	0.281	Nd
Desogestrel-ethinyl estradiol, 2 mg/Capsule	Marvelon (Organon.)	0.281	Nd
Dexamethasone, 1 mg/mL/Liquid	Pms-Dexamethasone (Pharmascience)	0.64	Nd
Dexamethasone, 4 mg/Tablet	Dexasone (ICN)	0.591	Nd
Dexamethasone, 500 µg/Tablet	Dexasone (ICN)	0.591	Nd
Dexamethasone, 750 µg/Tablet	Dexasone (ICN)	0.589	Nd
Dextromethorphan, bromhydrate, sugar free, 3 mg/mL/Liquid	Balminil DM (Rougier)	1.40	Nd
Dextromethorphan, bromhydrate-pseudoephedrine-guaifenesin, 3 mg + 6 mg + 20 mg/mL/Liquid	Novahistex DM expectorant decongestant (Hoechst Marion Roussel)	2.60	Nd
Dextromethorphan, bromhydrate-pseudoephedrine, 1.5 mg + 3 mg/mL/Liquid	Novahistine DM decongestant (Hoechst Marion Roussel)	3.00	Nd
Dextromethorphan, bromhydrate-pseudoephedrine, 3 mg + 6 mg/mL/Liquid	Novahistex DM decongestant (Hoechst Marion Roussel)	2.40	Nd
Dextromethorphan, bromhydrate, 3 mg/mL/Liquid	Balminil DM (Rougier)	2.40	Nd
Dextromethorphan, bromhydrate, 3 mg/mL/Liquid	Novahistex DM (Hoechst Marion Roussel)	2.40	Nd
Dextromethorphan, bromhydrate-pseudoephedrine-guaifenesin, 1.5 mg + 3 mg + 10 mg/mL/Liquid	Novahistine DM Expt Dcgt (Hoechst Marion Roussel)	2.44	Nd
Dextromethorphan, bromhydrate, 1.5 mg/mL/Liquid	Novahistine DM (Hoechst Marion Roussel)	3.00	Nd
Diazepam, 1 mg/mL/Liquid	Pms-diazepam (Pharmascience)	1.38	Nd
Diazepam, 10 mg/Tablet	Apo-Diazepam (Apotex)	Nd	0.59
Diazepam, 10 mg/Tablet	Valium Roche oral (Hoffman-La Roche)	Nd	0.7
Diazepam, 10 mg/Tablet	Novo-Dipam (Novopharm)	0.692	0.974

(continues)

Table 1
(Continued)

Drug, concentration, and presentation	Commercial name and company	Caloric content (kcal)	
		Carbohydrate[b]	Total[b]
Diazepam, 2 mg/Tablet	Apo-Diazepam (Apotex)	Nd	0.62
Diazepam, 2 mg/Tablet	Vivol (Carter Horner)	Nd	0.4
Diazepam, 2 mg/Tablet	Novo-Dipam (Novopharm)	0.710	0.744
Diazepam, 5 mg/Tablet	Apo-Diazepam (Apotex)	Nd	0.61
Diazepam, 5 mg/Tablet	Valium Roche Oral (Hoffman-La Roche)	Nd	0.7
Diazepam, 5 mg/Tablet	Novo-Dipam (Novopharm)	0.695	0.712
Diclofenac, 100 mg/Tablet	Novo-Difenac SR (Novopharm)	0.878	0.900
Diclofenac, 25 mg/Tablet	Novo-Difenac (Novopharm)	0.129	0.135
Diclofenac, 50 mg/Tablet	Novo-Difenac (Novopharm)	0.109	0.116
Diclofenac, 75 mg/Tablet	Novo-Difenac SR (Novopharm)	0.658	0.675
Dicyclomine, 10 mg/Tablet	Bentylol (Hoechst Marion Roussel)	0.369	Nd
Dicyclomine, 2 mg/mL/Liquid	Bentylol (Hoechst Marion Roussel)	4.00	Nd
Dicyclomine, 20 mg/Tablet	Bentylol (Hoechst Marion Roussel)	0.369	Nd
Diflunisal, 250 mg/Tablet	Novo-Diflunisal (Novopharm)	0.125	0.155
Diflunisal, 500 mg/Tablet	Novo-Diflunisal (Novopharm)	0.250	0.311
Digoxin, 0.05 mg/mL/Liquid	Lanoxin (Glaxo Wellcome)	1.93	2.30
Diltiazem, 120 mg/Tablet	Novo-Diltazem SR (Novopharm)	0.00	0.00
Diltiazem, 30 mg/Tablet	Novo-Diltazem (Novopharm)	0.623	0.641
Diltiazem, 60 mg/Tablet	Novo-Diltazem SR (Novopharm)	0.00	0.00
Diltiazem, 60 mg/Tablet	Novo-Diltazem (Novopharm)	1.246	1.282
Diltiazem, 90 mg/Tablet	Novo-Diltazem SR (Novopharm)	0.00	0.00
Dimenhydrinate, 15 mg/Tablet	Gravol (Carter Horner)	Nd	0.20
Dimenhydrinate, 15 mg/Chewable tablet	Gravol (Carter Horner)	Nd	1.40
Dimenhydrinate, 25 mg/Tablet	Gravol (Carter Horner)	Nd	0.30

Drug/Formulation	Brand (Manufacturer)		
Dimenhydrinate, 25 mg immediate + 50 mg, controlled release/Capsule	Gravol (Carter Horner)		1.20
Dimenhydrinate, 3 mg/mL/Liquid	Gravol (Carter Horner)	Nd	2.94
Dimenhydrinate, 3 mg/mL/Liquid	Pms-dimenhydrinate (Pharmascience)	1.5	Nd
Dimenhydrinate, 50 mg/Tablet	Gravol (Carter Horner)	Nd	1.40
Dimenhydrinate, 50 mg/Chewable tablet	Gravol (Carter Horner)	Nd	2.60
Diphenhydramine, 2.5 mg/mL/Liquid	Benadryl elixir (Warner-Lambert)	Nd	2.04
Diphenhydramine, 2.5 mg/mL/Liquid	PMS-diphenydramine (Pharmascience)	1.7	Nd
Diphenhydramine, 6.25 mg/mL/Liquid	Benadryl (Warner-Lambert)	Nd	1.57
Dipyridamole, 100 mg/Tablet	Novo-Dipiradol (Novopharm)	0.088	0.479
Dipyridamole, 25 mg/Tablet	Novo-Dipiradol (Novopharm)	0.022	0.153
Dipyridamole, 50 mg/Tablet	Novo-Dipiradol (Novopharm)	0.044	0.293
Dipyridamole, 75 mg/Tablet	Novo-Dipiradol (Novopharm)	0.066	0.379
Divalproex, sodium, 125 mg/Tablet	Epival (Abbot)	0.08	Nd
Divalproex, sodium, 250 mg/Tablet	Epival (Abbot)	0.17	Nd
Divalproex, sodium, 500 mg/Tablet	Epival (Abbot)	0.33	Nd
Docusate calcium, 240 mg/Capsule	Surfak (Hoechst Marion Roussel)	0.555	Nd
Docusate, calcium, 240 mg/Capsule	PMS-Docusate calcium (Pharmascience)	1.00	Nd
Docusate, calcium, 240 mg/Capsule	Soflax C (Pharmascience)	1.00	Nd
Docusate, sodium + casanthranol, 100 mg + 30 mg/Capsule	Peri-Colace (Roberts Pharmaceutical)	1.00	Nd
Docusate, sodium + sennosides, 50 mg + 8.6 mg/Tablet	Senokot-S (Purdue Frederick)	Nd	0.11
Docusate, sodium, 10 mg/mL/Liquid	Colace (Roberts Pharmaceutical)	Nd	2.40
Docusate, sodium, 10 mg/mL/Liquid	PMS-Docusate, sodium (Pharmascience)	1.7	Nd
Docusate, sodium, 100 mg/Capsule	Soflax (Pharmascience)	0.51	Nd
Docusate, sodium, 100 mg/Capsule	Colace (Roberts Pharmaceutical)	1.00	Nd
Docusate, sodium, 200 mg/Capsule	Soflax (Pharmascience)	0.51	Nd
Docusate, sodium, 4 mg/mL/Liquid	Docusate, Sodium (Technilab)	Nd	2.78
Docusate, sodium, 4 mg/mL/Liquid	Docusate Sodic (Taro Pharmaceuticals)	Nd	2.40
Docusate, sodium, 4 mg/mL/Liquid	PMS-Docusate, sodium (Pharmascience)	1.7	Nd

(continues)

Table 1
(Continued)

Drug, concentration, and presentation	Commercial name and company	Caloric content (kcal)	
		Carbohydrate[b]	Total[b]
Docusate, sodium, 4 mg/mL/Liquid	Colace (Roberts Pharmaceutical)	2.40	Nd
Docusate, sodium, 4 mg/mL/Liquid	Docusate, sodium, syrup (Altas)	2.40	Nd
Docusate, sodium, 50 mg/mL/Liquid	Pms-docusate sodium (Pharmascience)	1.05	Nd
Doxepin HCl, 100 mg/Capsule	Novo-Doxepine (Novopharm)	0.772	0.819
Doxepin HCl, 150 mg/Capsule	Novo-Doxepine (Novopharm)	0.923	0.990
Doxepin HCl, 25 mg/Capsule	Novo-Doxepine (Novopharm)	0.428	0.452
Doxepin HCl, 50 mg/Capsule	Novo-Doxepine (Novopharm)	0.694	0.735
Doxepin HCl, 75 mg/Capsule	Novo-Doxepine (Novopharm)	0.568	0.608
Doxycycline, hyclate, 100 mg/Capsule	Apo-Doxy (Apotex)	Nd	0.74
Doxycycline, hyclate, 100 mg/Capsule	Nu-Doxycycline (Nu-Pharm)	Nd	0.74
Doxycycline, hyclate, 100 mg/Capsule	Novo-Doxylin (Novopharm)	0.022	0.052
Doxycycline, hyclate, 100 mg/Capsule	Vibramycin (Pfizer)	0.956	Nd
Doxycycline, hyclate, 100 mg/Tablet	Apo-Doxy (Apotex)	Nd	0.44
Doxycycline, hyclate, 100 mg/Tablet	Nu-Doxycycline (Nu-Pharm)	Nd	0.44
Doxycycline, hyclate, 100 mg/Tablet	Vibra-Tabs (Pfizer)	0.516	Nd
Erythromycin base, 25 mg/mL/Liquid	Erythrocin (Abbott)	Nd	1.96
Erythromycin base, 250 mg/Capsule	Apo-Erythro E.C. (Apotex)	Nd	0.20
Erythromycin base, 250 mg/Capsule	Novo-Rythro Encap (Novopharm)	0.198	Nd
Erythromycin base, 250 mg/Tablet	Apo-Erythro Base (Apotex)	Nd	1.34
Erythromycin base, 250 mg/Tablet	Erythromid (Abbott)	0.00	Nd
Erythromycin base, 333 mg/Capsule	Eryc (Parke-Davis)	Nd	0.13
Erythromycin base, 333 mg/Capsule	Apo-Erythro E.C. (Apotex)	0.473	Nd
Erythromycin base, 333 mg/Tablet	PCE (Abbott)	0.64	Nd
Erythromycin base, 50 mg/mL/Liquid	Erythrocin (Abbott)	Nd	1.84
Erythromycin base, 500 mg/Tablet	Erybid (Abbott)	0.00	Nd

Drug	Brand (Manufacturer)		
Erythromycin, estolate , 25 mg/ml/Liquid	Ilosone (Eli Lilly)	Nd	1.8
Erythromycin, estolate , 50 mg/ml/Liquid	Ilosone (Eli Lilly)	Nd	1.42
Erythromycin, estolate, 25 mg/mL/Liquid	Novo-Rythro estolate (Novopharm)	1.37	1.37
Erythromycin, estolate, 250 mg/Capsule	Novo-Rythro Estolate (Novopharm)	0.266	0.330
Erythromycin, estolate, 50 mg/mL/Liquid	Novo-Rythro estolate (Novopharm)	1.37	1.37
Erythromycin, stearate, 25 mg/mL/Liquid	Erythrocin (Abbott)	Nd	1.96
Erythromycin, stearate, 250 mg/Tablet	Apo-Erythro S (Apotex)	Nd	0.87
Erythromycin, stearate, 250 mg/Tablet	Nu-Erythromycin-S (Nu-Pharm)	Nd	0.87
Erythromycin, stearate, 250 mg/Tablet	Novo-Rythro Stearate (Novopharm)	0.185	1.846
Erythromycin, stearate, 50 mg/mL/Liquid	Erythrocin (Abbott)	Nd	1.84
Erythromycin, stearate, 500 mg/Tablet	Apo-Erythro S (Apotex)	Nd	1.73
Erythromycin, succinate, 40 mg/mL/Liquid	EES 200 (Abbott)	2.63	Nd
Erythromycin, succinate, 600 mg/Tablet	Apo-Erythro-ES (Apotex)	Nd	1.39
Erythromycin, succinate, 600 mg/Tablet	EES 600 (Abbott)	0.17	Nd
Erythromycin, succinate, 80 mg/mL/Liquid	EES 400 (Abbott)	2.43	Nd
Erythromycin, succinate, 40 mg/mL/Liquid	Novo-Rythro Ethyl Succinate (Novopharm)	1.96	1.96
Erythromycin, succinate, 80 mg/mL/Liquid	Novo-Rythro Ethyl Succinate (Novopharm)	1.76	1.76
Erythromycin, sulfisoxazole, 40–120 mg/mL/Liquid	Pediazole (Abbott)	Nd	1.50
Ethosuximide, 50 mg/mL/Liquid	Zarontin (Parke-Davis)	Nd	3.00
Famotidine, 10 mg/Tablet	Novo-Famotidine (Novopharm)	0.066	0.075
Famotidine, 20 mg/Tablet	Novo-Famotidine (Novopharm)	0.132	0.149
Famotidine, 40 mg/Tablet	Novo-Famotidine (Novopharm)	0.132	0.149
Fenofibrate, 100 mg/Capsule	Novo-Fenofibrate (Novopharm)	0.554	0.566
Ferrous sulfate, 15 mg (elemental iron)/mL/Liquid	Pms-ferrous sulfate (Pharmascience)	2.71	Nd
Ferrous sulfate, 15 mg (elemental iron)/mL/Liquid	Fer-In-Sol (Mead Johnson)	2.76	Nd
Ferrous sulfate, 300 mg/Tablet	Apo-sulfate ferreux (Apotex)	Nd	0.30
Ferrous sulfate, 300 mg/Tablet	PMS-sulfate ferreux (Pharmascience)	0.57	Nd
Ferrous sulfate, 6 mg (elemental iron)/mL/Liquid	PMS-ferrous sulfate (Pharmascience)	1.22	Nd
Ferrous sulfate, 6 mg (elemental iron)/mL/Liquid	Fer-In-Sol (Mead Johnson)	5.00	Nd
Fluconazole , 10 mg/mL/Liquid	Diflucan (Pfizer)	2.72	Nd

(continues)

Table 1
(Continued)

Drug, concentration, and presentation	Commercial name and company	Caloric content (kcal)	
		Carbohydrate[b]	Total[b]
Flunarizine HCl, 5 mg/Capsule	Novo-Flunarizine (Novopharm)	0.576	0.583
Flouride, sodium, 5.56 mg/mL/Liquid	Fluor-A-Day (Pharmascience)	0	Nd
Fluoxetine, 4 mg/mL/Liquid	Prozac (Eli Lilly)	Nd	2.40
Fluoxetine, 10 mg/Capsule	Novo-Fluoxetine (Novopharm)	0.730	0.747
Fluoxetine, 20 mg/Capsule	Novo-Fluoxetine (Novopharm)	0.694	0.710
Fluoxetine, 4 mg/mL/Liquid	Apo-Fluoxetine (Apotex)	3.64	Nd
Fluphenazine, 0.5 mg/mL/Liquid	PMS-Fluphenazine (Pharmascience)	2.39	Nd
Flurazepam, 15 mg/Capsule	Novo-Flupam Novo-Flupam SP.C. (Novopharm)	1.193	1.236
Flurazepam, 30 mg/Capsule	Novo-Flupam Novo-Flupam SP.C. (Novopharm)	1.060	1.103
Flurbiprofen, 100 mg/Tablet	Novo-Flurprofen (Novopharm)	0.368	0.401
Flurbiprofen, 50 mg/Tablet	Novo-Flurprofen (Novopharm)	0.299	0.322
Flutamide, 250 mg/Tablet	Novo-Flutamide (Novopharm)	1.249	1.311
Furosemide, 10 mg/mL/Liquid	Lasix (Hoechst Marion Roussel)	1.913	Nd
Furosemide, 20 mg/Tablet	Novo-Semide (Novopharm)	0.179	0.187
Furosemide, 20 mg/Tablet	Lasix (Hoechst Marion Roussel)	0.211	Nd
Furosemide, 40 mg/Tablet	Novo-Semide (Novopharm)	0.360	0.377
Furosemide, 40 mg/Tablet	Lasix (Hoechst Marion Roussel)	0.420	Nd
Furosemide, 500 mg/Tablet	Lasix Special (Hoechst Marion Roussel)	0.466	Nd
Furosemide, 80 mg/Tablet	Novo-Semide (Novopharm)	0.719	0.751
Furosemide, 80 mg/Tablet	Lasix (Hoechst Marion Roussel)	0.840	Nd
Fusidic acid, 250 mg/Tablet	Fucidin (Leo Pharma)	Nd	0.29
Fusidic acid, 49.2 mg/ml/Liquid	Fucidin (Leo Pharma)	Nd	0.37
Fusidic acid, 50 mg/ ml/Liquid	Fucidin (Leo Pharma)	Nd	0.78
Gemfibrozil, 300 mg/Capsule	Novo-Gemfibrozil (Novopharm)	0.546	0.568
Gemfibrozil, 600 mg/Capsule	Novo-Gemfibrozil (Novopharm)	0.205	0.259

Glyburide, 2.5 mg/Tablet	Novo-Glyburide (Novopharm)	0.052	0.055
Glyburide, 5 mg/Tablet	Novo-Glyburide (Novopharm)	0.103	0.110
Grepafloxacin, chlorhydrate, 200 mg/Tablet	Raxar (Glaxo Wellcome)	0.00	Nd
Guaifenesin, 20 mg/mL/Liquid	Balminil E (Rougier)	Nd	1.60
Guaifenesin, 20 mg/mL/Liquid	Balminil E, sugar free (Rougier)	Nd	1.62
Haloperidol, 0.5 mg/Tablet	Novo-Peridol (Novopharm)	0.025	0.041
Haloperidol, 1 mg/Tablet	Novo-Peridol (Novopharm)	0.025	0.041
Haloperidol, 10 mg/Tablet	Novo-Peridol (Novopharm)	0.050	0.082
Haloperidol, 2 mg/Tablet	Novo-Peridol (Novopharm)	0.025	0.041
Haloperidol, 2 mg/mL/Liquid	Apo-Haloperidol (Apotex)	Nd	0.01
Haloperidol, 2 mg/mL/Liquid	Novo-Peridol (Novopharm)	0.00	0.00
Haloperidol, 2 mg/mL/Liquid	Pms-haloperidol (Pharmascience)	0.00	0.00
Haloperidol, 20 mg/Tablet	Novo-Peridol (Novopharm)	0.050	0.082
Haloperidol, 5 mg/Tablet	Novo-Peridol (Novopharm)	0.025	0.041
Hydralazine HCl, 10 mg/Tablet	Novo-Hylazin (Novopharm)	0.292	0.301
Hydralazine, 25 mg/Tablet	Novo-Hylazin (Novopharm)	0.182	0.189
Hydralazine, 50 mg/Tablet	Novo-Hylazin (Novopharm)	0.100	0.106
Hydrochlorothiazide, 25 mg/Tablet	Novo-Hydrazide (Novopharm)	0.238	0.247
Hydrochlorothiazide, 50 mg/Tablet	Novo-Hydrazide (Novopharm)	0.477	0.495
Hydrochlorothiazide/methyldopa, 250 + 15 mg/Tablet	Novo-Doparil-15 (Novopharm)	0.168	0.211
Hydrochlorothiazide/methyldopa, 250 + 25 mg/Tablet	Novo-Doparil-25 (Novopharm)	0.135	0.178
Hydromorphone HCl, 1 mg/mL/Liquid	Dilaudid (Knoll)	Nd	2.00
Hydromorphone HCl, 1 mg/mL/Liquid	Pms-hydromorphone (Pharmascience)	1.09	Nd
Hydroxyzine, 2 mg/mL/Liquid	Atarax (Pfizer)	Nd	3.20
Hydroxyzine, 10 mg/Capsule	Apo-Hydroxyzine (Apotex)	Nd	0.47
Hydroxyzine, 10 mg/Capsule	Novo-Hydroxyzin (Novopharm)	0.00	1.40
Hydroxyzine, 2 mg/mL/Liquid	PMS-hydroxyzine (Pharmascience)	2.37	Nd
Hydroxyzine, 25 mg/Capsule	Apo-Hydroxyzine (Apotex)	Nd	0.44
Hydroxyzine, 25 mg/Capsule	Novo-Hydroxyzin (Novopharm)	0.00	1.30
Hydroxyzine, 50 mg/Capsule	Apo-Hydroxyzine (Apotex)	Nd	0.44

(continues)

Table 1
(Continued)

Drug, concentration, and presentation	Commercial name and company	Caloric content (kcal)	
		Carbohydrate[b]	Total[b]
Hydroxyzine, 50 mg/Capsule	Novo-Hydroxyzin (Novopharm)	0.00	1.25
Ibuprofen, 20 mg/mL/Liquid	Advil (Whitehall-Robins)	2.76	Nd
Ibuprofen, 200 mg/Tablet	Novo-Profen (Novopharm)	0.180	0.215
Ibuprofen, 200 mg/Tablet (sugar coating)	Novo-Profen (Novopharm)	0.256	0.291
Ibuprofen, 300 mg/Tablet	Novo-Profen (Novopharm)	0.270	0.322
Ibuprofen, 300 mg/Tablet (sugar coating)	Novo-Profen (Novopharm)	0.373	0.425
Ibuprofen, 400 mg/Tablet	Novo-Profen (Novopharm)	0.360	0.429
Ibuprofen, 400 mg/Tablet (suger coating)	Novo-Profen (Novopharm)	0.463	0.532
Ibuprofen, 600 mg/Tablet	Novo-Profen (Novopharm)	0.540	0.593
Imipramine, 10 mg/Tablet	Novo-Pramine (Novopharm)	0.080	0.088
Imipramine, 25 mg/Tablet	Novo-Pramine (Novopharm)	0.080	0.088
Imipramine, 50 mg/Tablet	Novo-Pramine (Novopharm)	0.195	0.209
Indapamide, 2.5 mg/Tablet	Novo-Indapamide (Novopharm)	0.255	0.260
Indomethacin, 25 mg/Capsule	Novo-Methacin Novo-Methacin SP.C. (Novopharm)	0.887	0.910
Indomethacin, 50 mg/Capsule	Novo-Methacin Novo-Methacin SP.C. (Novopharm)	1.458	1.495
Isoniazid, 10 mg/mL/Liquid	Pms-isoniazid (Pharmascience)	0.89	Nd
Isosorbide dinitrate, 10 mg/Tablet	Novo-Sorbide (Novopharm)	0.160	0.174
Isosorbide dinitrate, 30 mg/Tablet	Novo-Sorbide (Novopharm)	0.420	0.442
Itraconazole, 10 mg/mL/Liquid	Sporanox (Jansen-Ortho)	0.50	Nd
Ketoconazole, 20 mg/mL/Liquid	Nizoral (Jansen-Ortho)	0.25	Nd
Ketotifen, fumarate, 0.2 mg/mL/Liquid	Apo-Ketotifen (Apotex)	2.562	Nd
Ketotifen, fumarate, 0.2 mg/mL/Liquid	Novo-Ketotifen (Novopharm)	3.31	3.31
Ketotifen, fumarate, 1 mg/Tablet	Novo-Ketotifen (Novopharm)	0.493	0.499
Ketotifen, fumarate, 0.2 mg/mL/Liquid	Zaditen (Novartis Pharma)	2.41	Nd
Lactose (placebo) /Capsule	Novo-Plus (Novopharm)	0.720	0.732

Lactulose, 666.7 mg/mL/Liquid	Gen-lac (Genpharm)	Nd	3.64
Lactulose, 666.7 mg/mL/Liquid	PMS-Lactulose (Pharmascience)	3.5	Nd
Lamivudine, 10 mg/mL/Liquid	3-TC (Glaxo Wellcome)	1.13	1.27
Lamotrigine, 100 mg/Tablet	Lamictal (Glaxo Wellcome)	0.428	Nd
Lamotrigine, 150 mg/Tablet	Lamictal (Glaxo Wellcome)	0.644	Nd
Lamotrigine, 25 mg/Tablet	Lamictal (Glaxo Wellcome)	0.107	Nd
Lidocaine, 2%/Liquid	PMS-Lidocaine, viscous (Pharmascience)	0.2	Nd
Lithium, carbonate, 60 mg/mL/Liquid	PMS-Lithium citrate (Pharmascience)	1.77	Nd
Loperamide, 0.2 mg/mL/Liquid	PMS-Loperamide (Pharmascience)	2.19	Nd
Loperamide, 2 mg/Tablet	Novo-Loperamide (Novopharm)	1.353	1.383
Loratadine, 1 mg/mL/Liquid	Claritin (Schering)	3.20	Nd
Lorazepam, 0.5 mg/Tablet	Apo-Lorazepam (Apotex)	Nd	0.19
Lorazepam, 0.5 mg/Tablet (sublingual)	Ativan (Wyeth-Ayerst)	Nd	0.14
Lorazepam, 0.5 mg/Tablet	Nu-Loraz (Nu-Pharm)	Nd	0.19
Lorazepam, 0.5 mg/Tablet	Novo-Lorazem (Novopharm)	0.049	0.049
Lorazepam, 1 mg/Tablet	Novo-Lorazem (Novopharm)	0.098	0.099
Lorazepam, 1.0 mg/Tablet	Apo-Lorazepam (Apotex)	Nd	0.38
Lorazepam, 1.0 mg/Tablet (sublingual)	Ativan (Wyeth-Ayerst)	Nd	0.59
Lorazepam, 1.0 mg/Tablet	Nu-Loraz (Nu-Pharm)	Nd	0.38
Lorazepam, 2 mg/Tablet	Novo-Lorazem (Novopharm)	0.110	0.112
Lorazepam, 2.0 mg/Tablet	Apo-Lorazepam (Apotex)	Nd	0.47
Lorazepam, 2.0 mg/Tablet (sublingual)	Ativan (Wyeth-Ayerst)	Nd	0.19
Lorazepam, 2.0 mg/Tablet	Nu-Loraz (Nu-Pharm)	Nd	0.47
Magaldrate, 96 mg/mL/Liquid	Riopan (Whitehall-Robins)	0	Nd
Magnesium, citrate, 15g/flacon/Liquid	Citro-Mag (Rougier)	Nd	1.05
Magnesium, hydroxide, 80 mg/mL/Liquid	Milk of magnesia (Atlas Laboratories)	0	Nd
Maprotiline HCl, 10 mg/Tablet	Novo-Maprotiline (Novopharm)	0.290	0.299
Maprotiline HCl, 50 mg/Tablet	Novo-Maprotiline (Novopharm)	0.266	0.279
Maprotiline HCl, 75 mg/Tablet	Novo-Maprotiline (Novopharm)	0.366	0.384
Medroxyprogesterone acetate, 10 mg/Tablet	Novo-Medrone (Novopharm)	0.428	0.433

(continues)

Table 1
(Continued)

Drug, concentration, and presentation	Commercial name and company	Caloric content (kcal)	
		Carbohydrate[b]	Total[b]
Medroxyprogesterone acetate, 2.5 mg/Tablet	Novo-Medrone (Novopharm)	0.380	0.384
Medroxyprogesterone acetate, 5 mg/Tablet	Novo-Medrone (Novopharm)	0.370	0.374
Meprobamate, 200 mg/Tablet	Novo-Mepro (Novopharm)	0.084	0.117
Meprobamate, 400 mg/Tablet	Novo-Mepro (Novopharm)	0.168	0.235
Methotrimeprazine maleate, 25 mg/Tablet	Novo-Meprazine (Novopharm)	0.023	0.035
Methotrimeprazine maleate, 50 mg/Tablet	Novo-Meprazine (Novopharm)	0.104	0.130
Methotrimeprazine, 40 mg/mL/Liquid	Nozinan (Rhône-Poulenc Rorer)	Nd	1.80
Methotrimeprazine, 5 mg/mL/Liquid	Nozinan (Rhône-Poulenc Rorer)	Nd	2.98
Methyldopa, 125 mg/Tablet	Novo-Medopa (Novopharm)	0.060	0.074
Methyldopa, 250 mg/Tablet	Novo-Medopa (Novopharm)	0.119	0.148
Methyldopa, 500 mg/Tablet	Novo-Medopa (Novopharm)	0.238	0.297
Metoclopramide, 1 mg/mL/Liquid	PMS-Metoclopramide (Pharmascience)	1.3	Nd
Metoclopramide, chlorhydrate, 1 mg/mL/Liquid	Maxeran (Hoechst Marion Roussel)	1.960	Nd
Metoclopramide, chlorhydrate, 10 mg/Tablet	Maxeran (Hoechst Marion Roussel)	0.361	Nd
Metoclopramide, chlorhydrate, 5 mg/Tablet	Maxeran (Hoechst Marion Roussel)	0.371	Nd
Metoprolol, 100 mg/Tablet, coated	Novo-Metoprol (Novopharm)	0.601	0.635
Metoprolol, 100 mg/Tablet, uncoated	Novo-Metoprol, uncoated (Novopharm)	0.601	0.631
Metoprolol, 50 mg/Tablet, coated	Novo-Metoprol, (Novopharm)	0.509	0.531
Metoprolol, 50 mg/Tablet, uncoated	Novo-Metoprol, uncoated (Novopharm)	0.301	0.340
Metronidazole, 250 mg/Tablet	Apo-Metronidazole (Apotex)	Nd	0.95
Metronidazole, 250 mg/Tablet	Novo-Nidazole (Novopharm)	0.585	0.620
Metronidazole, 500 mg/Capsule	Flagyl (Rhône-Poulenc Rorer)	0.00	Nd
Mexiletine, chlorhydrate, 100 mg/Granules	Novo-Mexiletine (Novopharm)	0.192	0.200
Mexiletine, chlorhydrate, 200 mg/Granules	Novo-Mexiletine (Novopharm)	0.383	0.401
Mineral oil 78% sugar-free jelly/Jelly	Lansoyl (Jouveinal)	Nd	0.27

Lansoyl (Jouveinal)	Mineral oil 78% gel/Jelly	Nd	0.60
Agarol (Warner-Lambert)	Mineral oil + glycerine./Liquid	Nd	0.65
Apo-Minocycline (Apotex)	Minocycline, chlorhydrate, 100 mg/Capsule	Nd	0.56
Minocin (Wyeth-Ayerst)	Minocycline, chlorhydrate, 100 mg/Capsule	Nd	1.0
Apo-Minocycline (Apotex)	Minocycline, chlorhydrate, 50 mg/Capsule	Nd	0.28
Minocin (Wyeth-Ayerst)	Minocycline, chlorhydrate, 50 mg/Capsule	Nd	1.0
Novo-Minocycline (Novopharm)	Minocycline, chlorhydrate, 100 mg/Capsule	0.608	0.625
Novo-Minocycline (Novopharm)	Minocycline, chlorhydrate, 50 mg/Capsule	0.524	0.536
Morphitec-1 (Technilab)	Morphine, 1 mg/mL/Liquid	Nd	2.23
M.O.S. (ICN)	Morphine, 1 mg/mL/Liquid	0.21	Nd
Morphitec-10 (Technilab)	Morphine, 10 mg/mL/Liquid	Nd	2.23
M.O.S. (ICN)	Morphine, 10 mg/mL/Liquid	1.00	Nd
Morphitec-20 (Technilab)	Morphine, 20 mg/mL/Liquid	Nd	2.23
Morphitec-5 (Technilab)	Morphine, 5 mg/mL/Liquid	Nd	2.23
M.O.S. (ICN)	Morphine, 5 mg/mL/Liquid	1.17	Nd
Novo-Nadolol (Novopharm)	Nadolol, 160 mg/Tablet	1.228	1.276
Novo-Nadolol (Novopharm)	Nadolol, 40 mg/Tablet	0.307	0.320
Novo-Nadolol (Novopharm)	Nadolol, 80 mg/Tablet	0.614	0.639
Novo-Naprox (Novopharm)	Naproxen, 125 mg/Tablet	0.037	0.061
Naprosyn (Hoffman-La Roche)	Naproxen, 25 mg/mL/Liquid	1.16	Nd
Novo-Naprox (Novopharm)	Naproxen, 250 mg/Tablet	0.075	0.122
Novo-Naprox (Novopharm)	Naproxen, 375 mg/Tablet	0.112	0.183
Novo-Naprox (Novopharm)	Naproxen, 500 mg/Tablet	0.149	0.245
Novo-Naprox, sodium (Novopharm)	Naproxen, sodium, 275 mg/Tablet	0.077	0.135
Novo-Naprox, sodium D.S. (Novopharm)	Naproxen, sodium, 550 mg/Tablet	0.154	0.270
Nitrazadon (ICN)	Nitrazepam, 10 mg/Tablet	0.47	Nd
Rho-Nitrazepam (Rhodiapharm)	Nitrazepam, 10 mg/Tablet	0.47	Nd
Mogadon (Hoffman-La Roche)	Nitrazepam, 10 mg/Tablet	0.70	0.80
Nitrazadon (ICN)	Nitrazepam, 5 mg/Tablet	0.233	Nd
Rho-Nitrazepam (Rhodiapharm)	Nitrazepam, 5 mg/Tablet	0.233	Nd

(continues)

Table 1
(Continued)

Drug, concentration, and presentation	Commercial name and company	Caloric content (kcal) Carbohydrate[b]	Total[b]
Nitrazepam, 5 mg/Tablet	Mogadon (Hoffman-La Roche)	0.35	0.40
Nitrofurantoin, 100 mg/Tablet	Novo-Furan (Novopharm)	0.146	0.172
Nitrofurantoin, 5 mg/mL/Liquid	Novo-Furan (Novopharm)	2.25	2.27
Nitrofurantoin, 50 mg/Capsule	Novo-Furantoin Capsules (Novopharm)	0.037	0.037
Nitrofurantoin, 50 mg/Tablet	Novo-Furan (Novopharm)	0.073	0.086
Norfloxacin, 400 mg/Tablet	Apo-Norflox (Apotex)	0.044	Nd
Norfloxacin, 400 mg/Tablet	Noroxin (Merck Sharp & Dohme)	0.00	Nd
Normethadone + ephedrine , 10 mg/mL/Liquid	Cophylac (Hoechst Marion Roussel)	0.80	Nd
Nilstat (Technilab)	Nilstat (Technilab)	—	3.00
Nystatin, 100,000 U/mL/Liquid	Mycostatin (Bristol-Myers Squibb)	2.41	Nd
Nystatin, 100,000 U/mL/Liquid	PMS-Nystatin (Pharmascience)	2.62	Nd
Nystatin, 100,000 U/mL/Liquid	Nadostine (Laboratoire Nadeau)	Nd	2.60
Nystatin, 100,000 IU/mL/Liquid	Nadostine (Laboratoire Nadeau)	Nd	0.42
Nystatin, 100,000 IU/mL/Liquid, sugar free	Nadostine (Laboratoire Nadeau)	Nd	0.43
Nystatin, 500,000 IU/Tablet	Mycostatin (Bristol-Myers Squibb)	0.35	Nd
Nystatin, 500,000 IU/Tablet	Apo-Oflox (Apotex)	0.096	Nd
Ofloxacin, 200 mg/Tablet	Apo-Oflox (Apotex)	0.15	Nd
Ofloxacin, 300 mg/Tablet	Apo-Oflox (Apotex)	0.21	Nd
Ofloxacin, 400 mg/Tablet	Alti-Orciprenalline (Altimed Pharmaceutical)	Nd	0.036
Orciprenaline, 2 mg/mL/Liquid	Apo-Orciprenaline (Apotex)	1.99	Nd
Orciprenaline, 2 mg/mL/Liquid	Novoxapam (Novopharm)	0.588	0.613
Oxazepam, 10 mg/Tablet	Novoxapam (Novopharm)	0.566	0.584
Oxazepam, 15 mg/Tablet	Choledyl (Parke-Davis)	Nd	3.66
Oxtriphylline, 10 mg/mL/Liquid	Novo-Triphyl (Novopharm)	0.104	0.170
Oxtriphylline, 100 mg/Tablet	Choledyl (Parke-Davis)	Nd	2.80
Oxtriphylline, 20 mg/mL/Liquid			

Drug	Product (Manufacturer)		
Oxtriphylline, 200 mg/Tablet	Novo-Triphyl (Novopharm)	0.134	0.220
Oxtriphylline, 300 mg/Tablet	Novo-Triphyl (Novopharm)	0.136	0.224
Oxybutinin, 1 mg/mL/Liquid	Apo-Oxybutinine (Apotex)	2.81	Nd
Oxybutinin, 1 mg/mL/Liquid	Ditropan (Procter & Gamble)	1.01	Nd
Oxybutinin, 5 mg/Tablet	Novo-Oxybutinin (Novopharm)	0.601	0.616
Penicillin G, 500,000 I.U./Tablet	Novo-Pen G-500 (Novopharm)	0.104	0.171
Penicillin VK, 25 mg/mL/Liquid	Apo-Pen VK (Apotex)	Nd	0.81
Penicillin VK, 300 mg/Tablet	Apo-Pen VK (Apotex)	Nd	0.09
Penicillin VK, 500,000 I.U./Tablet	Novo-Pen VK (Novopharm)	0.501	0.573
Penicillin VK, 60 mg/mL/Liquid	Apo-Pen VK (Apotex)	Nd	2.50
Penicillin VK, 60 mg/mL/Liquid	Novo-Pen VK (Novopharm)	2.028	2.112
Pericyazin, 10 mg/mL/Liquid	Neuleptil (Rhône-Poulenc Rorer)	Nd	1.00
Phenobarbital, 100 mg/Capsule	Novo-Pentobarb (Novopharm)	0.227	0.254
Phenobarbital, 15 mg/Tablet	Phenobarbital (Parke-Davis)	0.24	0.24
Phenobarbital, 30 mg/Tablet	Phenobarbital (Parke-Davis)	0.33	0.33
Phenobarbital, 5 mg/mL/Liquid	Phenobarbital elixir USP (Stanley Pharmaceuticals.)	3.78	Nd
Phenobarbital, 60 mg/Tablet	Phenobarbital (Parke-Davis)	0.35	0.35
Phenylbutazone, 100 mg/Tablet	Novo-Butazone (Novopharm)	0.053	0.060
Phenylephrine HCl-hydrocodone bitartrate-guaifenesin, 4 mg + 1 mg + 40 mg/mL/Liquid	Novahistex DH Expt (Hoechst Marion Roussel)	3.00	Nd
Phenylephrine HCl-hydrocodone bitartrate, 2 mg + 0.34 mg/mL/Liquid	Novahistine DH (Hoechst Marion Roussel)	1.38	Nd
Phenylephrine HCl-hydrocodone bitartrate, 4 mg + 1 mg/mL/Liquid	Novahistex DH (Hoechst Marion Roussel)	2.42	Nd
Phenylephrine HCl-codeine phosphate, 4 mg + 3 mg/mL/Liquid	Novahistex C (Hoechst Marion Roussel)	2.22	Nd
Phenytoin, sodium, 100 mg/Capsule	Dilantin (Parke-Davis)	0.48	0.60
Phenytoin, sodium, 30 mg/Capsule	Dilantin (Parke-Davis)	Nd	0.70
Phenytoin, 25 mg/mL/Liquid	Dilantin-125 (Parke-Davis)	1.14	Nd
Phenytoin, 50 mg/Tablet	Dilantin Infatabs (Parke-Davis)	1.92	Nd

(continues)

Table 1
(Continued)

Drug, concentration, and presentation	Commercial name and company	Caloric content (kcal)	
		Carbohydrate[b]	Total[b]
Pindolol, 10 mg/Tablet	Novo-Pindol (Novopharm)	0.055	0.063
Pindolol, 15 mg/Tablet	Novo-Pindol (Novopharm)	0.083	0.094
Pindolol, 5 mg/Tablet	Novo-Pindol (Novopharm)	0.050	0.056
Piroxicam, 10 mg/Capsule	Novo-Pirocam (Novopharm)	1.056	1.086
Piroxicam, 20 mg/Capsule	Novo-Pirocam (Novopharm)	1.056	1.086
Pivampicillin, 35 mg/mL/Liquid	Pondocillin (Leo Pharma)	1.62	1.62
Pivampicillin, 500 mg/Tablet	Pondocillin (Leo Pharma)	0.43	0.43
Pivmecillinam, chlorhydrate, 200 mg/Tablet	Selaxid (Leo Pharma)	0.00	Nd
Polyethylene glycol/electrolytes,/Liquid	Lyteprep (Therapex)	0.00	Nd
Polyethylene glycol/electrolytes,/Liquid	Colyte (Reed & Carrick)	0.00	Nd
Polyethylene glycol/electrolytes,/Liquid	PegLyte (Pharmascience)	0.00	Nd
Polyethylene glycol/electrolytes,/Powder	PegLyte (Pharmascience)	0.00	Nd
Polystyrene sulfonate/Liquid	Novo-Prazin (Novopharm)	0.202	0.208
Prazocin HCl, 2 mg/Tablet	Novo-Prazin (Novopharm)	0.253	0.260
Prazocin HCl, 5 mg/Tablet	Novo-Prazin (Novopharm)	0.471	0.484
Prednisolone, 1 mg/mL/Liquid	Pediapred (Rhône-Poulenc Rorer)	2.26	Nd
Prednisolone, 5 mg/Tablet	Novo-Prednisolone (Novopharm)	0.262	0.273
Prednisone, 5 mg/Tablet	Novo-Prednisone (Novopharm)	0.510	0.520
Prednisone, 50 mg/Tablet	Novo-Prednisone (Novopharm)	0.586	0.606
Primidone, 125 mg/Chewable tablet	Mysoline (Wyeth-Ayerst)	Nd	0.12
Primidone, 125 mg/Tablet	Apo-Primidone (Apotex)	Nd	0.17
Primidone, 250 mg/Foaming tablet	Mysoline (Wyeth-Ayerst)	Nd	0.23
Primidone, 250 mg/Tablet	Apo-Primidone (Apotex)	Nd	0.34
Prochlorperazine, 1 mg/mL/Liquid	Stemetil (Rhône-Poulenc Rorer)	3.18	Nd
Prochlorperazine, 10 mg/Tablet	Stemetil (Rhône-Poulenc Rorer)	0	Nd

Product (manufacturer)	Description		
Stemetil (Rhône-Poulenc Rorer)	Prochlorperazine, 5 mg/Tablet	0	Nd
PMS-Procyclidine (Pharmascience)	Procyclidine, 0.5 mg/mL/Liquid	1.16	Nd
Kemadrin (Glaxo Wellcome)	Procyclidine, 0.5 mg/mL/Liquid	2.30	Nd
Kemadrin (Glaxo Wellcome)	Procyclidine, 5 mg/Tablet	0.47	Nd
Pms-Promethazine (Pharmascience)	Promethazine, 2 mg/mL/Liquid	1.8	Nd
Novo-Propoxyn (Novopharm)	Propoxyphene, hydrochloride, 65 mg/Capsule	0.491	0.504
Novo-Pranol (Novopharm)	Propranolol, 10 mg/Tablet	0.434	0.451
Novo-Pranol (Novopharm)	Propranolol, 120 mg/Tablet	1.196	1.240
Novo-Pranol (Novopharm)	Propranolol, 20 mg/Tablet	0.352	0.374
Novo-Pranol (Novopharm)	Propranolol, 40 mg/Tablet	0.704	0.725
Novo-Pranol (Novopharm)	Propranolol, 80 mg/Tablet	0.819	0.861
Novo-Propoxyn compound (Novopharm)	Prpoxyphen HCl-ASA-caffeine/Capsule	0.371	0.396
Balminil Decongestionnant (Rougier)	Pseudoephedrin, 6 mg/mL/Liquid	Nd	1.88
PMS-Pseudoephedrine (Pharmascience)	Pseudoephedrin, 6 mg/mL/Liquid	3.70	Nd
Novo-Mucilax (Novopharm)	Psyllium, no flavor,/Powder	1.983/g	1.983/g
Novo-Mucilax (Novopharm)	Psyllium, sugar free,/Powder	0.000/g	0.000/g
Novo-Mucilax (Novopharm)	Psyllium, orange flavor /Powder	1.617/g	1.617/g
Metamucil (Procter & Gamble)	Psyllium, orange, smooth texture/Powder	7.76/g	7.76/g
Metamucil (Procter & Gamble)	Psyllium (hydrophilic viscous liquid for oral suspension) orange flavor, smooth texture, "sugar free"/Powder	3.45/g	3.45/g
Metamucil (Procter & Gamble)	Psyllium, no flavor,/Powder	1.98/g	1.98/g
Metamucil (Procter & Gamble)	Psyllium no flavor, sugar free, smooth texture,/Powder	3.45/g	3.45/g
Prodiem Plus (Novartis)	Psyllium + sene,/Granules	Nd	0.74/g
Prodiem Simple (Novartis)	Psyllium/Granules	Nd	0.72/g
Combantrin (Pfizer)	Pyrantel pamoate, 50 mg/mL/Liquid	3.24	Nd
Vitamin B$_6$ (Wampole)	Pyridoxine hydrochloride, 25 mg/Tablet	0.00	Nd
Vanquin (Warner-Lambert)	Pyrvinium pamoate, 10 mg/mL/Liquid	Nd	0.90
Novo-Quinidine (Novopharm)	Quinidine, 200 mg/Tablet	0.127	0.228
Novo-Quinine (Novopharm)	Quinine, 200 mg/Capsule	0.428	0.536
Zantac (Glaxo Wellcome)	Ranitidine, 15 mg/mL/Liquid	0.80	0.83

(continues)

Table 1
(Continued)

Drug, concentration, and presentation	Commercial name and company	Caloric content (kcal)	
		Carbohydrate[b]	Total[b]
Ranitidine, 150 mg/Tablet	Novo-Ranitidine (Novopharm)	0.00	0.138
Ranitidine, 150 mg/Tablet	Zantac (Glaxo Wellcome)	0.01	Nd
Ranitidine, 300 mg/Tablet	Novo-Ranitidine (Novopharm)	0.00	0.276
Ranitidine, 300 mg/Tablet	Zantac (Glaxo Wellcome)	0.01	Nd
Reserpine, 0.25 mg/Tablet	Novo-Reserpine (Novopharm)	0.607	0.613
Rifampin, 150 mg/Capsule	Rifadin (Hoechst Marion Roussel)	0.091	Nd
Rifampin, 300 mg/Capsule	Rifadin (Hoechst Marion Roussel)	0.181	Nd
Salbutamol, 0.4 mg/mL/Liquid	Ventolin (Glaxo Wellcome)	0.03	0.03
Salbutamol, 2 mg/Tablet	Novo-Salmol (Novopharm)	0415	0.430
Salbutamol, 4 mg/Tablet	Novo-Salmol (Novopharm)	0.829	0.860
Secobarbital, sodium, 100 mg/Capsule	Novo-Secobarb (Novopharm)	0.385	0.424
Selegiline, 5 mg/Tablet	Novo-Selegiline (Novopharm)	0.487	0.514
Sennosides, 1.7 mg/mL/Liquid	Senokot (Purdue Frederick)	Nd	3.04
Sennosides, 15 mg/5 mL (3 g)/Granules	Senokot (Purdue Frederick)	Nd	2.93/g
Sennosides, 8.6 mg/Tablet	Senokot (Purdue Frederick)	Nd	0.22
Sennosides, 119 mg/single dose (70 mL)/Liquid	X-Prep (Purdue Frederick)	Nd	212/70-mL bottle
Sennosides, 12 mg/Foaming tablet	Glysennid (Novartis)	Nd	0.36
Sennosides, 12 mg/Tablet	PMS-Sennosides (Pharmascience)	0.04	Nd
Sennosides, chocolate, 15 mg/Tablet	Ex-Lax, chocolates pieces (Novartis)	1.80	Nd
Sennosides, 15 mg/Tablet	Ex-Lax, foaming tablets (Novartis)	0.74	Nd
Sennosides, 157.5 mg (21 g)/Powder	X-Prep foaming (Purdue Frederick)	Nd	38/sachet
Sennosides, 25 mg/Tablet	Ex-Lax Extra-Fort, foaming tablets (Novartis)	0.74	Nd
Sennosides, 8.6 mg/Foaming tablet	Glysennid (Novartis)	Nd	0.34
Sennosides, 8.6 mg/Tablet	Pms-Sennosides (Pharmascience)	0.06	Nd

Simethicone, 40 mg/mL/Liquid	Ovol (Carter Horner)	Nd	0.30
Sodium citrate + citric acid, 1 mEq/mL/Liquid	PMS-Dicitrate sodium (Pharmascience)	0	Nd
Sodium phosphates, 2.4 g monobasic + 0.9 g dibasic/5 mL/Liquid	Fleet Phospho-Soda (Johnson & Johnson, Merck Consumer Pharmaceuticals)	0.05	Nd
Sodium phosphate 2.4 g monobasic + 0.9 g dibasic/5 mL/Liquid	PMS-Phosphate solution (Pharmascience)	0.2	Nd
Sotalol HCl, 80 mg/Tablet	Novo-Stalol (Novopharm)	0.241	0.253
Spiramycin, 250 mg/Capsule	Rovamycine (Rhône-Poulenc Rorer)	0.92	Nd
Spiramycin, 500 mg/Capsule	Rovamycine (Rhône-Poulenc Rorer)	1.84	Nd
Spironolactone/hydrochlorothiazide, 25/25 mg/Tablet	Novo-Spirozine (Novopharm)	1.154	1.188
Spironolactone/hydrochlorothiazide, 50/50 mg/Tablet	Novo-Spirozine (Novopharm)	2.308	2.377
Spironolactone, 100 mg/Tablet	Novo-Spiroton (Novopharm)	2.042	2.126
Spironolactone, 25 mg/Tablet	Novo-Spiroton (Novopharm)	0.895	0.929
Stavudine, 1 mg/mL/Liquid	Zerit (Bristol-Myers Squibb)	0.195	Nd
Stavudine, 15 mg/Capsule	Zerit (Bristol-Myers Squibb)	0.514	Nd
Stavudine, 20 mg/Capsule	Zerit (Bristol-Myers Squibb)	0.772	Nd
Stavudine, 30 mg/Capsule	Zerit (Bristol-Myers Squibb)	0.772	Nd
Stavudine, 40 mg/Capsule	Zerit (Bristol-Myers Squibb)	1.02	Nd
Sucralfate, 1000 mg/Tablet	Sulcrate (Hoechst Marion Roussel)	0.00	Nd
Sucralfate, 1000 mg/Tablet	Novo-Sucralate (Novopharm)	0.144	0.247
Sucralfate, 200 mg/mL/Liquid	Sulcrate Suspension Plus (Hoechst Marion Roussel)	1.04	Nd
Sulfapyridine, 500 mg/Tablet	Dagenan (Rhône-Poulenc Rorer)	2.053	Nd
Sulfinpyrazone, 100 mg/Tablet	Novo-Pyrazone (Novopharm)	0.060	0.086
Sulfinpyrazone, 200 mg/Tablet	Novo-Pyrazone (Novopharm)	0.603	0.629
Sulfisoxazole, 500 mg/Tablet	Novo-Soxazole (Novopharm)	0.518	0.616
	PMS-Sodium Polystyrene Sulfonate (Pharmascience)	0.94	Nd
Sulindac, 150 mg/Tablet	Novo-Sundac (Novopharm)	0.055	0.094
Sulindac, 200 mg/Tablet	Novo-Sundac (Novopharm)	0.102	0.126
Temazepam, 15 mg/Capsule	Novo-Temazepam (Novopharm)	0.781	0.795
Tenoxicam, 20 mg/Tablet	Novo-Tenoxicam (Novopharm)	0.635	0.645

(continues)

Table 1
(Continued)

Drug, concentration, and presentation	Commercial name and company	Caloric content (kcal)	
		Carbohydrate[b]	Total[b]
Terfenadine, 120 mg/Tablet	Seldane (Hoechst Marion Roussel)	1.732	Nd
Terfenadine, 6 mg/mL/Liquid	Seldane (Hoechst Marion Roussel)	1.44	Nd
Terfenadine, 60 mg/Tablet	Seldane (Hoechst Marion Roussel)	0.198	Nd
Terfenadine, 60 mg/Tablet	Novo-Terfenadine (Novopharm)	1.453	1.483
Tetracycline, 25 mg/mL/Liquid	Novo-Tetra (Novopharm)	1.98	1.98
Tetracycline, 250 mg/Capsule	Novo-Tetra (Novopharm)	0.163	0.217
Tetracycline, 250 mg/Tablet	Novo-Tetra (Novopharm)	0.064	0.110
Tetracycline, chlorhydrate, 250 mg/Capsule	Apo-Tetra (Apotex)	Nd	0.21
Tetracycline, chlorhydrate, 250 mg/Capsule	Nu-Tetra (Nu-Pharm)	Nd	0.21
Theophylline, 5.33 mg/mL/Liquid	Theophylline, elixir (Rougier)	Nd	2.82
Theophylline, 5.33 mg/mL/Liquid	Theolair (3M Pharmaceutical Products)	2.38	Nd
Theophylline anhydrate, 100 mg/Tablet	Novo-Theophyl SR (Novopharm)	0.00	0.003
Thioridazine, 10 mg/Tablet	Novo-Ridazine (Novopharm)	0.194	0.204
Thioridazine, 100 mg/Tablet	Novo-Ridazine (Novopharm)	0.083	0.117
Thioridazine, 2 mg/mL/Liquid	Mellaril Suspension (Novartis Pharma)	2.27	Nd
Thioridazine, 200 mg/Tablet	Novo-Ridazine (Novopharm)	0.080	0.106
Thioridazine, 25 mg/Tablet	Novo-Ridazine (Novopharm)	0.082	0.093
Thioridazine, 30 mg/mL/Liquid	Mellaril Solution (Novartis Pharma)	1.23	Nd
Thioridazine, 50 mg/Tablet	Novo-Ridazine (Novopharm)	0.103	0.133
Tiaprofenic acid, 200 mg/Tablet	Novo-Tiaprofenic (Novopharm)	0.039	0.061
Tiaprofenic acid, 300 mg/Tablet	Novo-Tiaprofenic (Novopharm)	0.059	0.092
Timolol maleate, 10 mg/Tablet	Novo-Timol (Novopharm)	0.213	0.228
Timolol maleate, 20 mg/Tablet	Novo-Timol (Novopharm)	0.427	0.456
Timolol maleate, 5 mg/Tablet	Novo-Timol (Novopharm)	0.107	0.114
Tolbutamide, 500 mg/Tablet	Novo-Butamide SP.C. (Novopharm)	0.527	0.615

338

Tolbutamide, 500 mg/Tablet	Novo-Butamide (Novopharm)	0.532	0.613
Tolmetine sodium, 400 mg/Capsule	Novo-Tolmetin (Novopharm)	0.303	0.329
Topiramate, 100 mg/Tablet	Topamax (Jansen-Ortho)	0.642	Nd
Topiramate, 200 mg/Tablet	Topamax (Jansen-Ortho)	0.350	Nd
Topiramate, 25 mg/Tablet	Topamax (Jansen-Ortho)	0.161	Nd
Trazadone, 100 mg/Tablet	Novo-Trazadone (Novopharm)	0.604	0.638
Trazadone, 150 mg/Tablet	Novo-Trazadone (Novopharm)	0.147	0.163
Trazadone, 50 mg/Tablet	Novo-Trazadone (Novopharm)	0.301	0.318
Triamterene/Hydrochlorothiazide, 50/25 mg/Tablet	Novo-Triamzide (Novopharm)	0.060	0.091
Triazolam, 0.125 mg/Tablet	Novo-Triolam (Novopharm)	0.312	0.320
Triazolam, 0.25 mg/Tablet	Novo-Triolam (Novopharm)	0.310	0.319
Trifluoperazine, 1 mg/Tablet	Novo-Fluorazine (Novopharm)	0.267	0.278
Trifluoperazine, 10 mg/Tablet	Novo-Fluorazine (Novopharm)	0.520	0.542
Trifluoperazine, 10 mg/mL/Liquid	PMS-trifluoperazine (Pharmascience)	2.6	Nd
Trifluoperazine, 2 mg/Tablet	Novo-Flurazine (Novopharm)	0.387	0.403
Trifluoperazine, 20 mg/Tablet	Novo-Flurazine (Novopharm)	0.523	0.545
Trifluoperazine, 5 mg/Tablet	Novo-Flurazine (Novopharm)	0.430	0.447
Trihexyphenidyl, 0.4 mg/mL/Liquid	Pms trihexyphenidyl (Pharmascience)	2.02	Nd
Trihexyphenidyl, 2 mg/Tablet	Novo-Hexidyl (Novopharm)	0.056	0.076
Trihexyphenidyl, 5 mg/Tablet	Novo-Hexidyl (Novopharm)	0.115	0.155
Trimeprazin, 0.5 mg/mL/Liquid	Panectyl 2.5 (Rhône-Poulenc Rorer)	3.22	Nd
Trimethoprim, 100 mg/Tablet	Proloprim (Glaxo Wellcome)	0.52	Nd
Trimethoprim, 200 mg/Tablet	Proloprim (Glaxo Wellcome)	0.12	Nd
Trimethoprim + sulfamethoxazole, 160/800 mg/Tablet	Apo-Sulfatrim DS (Apotex)	Nd	0.30
Trimethoprim + sulfamethoxazole, 160/800 mg/Tablet	Bactrim Roche (Hoffman-La Roche)	Nd	0.40
Trimethoprim + sulfamethoxazole, 160/800 mg/Tablet	Nu-Cotrimox (Nu-Pharm)	Nd	0.30
Trimethoprim + sulfamethoxazole, 160/800 mg/Tablet	Septra DS (Glaxo Wellcome)	Nd	0.08
Trimethoprim + sulfamethoxazole, 160/800 mg/Tablet	Novo-Trimel (Novopharm)	0.325	0.470
Trimethoprim + sulfamethoxazole, 20/100 mg/Tablet pediatric	Apo-Sulfatrim (Apotex)	Nd	0.04
Trimethoprim + sulfamethoxazole, 8/40 mg/mL/Liquid	Apo-Sulfatrim (Apotex)	Nd	2.47

(continues)

Table 1
(Continued)

		Caloric content (kcal)	
Drug, concentration, and presentation	Commercial name and company	Carbohydrate[b]	Total[b]
Trimethoprim + sulfamethoxazole, 8/40 mg/mL/Liquid	Nu-Cotrimox (Nu-Pharm)	Nd	2.47
Trimethoprim + sulfamethoxazole, 8/40 mg/mL/Liquid	Septra (Glaxo Wellcome)	Nd	2.60
Trimethoprim + sulfamethoxazole, 8/40 mg/mL/Liquid	Novo-Trimel (Novopharm)	0.011	0.011
Trimethoprim + sulfamethoxazole, 8/40 mg/mL/Liquid	Bactrim Roche (Hoffman-La Roche)	1.81	2.42
Trimethoprim + sulfamethoxazole, 80/400 mg/Tablet	Apo-Sulfatrim (Apotex)	Nd	0.15
Trimethoprim + sulfamethoxazole, 80/400 mg/Tablet	Bactrim Roche (Hoffman-La Roche)	Nd	0.20
Trimethoprim + sulfamethoxazole, 80/400 mg/Tablet	Nu-Cotrimox (Nu-Pharm)	Nd	0.15
Trimethoprim + sulfamethoxazole, 80/400 mg/Tablet	Septra (Glaxo Wellcome)	Nd	0.04
Trimethoprim + sulfamethoxazole, 80/400 mg/Tablet	Novo-Trimel (Novopharm)	0.163	0.235
Trimipramine, maleate, 100 mg/Tablet	Novo-Tripramine (Novopharm)	0.046	0.067
Trimipramine, maleate, 25 mg/Tablet	Novo-Tripramine (Novopharm)	0.012	0.017
Trimipramine, maleate, 50 mg/Tablet	Novo-Tripramine (Novopharm)	0.023	0.033
Trovafloxacin, 100 mg/Tablet	Trovan (Pfizer)	0.388	Nd
Trovafloxacin, 200 mg/Tablet	Trovan (Pfizer)	0.780	Nd
Valproic acid, 250 mg/Capsule	Depakene (Abbott)	0.00	Nd
Valproic acid, 250 mg/Capsule	PMS-Valproic Acid (Pharmascience)	0.71	Nd
Valproic acid, 250 mg/Capsule	Novo-Valproic (Novopharm)	0.90	Nd
Valproic acid, 50 mg/mL/Liquid	Alti-Valproic (AltiMed)	Nd	3.54
Valproic acid, 50 mg/mL/Liquid	PMS-Valproic acid (Pharmascience)	2.8	Nd
Valproic acid, 500 mg/Capsule	Depakene (Abbot)	0.00	Nd
Valproic acid, 500 mg/Capsule	PMS-Valproic acid E.C. (Pharmascience)	0.00	Nd
Valproic acid, 500 mg/Capsule	PMS-Valproic acid (Pharmascience)	0.71	Nd
Valproic acid, 500 mg/Capsule	Novo-Valproic (Novopharm)	0.88	Nd
Valproic acid, 50 mg/mL/Liquid	Depakene (Abbott)	2.97	3.54
Verapamil, 120 mg/Tablet	Novo-Veramil (Novopharm)	0.083	0.096

Verapamil, 80 mg/Tablet	Novo-Veramil (Novopharm)	0.055	0.064
Vigabat, 500 mg/Tablet	Sabril (Hoechst Marion Roussel)	0.056	0.579
Vitamin A B C D/Liquid	Infantol Drops (Carter Horner)	Nd	2.8
Vitamin A B C D/Liquid	Infantol Liquid (Carter Horner)	Nd	1.16
Vitamin A B C D/Liquid	Polyvisol (Mead Johnson)	3.40	Nd
Vitamin A C D/Liquid	Tri-vi-sol (Mead Johnson)	2.20	Nd
Vitamin A C D + fluorine./Liquid	Tri-vi-flor (Mead Johnson)	2.20	Nd
Vitamin A C D + fluorine./Liquid	Tri-vi-sol with fluorine (Mead Johnson)	2.20	Nd
Vitamin D, 400 U/mL/Liquid	D-vi-sol 400 U/0.6 mL (Mead Johnson)	2.20	Nd
Vitamin E, 50 U/mL/Liquid	Aquasol E (Novartis)	1.52	Nd
Vitamin E, 100 IU/Capsule	Aquasol E (Novartis)	1.44	Nd
Vitamin E, 400 IU/capsule	Vitamin E (Santé Naturelle Adrien Gagnon)	0.29	Nd
Vitamins, multi-,/Capsule	Fortamines-10 Capsule (Rougier)	0.36	Nd
Vitamins, multi-,/Tablet	Fortamines-10 (Rougier)	0.36	Nd
Vitamins, multi-,/Tablet	Maxi-10 (Rougier)	0.36	Nd
Zidovudine, 100 mg/Capsule	Novo-AZT (Novopharm)	0.060	0.074

[a] The caloric content indicated is for 1 mL, one tablet, or one capsule unless otherwise indicated.

[b] Nd = No data. When no data are available for caloric content provided by carbohydrates, we suggest the use of total Caloric content.

Table 2
Worst-Case Scenario Study Data

Medication[a]	Formulation	Active ingredient (mg)	Weight (g)	Excipient weight (g)	Caloric content, estimated (kcal)	Caloric content (kcal)	Difference (kcal)
Biaxin	Tablet	250	0.5196	0.2696	1.0784	0.210	0.868
Cipro	Tablet	250	0.3805	0.1305	0.522	0.171	0.351
Epival	Tablet	250	0.4975	0.2475	0.99	0.170	0.820
Lamictal	Tablet	25	0.0802	0.0552	0.2208	0.107	0.114
Novamoxin	Capsule	250	0.3824	0.1324	0.5296	0.082	0.448
Novamoxin	Capsule	500	0.7052	0.2052	0.8208	0.164	0.657
Novo-Carbamaz	Tablet	200	0.2568	0.0568	0.2272	0.031	0.196
Novo-Chlorocap	Capsule	250	0.5557	0.3057	1.2228	0.863	0.360
Novo-Chloroquine	Tablet	250	0.7868	0.5368	2.1472	0.824	1.323
Novo-Chlorpromazine	Tablet	100	0.3922	0.2922	1.1688	0.216	0.953
Novo-Cloxin	Capsule	250	0.3884	0.1384	0.5536	0.139	0.415
Novo-Cloxin	Capsule	500	0.6628	0.1628	0.6512	0.000	0.651
Novo-Dipiradol	Tablet	50	0.1844	0.1344	0.5376	0.044	0.494
Novo-Doxepin	Capsule	25	0.1987	0.1737	0.6948	0.428	0.267
Novo-Doxylin	Capsule	100	0.3478	0.2478	0.9912	0.022	0.969
Novo-Furan	Tablet	50	0.1784	0.1284	0.5136	0.073	0.441
Novo-Hydrazide	Tablet	25	0.1047	0.0797	0.3188	0.238	0.081
Novo-Hydroxyzin	Soft gelatin	10	0.229	0.219	0.876	0.000	0.876
Novo-Hylazin	Tablet	25	0.1522	0.1272	0.5088	0.182	0.327
Novo-Lexin	Tablet	250	0.3622	0.1122	0.4488	0.075	0.374
Novo-Methacin	Capsule	25	0.299	0.274	1.096	0.887	0.209
Novo-Naprox	Tablet	250	0.3695	0.1195	0.478	0.075	0.403
Novo-Nidazol	Tablet	250	0.5395	0.2895	1.158	0.585	0.573
Novo-Peridol	Tablet	2	0.1258	0.1238	0.4952	0.025	0.470

Novo-Pheniram	Tablet	4	0.2198	0.2158	0.8632	0.032	0.831
Novo-Pirocam	Capsule	10	0.3959	0.3859	1.5436	1.056	0.488
Novo-Pranol	Tablet	10	0.1345	0.1245	0.498	0.434	0.064
Novo-Prednisone	Tablet	50	0.218	0.168	0.672	0.586	0.086
Novo-Purol	Tablet	100	0.2989	0.1989	0.7956	0.458	0.338
Novo-Rythro Estolate	Capsule	250	0.5589	0.3089	1.2356	0.266	0.970
Novo-Semide	Tablet	40	0.1648	0.1248	0.4992	0.360	0.139
Novo-Spiroton	Tablet	25	0.262	0.237	0.948	0.895	0.053
Novo-Spiroton	Tablet	100	0.6475	0.5475	2.19	2.042	0.148
Novo-Sucralate	Tablet	1000	1.19	0.19	0.76	0.144	0.616
Novo-Tetra	Capsule	250	0.3566	0.1066	0.4264	0.163	0.263
Novo-Trimel	Tablet	480	0.5284	0.0484	0.1936	0.163	0.031
Novo-Triptyn	Tablet	50	0.239	0.189	0.756	0.082	0.674
Novo-Veramil	Tablet	80	0.2808	0.2008	0.8032	0.055	0.748
Novo-Zolamide	Tablet	250	0.4977	0.2477	0.9908	0.100	0.891
Phenobarbital	Tablet	15	0.081	0.066	0.264	0.240	0.024
Phenobarbital	Tablet	30	0.1207	0.0907	0.3628	0.330	0.033
Pms-Sodium Docusate	Capsule	100	0.4355	0.3355	1.342	0.510	0.832
Rifadin	Soft gelatin	300	0.4244	0.1244	0.4976	0.181	0.317
Vigabatrin	Tablet	500	0.6789	0.1789	0.7156	0.056	0.660
Stemetil	Tablet	5	0.0822	0.0772	0.3088	0.000	0.309
Vitamin E (Adrien Gagnon)	Capsule	294	0.5862	0.2922	1.1688	0.290	0.879

[a] Brand names.

Table 3
Differences in Caloric Content of Similar Drug Preparations in Canada
and the United States

Drugs	Caloric content (Canada)	Caloric content (US)
Acetaminophen (syrup)	1.78 kcal/mL	1.8 kcal/mL
Acetaminophen (325-mg tablet)	0.2 kcal/tablet	0.16 kcal/tablet
Carbamazepine (syrup)	1.79 kcal/mL	2.68 kcal/mL
Carbamazepine (200-mg tablet)	0.35 kcal/tablet	0.205 kcal/tablet
Phenytoin (syrup)	1.14 kcal/mL	0.832 kcal/mL
Phenytoin (30-mg capsule)	0.7 kcal/capsule	0.6 kcal/capsule
Valproic acid (syrup)	3.54 kcal/mL	3.456 kcal/mL

Finally, as shown in Table 3, the caloric content of these formulations may vary from country to country *(4)*. We believe that a comprehensive table should be developed in each country and updated every 5 yr.

REFERENCES

1. Huttenlocher PR. Ketonemia and seizures: metabolic and anticonvulsant effects of two ketogenic diets in childhood epilepsy. Pediatr Res 1976;10:419–423.
2. Wheless JW. The ketogenic diet: fa(c)t or fiction. J Child Neurol 1995;10:419–423.
3. Lebel D, Morin C, Laberge M, Achim N, Carmant L. The carbohydrate and caloric content of concomitant medications for children with epilepsy on the ketogenic diet. Can J Neurol Sci 2001;28:322–340.
4. Feldstein TJ. Carbohydrate and alcohol content of 200 oral liquid medications for use in patients receiving ketogenic diets. Pediatrics 1996:97:506–511.

Appendix B
Ketogenic Diet Resources

Carl E. Stafstrom and Jong M. Rho

PUBLICATIONS

Books

Freeman JM, Freeman JB, Kelly MT (2000)
The Ketogenic Diet: A Treatment for Epilepsy, 3rd edition
Demos Publications, New York
Phone: (212) 683-0072

Freeman JM, Vining EPG, Pillas D (1990)
Seizures and Epilepsy in Childhood: A Guide for Parents
Johns Hopkins University Press, Baltimore

Pennington J (1994)
Bowes and Church's Food Values and Portions Commonly Used, 16th edition
JB Lippincott, Philadelphia

Keto Klub Newsletter

To receive or contribute, write to:
Keto Klub
61557 Miami Meadows Court
South Bend, IN 46614

Low-Carb Cookery

A book of low-carbohydrate recipes
The author, Alex Haas, can be contacted at *alexhaas@wilmington.net*

ORGANIZATIONS

The Charlie Foundation
The Charlie Foundation to Help Cure Pediatric Epilepsy
1223 Wilshire Blvd #815
Santa Monica, CA 90403-5406
310-395-6751
Educational and informational videotapes about the diet available by calling:
1-800-367-5386

From: *Nutrition and Health*
Epilepsy and the Ketogenic Diet
Edited by: C. E. Stafstrom and J. M. Rho © Humana Press Inc., Totowa, NJ

The Epilepsy Foundation of America
Information and advocacy for persons with epilepsy
4351 Garden City Dr.
Landover, MD 20785
800-332-1000
http://www.epilepsyfoundation.org/

American Epilepsy Society
Professional society that provides information, support, and grants to physicians and
health-care workers in the field of epilepsy
342 N. Main St.
West Hartford, CT 06117
860-586-7505
http://www.aesnet.org

National Institute of Neurological Disorders and Strokes
Provides research funding for neurological disorders, including epilepsy
9000 Rockville Pike
Bethesda, MD 20892
www.ninds.nih.gov

Society for Neuroscience
Professional society that provides information and support to neuroscientists
11 Dupont Circle
Washington, DC 20036
202-462-6688
www.sfn.org

OTHER RESOURCES

Ketogenic Diet Resources on the Web
www.mynchen.demon.co.uk/Ketogenic_diet/Resources/Ketogenic_diet_resources.htm

Stanford University Ketogenic Diet Web Site
A web site packed with useful information about KD formulation, resources, and frequently asked questions. www.stanford.edu/group/ketodiet/

E-mail list for parents of people on the ketogenic diet

An e-mail listserve for families who have had experience with the ketogenic diet to
share ideas, recipes, and moral support. To subscribe to this e-mail list, change the
URL of your browser to *http://www.squish.com/rickloek/ketopages/*.

Parents Helping Parents

3041 Olcott St.
Santa Clara, CA 95054
1-408-727-5775
BBS 1-408-727-7227

SHS North America

SHS is a world leader in specialized clinical nutrition. The company produces a ready-made ketogenic diet formula called KetoCal.
9900 Belward Campus Dr., Ste. 100
Rockville, MD 20850
800-365-7354
www.shsna.com

Ketocalculator

Ketocalculator is a web-based computer program for calculating the ketogenic diet prescription, ketogenic meals, and snacks. Recipes are included with special meals. An annual user fee is required, and the use of the Ketocalculator is restricted to dietitians.

Index

A

Absence seizures, 182
Acetazolamide, 58, 108
Acetoacetate (AcAc), 43, 129, 138, 180, 181, 188, 206, 209, 217–226, 249, 295
Acetone, 104, 129–132, 138, 150, 217–226
N-acetyl-aspartate (NAA), 144, 150
Acetyl-CoA, 179–181, 189
Action potentials, 14, 19, 136, 230
Adenosine, 21, 170
Adenosine triphosphate (ATP), 144, 149, 182, 239, 258, 267, 294
Adrenocorticotrophic hormone (ACTH), 25, 27, 303
Adrenoreceptors, 269–271
Afterhyperpolarization (AHP), 14
Amino acids, 185–196, 209
Amygdala, 266–267, 281, 283, 290
Antidepressants, 268, 271
Antiepileptic drugs (AEDs) (*see also* specific drugs), 25–27, 229
Arachidonic acid (AA), 133
Arcuate nucleus of hypothalamus, 280
Astrocytes, 185, 186, 191, 202, 208–212
Atkins' diet, 107, 154
Audiogenic seizures, 236

B

Barbiturates, 117, 231
Benzodiazepines, 25, 231
Bible, 31, 248
Bicuculline, 136, 233–234, 267
Bipolar disorder (manic–depressive disorder), 154, 156
Bleeding abnormalities, 125
Brain-derived neurotrophic factor (BDNF), 15

C

Cable properties, 14
Calcium channels (*see* Channels, calcium),
Calorie restriction, 161, 168–170, 209, 229, 233, 237, 240, 247–259, 271, 309
Cancer, 154
Carbamazepine, 25, 136, 154, 231, 258, 270
Cardiovascular disease, 107, 125–126, 154, 155, 294

Carnitine, 59, 123–124, 179
Carnitine acyltransferase I, 179
Caspase-3, 292
c-fos, 266–267
Channels, ionic, 6, 12
    calcium, 12, 25, 231, 233–234, 238, 294
    chloride, 23
    potassium, 136, 238–239
        2P-domain, 165
        calcium-dependent, 14
        K-ATP, 238–239
    sodium, 12, 230, 238, 294–295
Charlie Foundation, 41
Cholesterol, 105–106, 155
Choline, 162–164
Ciprofibrate, 208
Clonidine, 269–270
Cobb, Stanley, 35–37
Conklin, Hugh W., 31–39, 96
Corpus callosum, 5
Corticotrophin releasing hormone, 15, 27
Cyclic AMP response element (CRE), 207

D

Dentate gyrus, 21, 170, 296–297
2-Deoxyglucose (2-DG), 267
Diabetes, 155, 156
Dibenzylamine, 224
Diuretics, 118
Docosahaxaenoic acid (DHA), 133, 164–167
Dopamine-β-hydroxylase knockout mouse, 270–273
Dysgenesis, cerebral, 112, 115

E

Eicosapentaenoic acid (EPA), 133
EL (epileptic) mouse, 249–259, 268, 293
Electroconvulsive therapy (ECT), 154
Electroencephalogram (EEG), 5, 7, 17, 95, 100–101, 183
Electroshock, 224–225, 229–237, 266 (*see also* Epilepsy models)
Electrotonic synapses, 13–14
Energy metabolism, cerebral, 15–16, 179–183, 185–186

About the Editors

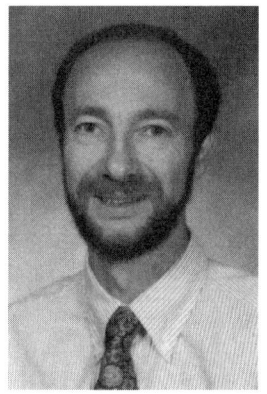

Carl E. Stafstrom, MD, PhD is Professor of Neurology and Pediatrics and Chief of the Division of Pediatric Neurology at the University of Wisconsin Medical School, Madison, WI. He received his AB from the University of Pennsylvania, followed by MD and PhD degrees (the latter in physiology and biophysics) from the University of Washington, Seattle. After completing a residency in pediatrics at the University of Washington Children's Hospital, Dr. Stafstrom trained in adult and pediatric neurology at Tufts-New England Medical Center in Boston, followed by fellowships in neurology research, epilepsy, and clinical neurophysiology at Children's Hospital, Harvard Medical School, Boston. Prior to his current position, he held faculty appointments at Duke University Medical Center and Tufts University School of Medicine.

Dr. Stafstrom's main research interests are the pathophysiological mechanisms of epilepsy in the developing brain, the consequences of seizures on cognition and behavior, and alternative epilepsy therapies such as the ketogenic diet. He actively pursues these interests in both the clinic and the laboratory.

Dr. Stafstrom is author of more than 100 publications on epilepsy and its mechanisms. He serves as chair of the scientific review committee of Partnership for Epilepsy Research and on the scientific advisory boards of the Epilepsy Foundation and the Charlie Foundation. He is the former chair of the Investigators Workshop Committee of the American Epilepsy Society. Dr. Stafstrom serves on the editorial boards of the journals *Epilepsia* and *Epilepsy Currents*. He is the recipient of numerous awards for teaching and research.

Jong M. Rho, MD is Associate Director of Child Neurology and Director of Pediatric Epilepsy Research at the Barrow Neurological Institute and St. Joseph's Hospital and Medical Center in Phoenix, Arizona. He received his BA at Yale University with a major in molecular biophysics and biochemistry, and completed his MD at the University of Cincinnati College of Medicine. He obtained residency training in pediatrics at the Los Angeles Children's Hospital, affiliated with the University of Southern California School of Medicine, and completed a neurology residency at the University of California Los Angeles School of Medicine. Dr. Rho then pursued a basic science fellowship in neuropharmacology in the Epilepsy Research Branch at the National Institute of Neurological Disorders and Stroke in Bethesda, Maryland. Prior to his current position, he was the director of the pediatric epilepsy program at the University of Washington School of Medicine and Seattle Children's Hospital and Regional Medical Center, as well as the

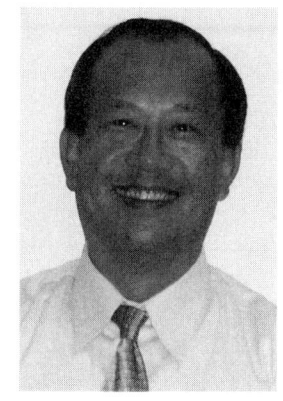

director of the University of California at Irvine Comprehensive Epilepsy Program for adults and children, where he was also an Associate Professor of pediatrics and neurology.

Dr. Rho's main research interests have been in anticonvulsant drug mechanisms, developmental animal models of epilepsy, and the basic mechanisms underlying the anticonvulsant and potentially neuroprotective actions of the ketogenic diet. His research has been funded for the past 8 years by the NIH, Epilepsy Foundation of America, and the Charlie Foundation. He has authored or co-authored more than 45 clinical and scientific publications, and has co-edited two additional books on the subject of epilepsy.

Dr. Rho is a recipient of several teaching awards, has been actively involved in resident and fellow education throughout the years, and has organized numerous clinical and scientific symposia and meetings at both national and international levels. He has served as an ad hoc reviewer on two NIH study sections, and is on the scientific advisory board of the Charlie Foundation.

About the Series Editor

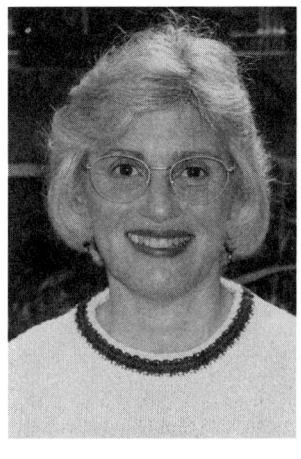

Dr. Adrianne Bendich is Clinical Director of Calcium Research at GlaxoSmithKline Consumer Healthcare, where she is responsible for leading the innovation and medical programs in support of TUMS and Os-Cal. Dr. Bendich has primary responsibility for the direction of GSK's support for the Women's Health Initiative intervention study. Prior to joining GlaxoSmithKline, Dr. Bendich was at Roche Vitamins Inc., and was involved with the groundbreaking clinical studies proving that folic acid-containing multivitamins significantly reduce major classes of birth defects. Dr. Bendich has co-authored more than 100 major clinical research studies in the area of preventive nutrition. Dr. Bendich is recognized as a leading authority on antioxidants, nutrition, immunity, and pregnancy outcomes, vitamin safety, and the cost-effectiveness of vitamin/mineral supplementation.

In addition to serving as Series Editor for Humana Press and initiating the development of the 15 currently published books in the *Nutrition and Health*™ series, Dr. Bendich is the editor of nine books, including *Preventive Nutrition: The Comprehensive Guide for Health Professionals.* She also serves as Associate Editor for *Nutrition: The International Journal of Applied and Basic Nutritional Sciences,* and Dr. Bendich is on the Editorial Board of the *Journal of Women's Health and Gender-Based Medicine,* as well as a past member of the Board of Directors of the American College of Nutrition.

Dr. Bendich was the recipient of the Roche Research Award, a *Tribute to Women and Industry* Awardee, and a recipient of the Burroughs Wellcome Visiting Professorship in Basic Medical Sciences, 2000–2001. Dr. Bendich holds academic appointments as Adjunct Professor in the Department of Preventive Medicine and Community Health at UMDNJ, Institute of Nutrition, Columbia University P&S, and Adjunct Research Professor, Rutgers University, Newark Campus. She is listed in *Who's Who in American Women.*